Chemical Dependence

H. Thomas Milhorn, Jr.

Chemical Dependence
Diagnosis, Treatment, and Prevention

With 11 Illustrations

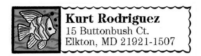

Kurt Rodriguez
15 Buttonbush Ct.
Elkton, MD 21921-1507

Springer-Verlag
New York Berlin Heidelberg London
Paris Tokyo Hong Kong Barcelona

H. Thomas Milhorn, Jr., M.D., Ph.D.
Department of Family Medicine
University of Mississippi Medical Center
Jackson, Mississippi 39216-4505
USA

Library of Congress Cataloging-in-Publication Data
Milhorn, Howard T.
    Chemical dependence : diagnosis, treatment, and prevention / H.
Thomas Milhorn
        p. cm.
    Includes bibliographical references.
    ISBN 0-387-97292-7 (alk. paper)
    1. Substance abuse. 2. Psychotropic drugs. I. Title.
    [DNLM: 1. Psychotropic Drugs—pharmacology. 2. Substance
Dependence. WM 270 M644C]
RC564M53 1990
616.86—dc20
DNLM/DLC
for Library of Congress   90-9708

Printed on acid-free paper.

Typeset by Publishers Service of Montana, Bozeman, Montana.
Printed and bound by Edwards Brothers, Ann Arbor, Michigan.
Printed in the United States of America.

9 8 7 6 5 4 3 2 1

ISBN 0-387-97292-7 Springer-Verlag New York Berlin Heidelberg
ISBN 3-540-97292-7 Springer-Verlag Berlin Heidelberg New York

Preface

Chemical dependence is a disease whose time has come. Alcoholism and other drug dependencies in our society have reached epidemic proportions. Physicians are in an excellent position to help prevent the disease, to diagnose it, to aid families in getting addicts into treatment, and to play an important role in long-term recovery. This text was written for medical students, interns, residents, and practicing physicians who daily come in contact with chemically dependent individuals and their families. It should also be helpful to physicians who treat chemical dependence, as well as to other health professionals, including psychologists, marriage and family therapists, social workers, and alcohol and drug counselors.

The introductory chapter covers basic definitions, concepts, and classification of psychoactive substances. After that the book is divided into three parts. Part One covers the basics—diagnosis, treatment, recovery, the family, and prevention. Part Two describes the basic principles of pharmacology and drugs of abuse (central nervous system depressants, opioids, central nervous system stimulants, cannabinoids, hallucinogens, phencyclidines, and inhalants). Part Three is devoted to chemical dependence in special groups—women, adolescents, the elderly, minority groups, the dual diagnosis patient, the patient infected with immunodeficiency virus, and the impaired physician. This book is my concept of what a medical school curriculum in chemical dependence should include.

I would especially like to thank Lyndell Gardner who did all the literature searches and typed the entire manuscript, all with an enthusiastic attitude. I would also like to thank my wife Kay for her patience and understanding during the many months of my partial absence while I worked on the manuscript.

H. THOMAS MILHORN, JR.
Jackson, Mississippi

Contents

Part II Psychoactive Substances

Part III Special Groups

CHAPTER I

Introduction

The Problem

The use of alcohol and other drugs has reached an epidemic level in the United States. The cost to the economy of such use is staggering. However, the cost in broken homes, damaged lives, and human suffering is beyond calculation.

Alcohol

The estimated consumption of alcohol in the United States is 2.65 gallons of pure ethanol per person each year. This is equivalent per person to approximately 50 gallons of beer, 20 gallons of wine, or more than 4 gallons of distilled spirits. Only 10 percent of the drinking population consumes half the alcohol drunk in the United States a year.[1] One-third of Americans report that alcohol has caused problems in their families.[2]

Alcohol is associated with a variety of physical and psychological disorders. The greatest chronic health hazard that results from the use of alcohol is liver disease. Cirrhosis of the liver is the ninth leading cause of death in the United States; most cirrhosis results from alcoholism.[1] Alcohol use is a factor in 10 percent of all deaths in the United States, accounting for 200,000 deaths a year. Almost 20,000 deaths a year are directly attributable to medically related alcohol problems, 24,000 are caused by motor vehicle accidents in which alcohol played a role, and 30,000 result from alcohol-related mishaps, such as falls, fires, and suicides.[3] In addition, almost 300,000 disabilities result each year from alcohol use.[4] The incidence of alcohol abuse and dependence is 1.5 times that of diabetes.[2]

Nearly half of convicted jail inmates were under the influence of alcohol at the time they committed their crimes. More than half of people convicted of violent crimes had been drinking at the time of their offenses.[1]

Of high school seniors, 91 percent have tried alcohol at least once, 66 percent use it in any one month, and 5 percent use it daily. Daily drinking is reported to be the same (5 percent) among college students; however, heavy drinking is much higher—at 45 percent. This number increases to 57 percent for men. Abuse of alcohol or other drugs is involved in 50 percent of young suicides, and drinking is involved in 80 to 90 percent of automobile accidents among those aged 16 to 20.[5,6]

The total yearly cost of alcoholism in the United States is estimated to be $116.7 billion. The largest portion ($71.2 billion) is the indirect cost of reduced productivity and lost employment. The next most costly category is alcohol-related premature deaths ($18.7 billion), followed by medical treatment costs ($12.8 billion).[3]

Other Drugs

An estimated 5.2 million Americans are dependent on prescription sleeping pills, tranquilizers, stimulants, and pain medication.[5] Although smoking is on the decline in the United States, 26.5 percent of adults still smoke, and 350,000 die from smoking annually. Total costs of smoking-related healthcare and lost productivity in the United States amount to approximately $65 billion each year.[7] Approximately 6 million people regularly use cocaine in the United States.[5]

Among American high school seniors, 17 percent admit to having tried cocaine, and 5 percent use it in any one month; 51 percent admit to having tried marijuana, and 4 percent use it daily.[6] Statistics are not available for alcohol or other drug use among those who drop out of school before their senior year. Because a large percentage of dropouts are substance abusers, the numbers would be expected to be higher even than those for high school seniors.

The international drug industry is the largest growth industry in the world, having an estimated annual revenue of $500 billion—more than the gross national products of all but a half-dozen major industrial nations. Illegal drug transactions in the United States are estimated to involve more than $100 billion annually. Drug abuse is thought to cost $177 billion in lost work time, accidents, treatment, legal assistance, and law enforcement, and 75 percent of all crime is related to drug use, drug selling, or related criminal activity.[5]

Medical Education

One out of every five to six patients physicians see is affected by alcohol or other drug problems. Such patients are heavy consumers of healthcare: They make more office visits and require more frequent hospitalizations. Despite this, healthcare professionals recognize alcohol or other drug problems in fewer than 20 percent of patients who have them, and refer for treatment as few as 10 percent. The primary reason for this is inadequate substance abuse education in medical schools. Medical education simply does not adequately address physicians' prejudices or prepare them to care for patients with substance abuse problems and the families of those patients. Of the 1 percent of curriculum time devoted to teaching substance abuse in U.S. medical schools, most consists of didactic lectures that address the medical complications of alcoholism. Schools rarely offer clinical experience in managing the primary problem of substance abuse.[2] This major deficiency in medical education needs to be addressed by individual medical schools.

Basic Definitions

Terminology in the field of substance abuse is not well standardized. Therefore, it is important that we define some basic terms as they will be used in this book. A *psychoactive substance* is defined as a chemical that exerts a mood-altering effect on the central nervous system and that can potentially produce dependence. The terms *psychoactive substance* and *drug* will be used interchangeably. The term *drug* will include alcohol. The terms *dependence* and *addiction* will also be used interchangeably. In addition, *substance dependence* and *chemical dependence* will be considered to have the same meaning.

An *addict* is defined as a person who is presently or has been dependent on one or more drugs, such as alcohol, heroin, cocaine, or marijuana. It is customary to divide addicts into those whose dependence involves alcohol (*alcoholic*) and those whose dependence involves drugs other than alcohol (*drug addict*). In reality most addicts, especially younger ones, use both alcohol and other drugs. An addict living a life of sobriety is said to be in *recovery*.

Chemical Dependence

A number of definitions of chemical dependence exist. The most helpful one to physicians is based on the American Medical Association's description of alcoholism. In addition, the American Psychiatric Association (APA) has established criteria for the diagnosis of chemical dependence.

Definition

In 1956 the American Medical Association (AMA) declared alcoholism to be an illness; in 1987 it extended the declaration to dependence on all drugs of abuse.[9] Based on the AMA's statement, we arrived at the following definition: *Chemical dependence is a chronic, progressive disease characterized by significant impairment that is directly associated with persistent and excessive use of a psychoactive substance. Impairment may involve physiological, psychological, or social dysfunction.*

This definition implicitly states several things, which are outlined in Table 1.1: (1) chemical dependence is a disease; (2) it is chronic—that is, it takes place over a period of time (months to years); (3) it is progressive—that is, it gets worse over time if untreated; and (4) it causes significant impairment from physiological, psychological, or social dysfunction. Physiological dysfunction consists of medical problems (such as alcoholic hepatitis or pancreatitis); psychological dysfunction consists of pathological mood states (such as anxiety, insomnia, or depression); and social dysfunction involves problems with personal relationships (for example, with family, friends, job, law). The impairment must be directly related to persistent and excessive use of a psychoactive substance.

However, the definition does not explain several things. Persistent is not defined. Drug use every weekend is certainly persistent, and a person does not have to use a drug daily to be chemically dependent. Excessive is also not

TABLE 1.1. Definition of chemical dependence.

Implicitly stated	Explicitly implied
1. Chemical dependence is a disease.	1. Persistent is not defined. Heavy use every weekend is certainly persistent. One does not have to use a drug daily to be chemically dependent on it.
2. It is chronic; i.e., a time factor is involved.	
3. It is progressive; untreated, it gets worse with time.	
4. Significant impairment from physiological, psychological, or social dysfunction must occur.	2. Excessive is not defined. It is the quantity of psychoactive substance, used in a persistent fashion, sufficient to cause significant impairment.
5. The impairment must result from persistent and excessive use of a psychoactive substance.	3. Occurrence of withdrawal symptoms on cessation of drug use may occur, but they are not required for a person to be considered chemically dependent.

defined. It suggests a quantity of a psychoactive substance that, when used persistently, is sufficient to cause significant impairment in one of the three major areas of life already discussed. Users may suffer withdrawal symptoms when they stop using the psychoactive substance, but such symptoms are not required for the diagnosis of chemical dependence.

APA Criteria

The APA's criteria for substance dependence, from the *Diagnostic and Statistical Manual of Mental Disorders*, Third Edition Revised (DSM-III-R), are given in Table 1.2. Three of the nine criteria must be met to make the diagnosis. In addition, some symptoms must have been present for at least a month or must have occurred repeatedly over a longer period of time.[10]

Both the AMA-based definition and the APA criteria are sufficient, and for the most part compatible, for making the diagnosis of chemical dependence.

Physical and Psychological Dependence

Traditionally, dependence has been subdivided into physical dependence and psychological dependence. *Physical dependence* is characterized by an unpleasant and sometimes life-threatening abstinence (withdrawal) syndrome. It may occur from repeated use of some drugs, but not from all. It generally occurs in two phases: Phase one consists of acute symptoms that usually last only a few days; phase two consists of milder symptoms that may last for several weeks to a year or more. Phase two is often referred to as the *postacute withdrawal syndrome*. The term *psychological dependence* developed because physicians observed that stopping the use of some drugs was not associated with an abstinence syndrome.[11] Because of this, it would probably be better to divide psychoactive substances into those that do and those that do not cause abstinence

TABLE 1.2. DSM-III-R diagnostic criteria for substance dependence.

A. At least three of the following:
  (1) substance often taken in larger amounts or over a longer period than the person intended
  (2) persistent desire or one or more unsuccessful efforts to cut down or control substance use
  (3) a great deal of time spent in activities necessary to get the substance (e.g., theft), taking the substances (e.g., chain smoking), or recovering from its effects
  (4) frequent intoxication or withdrawal symptoms when expected to fulfill major role obligations at work, school, or home (e.g., does not go to work because hung over, goes to school or work "high," intoxicated while taking care of his or her children), or when substance use is physically hazardous (e.g., drives when intoxicated)
  (5) important social, occupational, or recreational activities given up or reduced because of substance use
  (6) continued substance use despite knowledge of having a persistent or recurrent social, psychological, or physical problem that is caused or exacerbated by the use of the substance (e.g., keeps using heroin despite family arguments about it; cocaine-induced depression; or having an ulcer made worse by drinking)
  (7) marked tolerance: need for markedly increased amounts of the substance (i.e., at least a 50% increase) in order to achieve intoxication or desired effect, or markedly diminished effect with continued use of the same amount
  [Note: The following items may not apply to cannabis, hallucinogens, or phencyclidine (PCP):]
  (8) characteristic withdrawal symptoms
  (9) substance often taken to relieve or avoid withdrawal symptoms

B. Some symptoms of the disturbance have persisted for at least one month, or have occurred repeatedly over a longer period of time.

From *Diagnostic and Statistical Manual of Mental Disorders*, Third Edition, Revised (DSM-III-R), American Psychiatric Association, Washington, D.C., 1987, pp. 167–168.

syndromes, rather than saying they cause physical or psychological dependence. However, these last two terms are ingrained in the literature and will probably remain in use.

Physical dependence is not synonymous with the disease of chemical dependence; in fact, it is not a necessary part of the definition. The legitimate use of a narcotic opioid for several days following surgery, for example, can produce physical dependence, characterized by an abstinence syndrome. Such patients do not act as or become drug addicts. Narcotic addicts who blame their dependence on a past injury that required pain medication have a naive understanding of chemical dependence. Chemical dependence is complex, involving social, psychological, physiological, and pharmacological factors.

Substance Abuse and Use

Substance abuse is defined as the persistent and excessive use of a psychoactive substance that does not result in significant impairment from physiological, psychological, or social dysfunction. Some degree of dysfunction may occur, such as minor medical or social problems, but the substance use does not greatly affect the quality of the life of the person or of his or her family.

Substance use is defined as regular or intermittent, but not excessive, use of a psychoactive substance, such as social drinking or recreational drug use.

Some believe that any use of an illegal substance is abuse. The potential is certainly there for problems with legal authorities. The illegal use of any legal drug, such as prescription medication, could also be considered abuse.

Progression to Chemical Dependence

People who do not try drugs never get addicted. Fortunately, many people who do try them do not like being under their influence and stop using them after a few times. Others, however, find that they like the feeling they get from drugs and continue to use them for years without becoming addicted. Others, unfortunately, eventually develop the disease of chemical dependence. The course from drug use to drug dependence is a smooth progression over a period of time, usually from months to years. It is convenient, however, to categorize this process into three discrete but somewhat arbitrary stages: use, abuse, and dependence.

Use

Drug use most commonly begins in adolescence with nicotine, generally from cigarettes. Lately, however, smokeless tobacco is becoming very popular among adolescent boys. Alcohol or marijuana use, or both, soon follows. Initially, use is limited to weekends, but later some use during the week begins to take place. Users learn that the drug will provide the feeling they desire every time and learn to control the degree of the feeling by regulating the amount of the drug they use. With the exception of alcohol, few people use one drug exclusively. Drug use in this stage takes place with friends, and users can take the drug or leave it. Therefore, this stage is sometimes referred to as social use.

Abuse

Here, the frequency of drug use escalates. Users begin to maintain their own supplies and may begin to use drugs when alone rather than with friends. In this stage, drugs are generally used only at night or on weekends. Users do not show up at school or work intoxicated and can usually control the time, amount, and outcome of drug use. They develop some degree of tolerance and increase the quantity of drugs they take. They may start to develop some guilt about their use and occasionally suffer blackouts—not remembering what happened when taking drugs. They may occasionally suffer some medical problems, such as alcoholic gastritic or hangover, or have occasional spats with their spouses about the magnitude of their use. They may at times have conflicts with the police when intoxicated.

Dependence

Here, most chemically dependent people use drugs almost every day, if not daily. Tolerance increases to the point that very large quantities of a drug are required for users to obtain the desired feeling. Blackouts become more frequent, users prefer to take drugs by themselves rather than with friends, and drugs become the major focus of users' lives, which revolve around getting, keeping, and using the drugs. Almost all activities involve drugs and drug-using friends. When family members or friends confront them, addicts deny having a problem. Family relationships, school and job performance, and health are destroyed. Users may be arrested for driving under the influence, possessing controlled substances, drunk and disorderly conduct, or even dealing drugs.

For many drugs, if users stop taking them in this stage, withdrawal may set in. Users have severe cravings for the drug and have to use it to feel normal. They lose control of their drug use, and the compulsion to take the drug is overwhelming. Users' abnormal behavior is masked by a denial system, and they suffer significant impairment from physiological, psychological, or social dysfunction. Drug use continues despite adverse consequences.

Crossing the Wall

Progression from abuse to dependence is often referred to as crossing the wall (Figure 1.1) because in the use and abuse stages an individual can cut back or stop using as circumstances dictate. However, once a person develops dependence, taking a drug is no longer a matter of choice. Trying to quit using a drug, once addicted to it, is said to be like beating your head against a brick wall: It is very difficult to do without help.

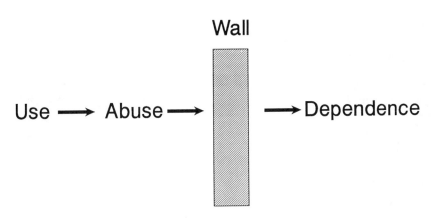

FIGURE 1.1. Crossing the wall.

Denial

Denial is most simply defined as not recognizing or admitting a problem, even in the face of significant adverse consequences and despite the fact that the problem is evident to others. Addicts' denial, and that of their families as well, is the primary reason many people are addicted for years.[12]

People get addicted to feelings, rather than to drugs per se. Dependence, then, is a repeated effort to obtain a specific feeling. Feelings originate in the limbic system, which controls emotions and motivation. It is composed of, among other things, the hypothalamus, the amygdala, and the septum. The hypothalamus contains the body's pleasure center, where many drugs exert their psychoactive effects.[12]

Drug addicts know that they are hurting themselves and others, but once they develop dependence, driven by impulses from the limbic system, they continue to use drugs (Figure 1.2). The logic center of the brain (the cerebral cortex) is unable to control the intense craving for a drug that originates in the limbic system. As a result, addicts develop behaviors (manipulation, lying, self-pity, irresponsibility) that enable them to keep using drugs. As one might expect, over a period of time addicts develop guilt over drug use, the inability to control it, and their addictive behaviors. Normally, guilt would reduce the drug use (indicated by the broken line in Figure 1.2); it does not once dependence develops. To protect the mind from the psychological pain of the internal conflict between drug use and guilt, an elaborate denial system evolves to separate the logic center from the feeling center and, thereby, to relieve guilt. Unfortunately, the denial system serves to perpetuate addiction.[12-13]

Addicts use at least eight tools to achieve denial: (1) *rationalization* — using socially acceptable but untrue explanations for inappropriate behavior; (2) *projection* — blaming others for one's own failings and inadequacies; (3) *minimization* — underestimating the magnitude of one's drug use; (4) *repression* —

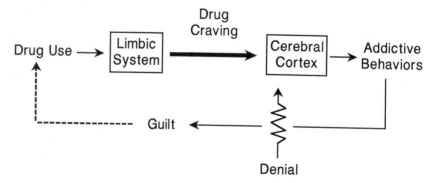

FIGURE 1.2. Mechanism of denial.

unconsciously excluding from one's conscious mind unbearable thoughts, experiences, or feelings; (5) *suppression*—consciously pushing away feelings and events into the background; (6) *isolation*—deliberately avoiding relationships and communication with others that might threaten the ability to use a drug; (7) *regression*—reverting to a level of emotional maturity appropriate to an earlier stage in life; and (8) *conversion*—expressing emotional conflict through physical symptoms. This last tool allows addicts to focus on physical symptoms so as to avoid dealing with the underlying cause of them, which is chemical dependence.[12]

Etiology of Chemical Dependence

Theories on the etiology of chemical dependence abound.[14] Although most of them involve many factors, their basic perspectives can be categorized into three general models—psychological, social, and biological.

Psychological Model

The psychological model argues that certain personality types, personality traits, or other psychopathology predispose individuals to chemical dependence and that underlying psychopathology generates aversive emotional states a person then relieves by substance use. Chemical dependence is viewed as a form of self-medication and, thus, is considered to be only symptomatic of the true, underlying psychological disorder. According to this model, substance abuse would be expected to stop once its cause has been effectively treated.[15]

Support for this position rests on studies showing significantly increased incidences of psychological pathologies among chemically dependent people. However, the vast majority of these studies were conducted on addicts after they had already become chemically dependent, so that their psychopathologies are at least as likely to be the product of substance abuse as its cause. In general, studies looking at personality characteristics in individuals before and after development of chemical dependence show little or no difference between those who subsequently become chemically dependent and those who do not. Personality characteristics, however, probably do play a role in the development of chemical dependence in some individuals. Some studies have reported higher incidences of antisocial tendencies before, as well as after, the development of chemical dependence in some people. However, these individuals account only for a small portion of the chemically dependent population. Traditional psychotherapy, especially when aimed at psychopathology other than chemical dependence itself, has not generally been successful in eliminating chemical dependence.[15]

Social Model

Sociological theories of chemical dependence argue that substance abuse is learned from environmental influences and experiences, much in the way that language and social customs are learned. Such behavior is then considered to be maintained by the positive reinforcement of the drug use itself. This behavior is considered to be predominantly controlled by external, environmental stimuli, such as underemployment, poverty, marital discord, and job stress. Social models have difficulty explaining middle-class and upper-class drug abusers.[15]

Children growing up in families with addicted parents are more apt to become chemically dependent than others in the general population. The social model considers drug abuse to be a learned behavior. Similarly, peer pressure is overwhelmingly important in the initiation of drug use and abuse. Why some individuals go on to become chemically dependent and others do not is poorly understood.[14]

Biological Model

The fundamental etiological assumption of the biological model of chemical dependence is that individuals who become addicts are in some significant way biologically different from people who do not become addicts. This factor, whatever it is, makes these individuals more susceptible to addiction. To date, although promising studies are in progress, this predispositioning factor has not been identified.[15]

Evidence from studies of twins and adopted children strongly implicates genetic predisposition as a contributing factor in some alcoholics. Comparative studies have reported a higher rate for alcoholism in identical twins than in fraternal twins. The strongest support of the genetic model of alcoholism, however, comes from adoption studies. Male adopted children who have alcoholic natural fathers are almost four times as likely to become alcoholic than are male adopted children who do not have alcoholic fathers. Further, when sons of alcoholics who have been reared by adoptive parents are compared to brothers who have been reared by biological, alcoholic fathers, the incidence of alcoholism is about the same. A significant number of people with no apparent genetic predisposition (no parental addiction) also develop alcoholism, indicating that, although genetic predisposition may make it easier to become chemically dependent, it is not necessary. Because many people who would be expected to have a genetic predisposition for alcoholism never drink, it is also not a sufficient criterion by itself. Other factors must be involved. Studies are in progress regarding possible genetic predispositions to other abused drugs.[15]

Disease Model

There is a growing consensus that chemical dependence is a disease, because it is a pathological state with characteristic signs and symptoms and a predictable course and outcome if untreated. This model holds that the etiology of chemical dependence involves an interplay of all three factors—biological, psychological, and social. Thus, chemical dependence is considered to be a biopsychosocial disease, characterized by compulsion to use a drug, loss of control over its use, and continued use despite adverse consequences. The model further holds that once individuals develop the disease of chemical dependence, they cannot return to controlled use of a psychoactive substance. Abstinence in recovery (living a comfortable and responsible life without alcohol or other drugs) is the most effective long-term treatment of the disease.[9]

Specialists in addictive medicine currently regard the disease model as the best for understanding and treating chemical dependence. It allows physicians to use familiar techniques to make a diagnosis, form a treatment plan, educate a patient, and discuss prognosis. It helps differentiate chemical dependence from a bad habit, moral weakness, or lack of willpower. Perhaps most important, it obligates physicians to address the problem of chemical dependence in a nonjudgmental way.[16]

Classification of Drugs by Their Effects on the Central Nervous System

In this book we will classify drugs of abuse according to how they most prominently affect the central nervous system (CNS) (Table 1.3). This classification is most useful to physicians.

1. *CNS depressants:* These drugs depress excitable tissues in the brain. They decrease inhibitions, relieve anxiety, intoxicate, and sedate. This group of drugs includes alcohol, barbiturates (amobarbital, phenobarbital, secobarbital), barbiturate-like drugs (glutethimide, methyprylon, methaqualone), carbamate compounds (meprobamate), benzodiazepines (diazepam, chlordiaz-

TABLE 1.3. Classification of drugs by their effects on the central nervous system.

Drug group	Examples	Effects on CNS
CNS depressants	alcohol, barbiturates, benzodiazepines	decrease inhibitions, relieve anxiety, intoxicate, sedate
Opioids	heroin, morphine, codeine, hydromorphone, fentanyl	reduce pain, cause euphoria, sedate
CNS stimulants	cocaine, amphetamines, phenmetrazine	cause excitement, produce euphoria, depress appetite, decrease need for sleep
Cannabinoids	marijuana, hashish	produce sense of detachment, euphoria, and altered time perception
Hallucinogens	LSD, psilocybin, mescaline, MDMA	produce hallucinations (usually visual but may be auditory or olfactory)
Phencyclidines	PCP, ketamine	produce intoxication, muscular rigidity, and reduced pain
Inhalants	gasoline, amyl nitrite, nitrous oxide	produce euphoria, sedate

epoxide, lorazepam), and several others (chloral hydrate, paraldehyde). Drugs in this group are also known as sedative-hypnotics. Sedatives produce calm and relaxation; hypnotics induce sleep.[17]

2. *Opioids:* Also called narcotic analgesics, the opioids are used clinically to reduce pain. They also produce euphoria and sedation. They are classified as naturally occurring (morphine, codeine), semisynthetic (heroin, hydromorphone, oxycodone), and synthetic (meperidine, methadone, propoxyphene). The agonist-antagonist opioids (pentazocine, nalbuphine) are also synthetic.[17]

3. *CNS stimulants:* The most prominent effect of these drugs is their ability to stimulate the CNS, causing excitement, euphoria, decreased appetite, and decreased need for sleep. Aside from caffeine and nicotine, the stimulants most commonly encountered in clinical situations are amphetamines and cocaine.[17]

4. *Cannabinoids:* The cannabinoids (marijuana, hashish) produce a sense of detachment, euphoria, and altered time. Their principle active ingredient is delta-9-tetrahydrocannabinol (THC).[17]

5. *Hallucinogens:* These substances produce hallucinations, usually visual, but some auditory or olfactory. Drugs in the hallucinogen class include lysergic acid diethylamide (LSD), mescaline (peyote cactus), and psilocybin (mushrooms).[17]

6. *Phencyclidines:* There are at least 60 active precursors, derivatives, and analogs related to phencyclidine (PCP). Although PCP now has no legal use, a related drug, ketamine, is still used as a dissociative anesthetic. PCP and its related compounds produce intoxication and muscle rigidity and reduce pain.[18]

7. *Inhalants:* These drugs are volatile, liquid substances whose fumes are inhaled directly or are gases that are inhaled. They include solvents (gasoline, glues, paint thinners), nitrites (amyl nitrite, butyl nitrite), and nitrous oxide. They produce altered states of consciousness, primarily light-headedness or euphoria and confusion. Nitrous oxide (laughing gas) is used legally as a dental anesthetic.[17]

Controlled Substance Act Classification of Drugs

Another important classification of abused drugs is that of the Federal Comprehensive Drug Abuse Prevention and Control Act, passed in 1970 to regulate the manufacture, distribution, and dispensing of controlled substances. The act established five schedules of controlled drugs, with varying degrees of control for each schedule. Drugs were placed in appropriate schedules based on three main criteria: (1) potential for abuse, (2) accepted medical use, and (3) potential to produce dependence.[19]

Schedule I. Drugs in this class have a high potential for abuse and have no currently accepted medical use. They are considered unsafe for use, even under medical supervision. Drugs listed in Schedule I include heroin, LSD, and marijuana.[19]

TABLE 1.4. Abbreviated schedule of controlled substances.

Schedule I	Schedule II	Schedule III	Schedule IV	Schedule V
Narcotic Analgesics	*Narcotic Analgesics*	*Narcotic Analgesics*	*Narcotic Analgesics*	Mixtures containing limited quantities of narcotic drugs, with non-narcotic active medicinal ingredients; generally for antitussive and antidiarrheal purposes
acetylmethadol (LAAM)	codeine	acetaminophen + codeine	pentazocine	
heroin	dihydrocodeine	APC + codeine	propoxyphene	
Stimulants	fentanyl	aspirin + codeine	*Depressants*	
amphetamine variants	hydrocodone	nalorphine	barbital	
Hallucinogens	hydromorphone	paregoric	chloral hydrate	
ibogaine	levorphanol	*Depressants*	chlordiazepoxide	
lysergic acid-25 (LSD)	meperidine	any compound containing	clonazepam	
mescaline	methadone	an unscheduled drug and:	chlorazepate	
peyote	morphine	amobarbital	diazepam	
psilocybin, psilocyn	opium	secobarbital	ethchlorvynol	
Cannabinoids	oxycodone	pentobarbital	ethinamate	
marijuana	oxymorphone	glutethimide	fenfluramine	
hashish	*Depressants*	methyprylon	flurazepam	
THC	amobarbital	*Stimulants*	meprobamate	
Phencyclidines	methaqualone	benzphetamine	mephobarbital	
Analogs of	Secobarbital	mazindol	oxazepam	
phencyclidines	pentobarbital	phendimetrazine	paraldehyde	
	Stimulants		phenobarbital	
	amphetamine		prazepam	
	cocaine		*Stimulants*	
	methamphetamine		diethylpropion	
	methylphenidate		phentermine	
	phenmetrazine		pemoline	
	Pencyclidines			
	phencyclidine			

Based on the Federal Comprehensive Drug Abuse Prevention and Control Act of 1970 and subsequent revisions. State laws may vary.

Schedule II. Drugs in this class also have a high potential for abuse; however, they have a currently accepted medical use. Abuse of one of these drugs may lead to severe dependence. Drugs listed in Schedule II include morphine, cocaine, and PCP.

Schedule III. Drugs in this class have a lower potential for abuse than the drugs in Schedules I and II. They also have currently accepted medical uses. Abuse of these drugs may lead to moderate to low physical dependence or high psychological dependence. They include paregoric, glutethimide (Doriden), and benzphetamine (Didrex).

Schedule IV. Drugs in this class have a low potential for abuse compared to drugs in Schedule III. They have currently accepted medical uses and may lead to limited dependence. They include diazepam (Valium), phenobarbital (Luminal), and pemoline (Cylert).

Schedule V. Drugs in this class have a low potential for abuse compared to drugs in Schedule IV. They have currently accepted medical uses and may lead to limited dependence. They are mixtures containing limited quantities of narcotics and nonnarcotic active medicinal ingredients. They are generally antitussives and antidiarrheals. Examples are diphenoxylate plus atropine (Lomotil) and hydrocodone plus phenyltoloxamine (Tussionex).[19]

Examples of abused drugs in each of the five schedules are given in Table 1.4.

References

1. *Epidemiology in Alcohol and Health.* DHHS Publication Number (ADM) 87-1519, U.S. Department of Health and Human Services, Rockville, Maryland, 1987, pp. 1–27.
2. Delbanco, T. L., and H. N. Barnes. The epidemiology of alcohol abuse and the response of physicians. In *Alcoholism: A Guide for the Primary Care Physician.* Ed. by H. N. Barnes, M. D. Aronson, and T. L. Delbanco. Springer-Verlag, New York, 1987, pp. 3–8.
3. Stoudemire, A., L. Wallack, and N. Hedenark. Alcohol dependence and abuse. In *Closing the Gap: The Burden of Unnecessary Illness.* Ed. by R. W. Amler and H. B. Dull. Oxford University Press, New York, 1987, pp. 9–18.
4. Milhorn, H. T., Jr. The diagnosis of alcoholism. *American Family Physician,* 37:175–183, 1988.
5. Van Cleave, S., W. Byrd, and K. Revell. The equal opportunity destroyer: The magnitude of the drug abuse epidemic. In *Counseling for Substance Abuse and Addiction.* Word Book, Waco, Texas, 1987, pp. 55–74.
6. Johnston, L. D., P. M. O'Malley, and J. G. Bachman. Drug use by high school seniors—class of 1986. U.S. Department of Health and Human Services, Rockville, Maryland, 1987.
7. Milhorn, H. T., Jr. Nicotine dependence. *American Family Physician,* 39:214–224, 1989.
8. Milhorn, H. T., Jr. Chemical dependency: Is medical education falling short? *Mississippi State Medical Association Impaired Physicians' Newsletter,* April, 1989.
9. Wilford, B. B. (Ed.). Etiology. In *Review Course Syllabus,* American Medical Society on Alcoholism and Other Drug Dependencies, New York, 1987, pp. 107–112.

10. Psychoactive substance use disorders. In *Diagnostic and Statistical Manual of Mental Disorders, Third Edition Revised (DSM-III-R)*, American Psychiatric Association, Washington, D.C., 1987, pp. 165–185.
11. Wilford, B. B. (Ed.). Nosology. In *Review Course Syllabus*, American Medical Society on Alcoholism and Other Drug Dependencies, New York, 1987, pp. 1–12.
12. Van Cleave, S., W. Byrd, and K. Revell. If drugs are so bad, why do people keep using them: How denial and guilt perpetuate drug abuse. In *Counseling for Substance Abuse and Addiction*. Word Books, Waco, Texas, 1987, pp. 63–87.
13. Milhorn, H. T., Jr. Introduction to physiological control systems. In *The Application of Control Theory to Physiological Systems*. W. B. Saunders, Philadelphia, 1966, pp. 113–137.
14. Lettieri, D. J. Drug abuse: A review of explanations and models of explanation. In *Alcohol and Substance Abuse in Adolescence*. Ed. by B. Stimmel, Haworth, New York, 1985, pp. 9–40.
15. Alford, G. S. Psychoactive substance use disorders. In *Recent Developments in Adolescent Psychiatry*. Ed. by L. K. G. Hsu and M. Hersen. Wiley, New York, 1989, pp. 309–331.
16. Aronson, M. D. Definition of alcoholism. In *Alcoholism: A Guide for the Primary Care Physician*. Ed. by H. N. Barnes, M. D. Aronson, and T. L. Delbanco. Springer-Verlag, New York, 1987, pp. 9–15.
17. Wilford, B. B. (Ed.). Major drugs of abuse. In *Drug Abuse: A Guide for Primary Care Physicians*. AMA, Chicago, 1981, pp. 21–84.
18. Milhorn, H. T., Jr. Diagnosis and management of phencyclidine intoxication. *American Family Physician*, in press.
19. Wilford, B. B. (Ed.). Prescribing practices and drug abuse. In *Drug Abuse: A Guide for Primary Care Physicians*, AMA, Chicago, 1981, pp. 263–284.

Part I   The Basics

Kurt A. Rodriguez
#5 Chase Hall
English Village Apts.
Newark, DE 19711

CHAPTER 2

Diagnosis

Introduction

Many physicians underdiagnose chemical dependence for various reasons. They may feel that chemical dependence is a weakness rather than a disease or may believe that addicts differ in appearance from other patients. Patients, family members, and personal physicians frequently deny the existence of a problem. Some physicians are reluctant to make the diagnosis of a disorder they don't know how to treat. Diagnosis depends mainly on a patient's medical, psychological, and social history, although a patient's presentation, physical examination, and laboratory findings can be helpful. Questionnaires are useful for routine screening of patients. As with any chronic progressive disease, the earlier in its course the diagnosis of chemical dependence is made, the better is the outcome.

Problems in Diagnosis

Common problems that interfere with a physician's making the diagnosis of chemical dependence include undereducation, false beliefs, denial, and feelings of inadequacy.

Undereducation

Physicians and patients are products of the same culture, one in which most people believe that chemical dependence is a weakness rather than a disease. As a result, many physicians believe that when they recognize addiction in a patient, they are accusing the patient of bad behavior rather than making a medical diagnosis. The belief largely results from inadequate education about chemical dependence in medical schools. Only about 3 percent of the nation's medical schools offer a separate course in chemical dependence, and physicians generally receive little training in the behavioral sciences, including family function and dysfunction. As a result of this inadequate education, medical students have been found to have less expertise in substance abuse than in other areas.[1-3]

Most physicians can recognize the late-stage symptoms of addiction (gastrointestinal bleeding, jaundice, ascites) but are unable to recognize the early symptoms, which are behavioral. Because chemical dependence is a chronic, progressive disease that responds well to early detection and early treatment, the failure to recognize the early symptoms of addiction represents a major oversight on the part of medical professionals. In most cases, this failure to diagnose addiction early in its course ensures that the chemically dependent person's disease will progress to more advanced, less treatable stages, even while under the care of a physician. Effective physician education has been found to increase the diagnosis of chemical dependence.[1,4]

False Beliefs

There is a common belief that chemically dependent people differ from other patients in appearance. The myth persists that most chemically dependent people can be recognized as skid row bums. In actuality, these individuals may account for as few as 3 percent of chemically dependent people. The other 97 percent, for the most part, are employed and on the surface appear to be doing well. Having accepted popular views of addiction and the resulting social stigma, physicians may be less likely to make diagnoses that they perceive to be embarrassing or demeaning to patients.[5-6]

The false perception that alcoholism and other drug dependencies are hopeless conditions may prevent many physicians from making a diagnosis of addiction and taking the steps to get a chemically dependent person the professional help he or she needs. Studies have shown that interns and residents are significantly more pessimistic about the outcome of treatment for alcoholics than first-year medical students. This general pessimism arises from unpleasant experiences on clinical wards with intoxicated individuals going through withdrawal, who are immediately discharged from the hospital once they are stable. Interns and residents, for the most part, have little or no experience with chemically dependent people with years of recovery. A number of studies have shown that many patients completing treatment are still drug-free after two years. Physicians need to be informed of these encouraging statistics and need to become aware of treatment programs in their local areas. Treatment offers hope for chemically dependent people and their families.[4-6]

Denial

Diagnosis is further complicated by denial, a hallmark of chemical dependence. Addicts may firmly believe that their problem is not drugs and continue to use them in spite of medical, psychological, or social problems. Denial is a subconscious defense mechanism; it is not pathological lying, but a predictable symptom of addiction. It is not used only by chemically dependent people. Frequently, spouses and children cover up for addicts out of misguided love and a reluctance to face the embarrassment of admitting the truth. Physicians must be careful not to become part of this denial system.

When patients refuse to acknowledge their illness, physicians face a considerably more difficult task. They need to be aware of the scope and subtleties of addictive denial so that they are not misled by addicts' manipulative behavior or caught off guard by addicts' persuasiveness, congeniality, or defensiveness. When physicians recognize that chemically dependent people are trapped within their own chemically altered perceptions, they can more easily maintain the emotional detachment that is necessary to make diagnoses and direct patients to the professional help they need.[5-7]

Feelings of Inadequacy

Many physicians face an additional problem: They are uncomfortable diagnosing an illness they don't know how to treat. Consequently, they limit their responsibility to treating the late medical stages of addiction and only warn patients that the offending agents are damaging their bodies and that they should quit using them. Physicians frequently do not realize that the problem is not that simple. Addicted people cannot stop on their own. If they could, they would.[6-7]

Making the Diagnosis

A number of diagnostic tools are available to help physicians diagnose addiction to chemical substances. These include screening questionnaires, a patient's personal and family history, a physical examination, and laboratory tests. Also, a patient's behavior during an office or emergency room visit may be a clue to the possibility of chemical dependence.

Definition of Chemical Dependence

As we saw in Chapter 1, chemical dependence can be defined as a chronic, progressive disease characterized by significant impairment that is directly associated with persistent and excessive use of a psychoactive substance. Impairment may involve physiological, psychological, or social dysfunction. Basically, patients who meet this definition are considered to have the disease of chemical dependence.[8]

Screening Questionnaires

Alcoholism

Anyone who consumes alcoholic beverages is at risk for developing alcoholism. Therefore, anyone who answers "yes" to the question "Do you drink?" should be screened. Ideally, screening should be part of every new patient's medical history and part of what is added to that history with each periodic physical examination.

Two short, self-administered questionnaires are suitable for this—the Short Michigan Alcohol Screening Test (SMAST) and the CAGE questionnaire.

The SMAST (Table 2.1) is a shortened, 13-question version of the original 24-question Michigan Alcohol Screening Test (MAST).[9-10] The SMAST has been shown to be as effective as the MAST and to have greater than 90 percent sensitivity.[9] It can be administered to a patient or the patient's spouse. As with all screening tests, some false positive results do occur. The SMAST deals with the consequences of drinking rather than the quantity, frequency, or duration of drinking.[9,11]

The CAGE questionnaire (Table 2.2) is even shorter and easier to administer than the SMAST; however, it is more likely to give false positive results. Like the SMAST, it has a high degree of sensitivity.[12-13] Either test is acceptable as a screening tool.

Because screening questionnaires have been developed for people in middle age, they are less appropriate for use with adolescents and the elderly.[14]

Other Drug Dependencies

Screening questionnaires for drugs other than alcohol have not been studied to the extent that the MAST, SMAST, and CAGE have. Less is known about their sensitivity and specificity. One such test is given in Table 2.3.[15]

TABLE 2.1. Short Michigan Alcoholism Screening Test (SMAST).*

1. Do you feel you are a normal drinker? (by normal we mean you drink less than or as much as most other people) (No)
2. Does your wife, husband, a parent or other near relative ever worry or complain about your drinking? (Yes)
3. Do you ever feel guilty about your drinking? (Yes)
4. Do friends or relatives think you are a normal drinker? (No)
5. Are you able to stop drinking when you want to? (No)
6. Have you ever attended a meeting of Alcoholics Anonymous? (Yes)
7. Has drinking ever created problems between you and your wife, husband, a parent or other near relative? (Yes)
8. Have you ever gotten into trouble at work because of your drinking? (Yes)
9. Have you ever neglected your obligations, your family, or your work for two or more days in a row because you were drinking? (Yes)
10. Have you ever gone to anyone for help about your drinking? (Yes)
11. Have you ever been in a hospital because of drinking? (Yes)
12. Have you ever been arrested for drunken driving, driving while intoxicated, or driving under the influence of alcoholic beverages? (Yes)
13. Have you ever been arrested, even for a few hours, because of other drunken behavior? (Yes)

* Answers related to a diagnosis of alcoholism are shown in parentheses after each question. Three or more of these answers indicate a diagnosis of alcoholism; two such answers indicate the possibility of alcoholism; fewer than two answers indicate that alcoholism is not likely.
Reprinted with permission from M.A. Selzer, A. Vinokur, and L. Van Rooijen, A self-administered Short Michigan Alcohol Screening Test, *Journal of Studies on Alcohol* 36:117–126, 1975. Copyright by Journal of Studies on Alcohol, Inc. Rutgers Center of Alcohol Studies, New Brunswick, N.J. 08903.

TABLE 2.2. CAGE questionnaire.

1. Have you ever felt you ought to Cut down on your drinking?
2. Have people Annoyed you by criticizing your drinking?
3. Have you ever felt bad or Guilty about your drinking?
4. Have you ever had a drink first thing in the morning (Eye opener) to steady your nerves or get rid of a hangover?

* Two or more affirmative answers indicate probable alcoholism. Any single affirmative answer deserves further evaluation.
From J.A. Ewing, Detecting alcoholism: The CAGE questionnaire, *Journal of the American Medical Association*, 252:1905–1907. Copyright 1984, American Medical Association.

TABLE 2.3. Drug abuse screening test.

1. Have you used drugs other than those required for medical reasons?
2. Have you abused prescription drugs?
3. Do you abuse more than one drug at a time?
4. Can you get through the week without using drugs?
5. Are you always able to stop using drugs when you want to?
6. Have you had blackouts or flashbacks as a result of drug use?
7. Do you ever feel bad or guilty about your drug use?
8. Does your spouse (or parents) ever complain about your involvement with drugs?
9. Has drug abuse created problems between you and your spouse or your parents?
10. Have you lost friends because of your use of drugs?
11. Have you neglected your family because of your use of drugs?
12. Have you been in trouble at work because of drug abuse?
13. Have you lost a job because of drug abuse?
14. Have you gotten into fights when under the influence of drugs?
15. Have you engaged in illegal activities in order to obtain drugs?
16. Have you been arrested for possession of illegal drugs?
17. Have you ever experienced withdrawal symptoms (felt sick) when you stopped taking drugs?
18. Have you had medical problems as a result of your drug use (e.g., memory loss, hepatitis, convulsions, bleeding, etc.)?
19. Have you gone to anyone for help for a drug problem?
20. Have you been involved in a treatment program especially related to drug use?

Scoring key: Score one point for each Yes answer, in questions 1–3, 6–20; score one point for each No answer on questions 4 and 5.

Score	Degree of drug abuse problem
0	none
1–5	low level
6–10	moderate level
11–15	substantial level
16–20	severe level

A low score does not necessarily mean that a person is free of drug-related problems. Any positive response may mean that you or someone you know needs help.

From S. Van Cleave, W. Byrd, and K. Revell, *Counseling for Substance Abuse and Addiction,* Word Books, Waco, Texas, 1987.

Personal and Family History

As part of a personal history related to chemical dependence, physicians should cover the following areas: (1) alcohol history, (2) other drug history (including prescription drugs), (3) social functioning, (4) psychological functioning, and (5) sexual functioning. In addition, a standard medical history should be taken, with special attention paid to medical problems associated with alcoholism and other drug addictions. The review of systems may also identify problems directing attention to chemical dependence. Family history may be helpful.[15]

Questions about substance use should begin with the least threatening subjects. Thus, start with questions about substances that are culturally acceptable, such as the number of cups of coffee a patient drinks a day. This can progress to the number of cigarettes a patient smokes a day and then to the patient's daily intake of alcohol and other drugs. A change in a patient's style of response can be a clue to addiction. Patients will freely tell you how many cups of coffee they drink a day or how many cigarettes they smoke, but when asked about alcohol or other drugs, chemically dependent people often switch from precise answers to vague ones such as "I drink a few beers now and then," "I drink socially," or "I've tried cocaine once or twice." Anger, evasiveness, or glib conversation from patients giving their substance use history should be regarded as suspicious.[8]

Information about substance use that may be helpful includes when a patient last drank or used drugs; how much the person drank or used on that occasion; if the person drinks or uses drugs every day and, if not, how often he or she does so; how much the person averages drinking or using on these occasions; how long the person has been drinking or using drugs in this manner; and how old the person was when he or she took a first drink or tried another drug. How much a patient is willing to admit depends to a great extent on the examiner's attitude. It should be emphasized that answers to these kinds of questions are only of secondary importance. The most important questions relate to what substance abuse is doing to a patient's life.[8,16]

A variety of findings may reveal psychological problems, such as insomnia, anxiety, depression, and suicide attempts or gestures. A social history should include questions about a patient's work, family, interpersonal relationship, and legal problems.[8] Psychological and social findings that may indicate chemical dependence are given in Table 2.4.

Chemical dependence is notorious for causing sexual problems, especially impotence in men and menstrual irregularities and infertility in women. Decreased interest in sex may occur in either sex. Questions about sexual functioning should be part of every medical history.[17]

Family history may also give physicians useful information. The tendency to become an alcoholic runs in families and is thought to be genetically transmitted. A male patient whose father was an alcoholic, for example, may have almost a fourfold increase in risk of becoming an alcoholic than someone in the general public.[18] Genetic transmission for other drugs has not been studied to the same extent as it has for alcoholism. It is likely that a tendency to chemical dependence, per se, will be found to have genetic transmission.

TABLE 2.4. Psychological and social findings that may indicate chemical dependence.

Anxiety, insomnia, depression, suicide gestures or attempts
Social isolation
Change in mood, including unpredictability and impulsivity
Self-medication, regular or prolonged use of sleeping pills or tranquilizers or repeated requests for
    them
Repeated requests for narcotics or stimulants
Visiting many physicians, or doctor hopping
Divorce or separation
Interpersonal problems at work or school
Other job or school problems (tardiness, calling in sick, absenteeism)
Frequent job changes
Frequent moves to new areas (geographic cure)
Underemployment for educational level
Decreased school performance
Decreased goal-directed drives (amotivational syndrome)
Change in choice of friends or associates
Child or spouse abuse
Children doing poorly in school, disturbed or runaway children
Preoccupation with recreational drinking or using
Binge drinking
Gulping the first two or three drinks
Use of alcohol before any office visit
Loss of interest in nondrinking or nonusing activities
Drinking before a party (just in case there's not enough to drink at the party)
History of increased tolerance to alcohol or other drugs; loss of tolerance in older indi-
    viduals
Repeated attempts to stop drinking or using (patients claim *they* can quit anytime)
Any alcohol or other drug-related arrests or driving under the influence
Blackouts (not remembering what happened during a drinking or using spell)
Loss of interest in personal hygiene or appearance
Complaints by family members about behavior related to use of alcohol or other drugs
Continued drinking or using despite medical, psychological, or social contraindications

Patient Presentation

Addicts often try to get drugs from physicians. Certain behaviors are common
among such patients, such as describing a dramatic and compelling but vague
complaint; making subjective complaints not accompanied by the usual objective
signs; offering a diagnosis and specifically requesting a certain drug, often claiming to be allergic to less potent ones; showing no interest in a diagnosis, failing
to keep appointments for X rays or laboratory tests, or failing to see another physician for a consulting opinion; and rejecting all treatments that do not include
psychoactive drugs.[19]

Patient hustlers use many manipulative approaches. These include feigning
physical problems. For example, those seeking narcotics often complain of renal
colic, toothache, or tic douloureux. They generally can simulate symptoms
exceptionally well. Those feigning renal colic may even prick their fingers to put

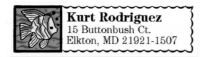

drops of blood in their urine. Those feigning toothache often claim to have an out-of-town dentist and to have left prescribed pain medication at home.

Hustlers also may feign psychological problems, such as anxiety, insomnia, or fatigue. Most such drug seekers want tranquilizers, sleeping pills, or stimulants. Often they are deceptive, complaining that their medication was lost, stolen, or accidentally dropped in the toilet. They may steal, alter, or forge prescriptions, request refills in a shorter period of time than was originally prescribed, or phone physicians on call and claim to be patients of their partners. Patients may also pressure physicians, to elicit sympathy or guilt. One way they do this is by suggesting that medical treatment caused their addiction. They may admit to being addicted and pressure physicians to detoxify them as outpatients, although they have no intention of giving up their drug use. Alcoholics commonly seek prescriptions for minor tranquilizers either to help them quit drinking or to treat the anxiety and insomnia associated with alcoholism. Such outpatient detoxification is usually not advisable for most drugs and is illegal for narcotics. Patients may directly threaten physicians with physical, legal or financial harm, may try to bribe them, or may use the names of influential people, claiming them to be relatives or friends.[19]

Physical Examination

Patients with chemical addictions may have a variety of physical signs that should prompt physicians to ask questions about alcohol or other drug use.

Alcoholism

All physicians are familiar with the signs and symptoms of late-stage alcoholism, such as cirrhosis of the liver, ascites, chronic pancreatitis (with or without pseudocysts), cardiomyopathy, and esophageal varicose, and they are experts at managing these conditions. The real challenge is to diagnose alcoholism in patients early in its course to prevent them from reaching advanced stages.

Physicians can find many clues to alcoholism in physical examinations. Acute intoxication causes sedation, confusion, disorientation, slurred speech, faulty judgment, and many other symptoms. Physicians may smell alcohol on a patient's breath. Chronic alcohol use leads to untidiness in personal habits and to depression.[16]

Alcoholics may have slightly bloated and plethoric faces. They may even have parotid swelling and in general, a cushingoid look. They may have small bruises in a variety of places and in a variety of colors, depending on how long ago they were acquired. This is particularly true of women alcoholics, who tend to bump into furniture and door knobs while doing housework. Cigarette burns on patients' fingers, chests, or legs may indicate alcoholism. Severe periodontal disease, despite an otherwise neat and clean appearance, is another clue.[20]

Mild to moderate hypertension is very common among alcoholics. This usually disappears in a few days to a week after they stop drinking. Alcoholics are frequently admitted to treatment centers on hypertensive medications. Many are later discharged on no medications and with good blood pressure control.[20] Cardiac arrhythmias, as well as abnormal ST-T findings, are also common in alcoholics.[21]

Elevated uric acid levels precipitate gouty attacks in some alcoholics. The attacks dissipate once patients stop drinking and their uric acid levels return to normal. Gout may be particularly difficult to control in alcoholics.[21]

Grand mal seizure in adults should make physicians think of alcoholism, especially if patients tell them they stopped drinking in the past 72 hours. A seizure within a few days of a patient's being admitted to a hospital may be a clue to alcohol withdrawal.[20]

Patients diagnosed with cancer of virtually any segment of the gastrointestinal tract should be questioned about drinking. Alcoholics have a higher incidence of cancers of the oral cavity, tongue, pharynx, larynx, esophagus, stomach, liver, pancreas, colon, and rectum than do nonalcoholics. Alcohol appears to act synergistically with cigarette smoking in this regard.[21]

Multiple rib fractures that show different stages of healing on chest X rays should also be a tip-off to alcoholism. Fractured ribs are the most common abnormalities on chest X rays in alcoholics. Alcohol use is frequently involved in motor vehicle accidents, drownings, accidental falls, beatings, shootings, and stabbings.[20]

Gastrointestinal problems are the most common medical complaints of alcoholics. Alcohol irritates the gastric mucosa and can cause gastritis, ulcers, duodenitis, ileitis, irritable bowel syndrome, and pancreatitis.[21] Alcoholics commonly show up at treatment centers on one or more stomach medications, some of which they have been on for years. These same patients are rarely discharged still needing these medications.

Some alcoholics' cushingoid appearance, along with the hypertension and glucose intolerance caused by alcohol, occasionally prompts physicians to do endocrine work-ups without first considering alcoholism. Similarly, physicians may confuse the combination of the mild tremors of minor alcohol withdrawal, hypertension, and occasional cardiac arrhythmias with hyperthyroidism.[20]

Physical findings that may indicate alcoholism are given in Table 2.5.

Other Drug Dependencies

Restlessness or agitated behavior most commonly suggests that patients are using stimulants or hallucinogens or are withdrawing from depressants or opioids. Marijuana use occasionally produces a similar response. Quiet, withdrawn behavior may indicate recent use of depressants, opioids, or hallucinogens. Withdrawal from stimulants may be characterized by apathy, somnolence, and depression. Depression can also occur with chronic use of depressants.[8]

Disorientation most often occurs with the use of hallucinogens and phencyclidines but may also occur with the use of stimulants, depressants, or cannabinoids. Depressants and stimulants are the drugs that most frequently cause psychotic

TABLE 2.5. Physical findings that may indicate alcoholism.

Acute/chronic use

Nervous system: sedation, confusion, disorientation, slurred speech, difficulty thinking, slowness of speech and comprehension, dizziness, poor memory, faulty judgment, narrowed range of attention, emotional lability, irritability, quarrelsomeness, hallucinosis, untidiness in personal habits, depression and suicide attempts, ataxia, impaired psychomotor performance, peripheral neuropathy, cerebellar degeneration, subdural hematoma, cerebral atrophy in a relatively young person, optic neuropathy, seizure disorder

Head, eyes, ears, nose, throat: poor dentition, oropharyngeal lesions, hoarseness, plethoric faces, parotid enlargement, injected conjunctiva, flushed skin, head trauma, alcohol on breath

Chest: repeated upper respiratory and bronchial infections, signs and symptoms of aspiration pneumonia, appearance of lobar pneumonias particularly Klebsiella and pneumococcus, tuberculosis, fractured ribs

Cardiovascular system: cardiac arrhythmias, sinus tachycardia, hypertension, cardiomyopathy

Abdomen and gastrointestinal system: nausea, vomiting, ascites, large or small liver, caput medusa, palpable spleen, abdominal tenderness due to gastritis, ulcers, duodenitis, esophagitis, ileitis, irritable bowel syndrome or pancreatitis, findings compatible with advanced liver disease such as loss of secondary sex characteristics, hemorrhoids, spider angiomata, or gynecomastia, positive hemocult stools

Musculoskeletal system: gout, especially if it is difficult to control, trauma, avascular necrosis of the femoral head in a young adult, myopathy primarily in shoulders and hips

Dermatological system: cigarette burns, bruises, seborrheic dermatitis, rosacea, palmar erythema

Genitourinary system: impotence, menstrual disturbances, infertility, testicular atrophy, feminization in men, masculinization in women

Overdose

stupor, respiratory depression, coma, death

Withdrawal

insomnia, anxiety, tremor, nausea, vomiting, elevated blood pressure and pulse rate, agitation, sweating, hyperactive reflexes, grand mal seizures, delirium tremens

reactions, although they may also occur with the use of hallucinogens, phencyclidines, or cannabinoids. Withdrawal from depressants may precipitate psychotic episodes. Stimulant users are often paranoiac.[8]

Slurred speech is characteristic of depressant intoxication, although any abused drug may alter speech patterns. Resting tremor may indicate stimulant or hallucinogen use or withdrawal from depressants or opioids. Grand mal seizures may result from stimulant or opioid (meperidine, propoxyphene) use or occur during withdrawal from depressants. Seizures may not occur until one week after the last dose of a long-acting benzodiazepine such as diazepam (Valium). They may also occur after overdoses of hallucinogens or phencyclidines. Hyperreflexia occurs most often with stimulant use or withdrawal from depressants or opioids.[8]

Flashbacks occur most often with hallucinogens, although they have been reported with phencyclidines and cannabinoids. Panic reactions most commonly occur with use of stimulants, hallucinogens, or cannabinoids, but they may also occur during withdrawal from depressants. Physicians should rule out other causes, such as myocardial infarction, hyperthyroidism, or various neuroses.

Elevated blood pressure most commonly occurs with stimulant use, but it may also occur with phencyclidine or hallucinogen use or with withdrawal from depressants or opioids. Pulse irregularities suggest the use of stimulants or inhalants. Tachycardia is present in most acute drug reactions and in withdrawal from depressants or opioids.[8]

Elevated temperature may occur with the use of stimulants or hallucinogens or in withdrawal from depressants or opioids. It may also occur with phencyclidine overdose. Malignant hyperthermia may occur with stimulant overdose.[8]

Sweating accompanies most acute drug reactions and can occur with withdrawal from depressants and opioids. It is a common complaint of those on methadone. Piloerection (gooseflesh) is a classic sign of opioid (heroin) withdrawal and may also occur in acute LSD reactions. Needle tracks most commonly indicate use of an opioid, although stimulants and depressants may also be injected intravenously. Patients may wear long-sleeved clothing in warm weather to cover up needle tracks.[8]

Excessive lacrimation, as well as rhinorrhea and dilated pupils, is a manifestation of opioid withdrawal. Opioid use, as a rule, constricts pupils. Stimulants, hallucinogens, cannabinoids, and sometimes meperidine (Demerol) dilate pupils. Depressants usually make pupils midpoint and slowly reactive, except glutethimide (Doriden), which tends to enlarge pupils. Horizontal nystagmus frequently occurs with barbiturate use or withdrawal. Horizontal or vertical nystagmus may occur with phencyclidine use. An exaggerated blink reflex is commonly associated with barbiturate withdrawal. Marijuana use produces conjunctival injection. Patients may wear sunglasses to hide this.[8]

Respiratory depression may indicate use of opioids or depressants, particularly barbiturates. Pulmonary edema and pulmonary fibrosis may be caused by use of intravenous heroin or some of its contaminants. Bronchial irritation may indicate recent heavy marijuana smoking.[8]

The occurrence together of pinpoint pupils, depressed respiration, and coma strongly suggests opioid overdose. Opioids depress the cough reflex, and stuporous abusers may aspirate. A similar syndrome may be found in users of depressants. Crampy abdominal pain and diarrhea occurs with opioid withdrawal.[8]

Glutethimide overdose is marked by cyclic central nervous system depression. Ethchlorvynol overdose can produce prolonged coma, particularly in individuals with liver disease.[8]

Phencyclidine use produces a combination of sympathetic (increased blood pressure, pulse rate, and reflexes) and cholinergic (sweating, drooling, flushing) overactivity. The combination of a comalike state, open eyes, decreased perception of pain, periods of temporary excitation, and bodily rigidity should lead a physician to suspect phencyclidine overdose. Toxic reaction to phencyclidine is not only life-threatening but tends to be the longest-lasting symptom caused by any abused drug.[22]

Inhalant abuse may produce respiratory depression, cardiac arrhythmias, rapid loss of consciousness, and death. In typical reported cases, young people inhale a volatile hydrocarbon and feel an urge to run. After sprinting a short distance, they fall to the ground dead, usually, it is thought, from cardiac arrhythmia. Individuals who inhale drugs from plastic bags placed over their heads can also die of suffocation. Inhalants sometimes cause rashes on the hands or around the mouth or nose and can also irritate mucous membranes.

Trauma, such as head injuries, limb fractures, stab wounds, and gunshot wounds, are not uncommon in chemically dependent people. Weight loss and malnutrition may accompany chronic, heavy use of any drug.[8]

Snorting stimulants (amphetamines, cocaine) can produce rhinitis, nasal bleeding, sinus problems, hyperemic nasal turbinates, abuse of nasal sprays, hoarseness, and difficulty swallowing. Snorting cocaine can lead to septal perforation.[8]

Drug inhalation (cocaine, marijuana) can produce a variety of conditions, including decreased pulmonary function, wheezing, chronic cough, pharyngitis, uveitis, sinusitis, bronchitis, and hemoptysis.[8]

Physical findings that may indicate addiction to specific drug groups are given in Table 2.6.

A variety of physical signs may indicate subcutaneous, intramuscular, or intravenous drug injection. Signs of such injections include needle marks, local infections, and scars. Signs of systemic infection (hepatitis B, infective endocarditis, osteomyelitis, AIDS) may be present. Physical signs indicating that patients may be injecting drugs are given in Table 2.7.

Laboratory Tests

Abnormal laboratory values are not diagnostic of chemical dependence; however, they should arouse suspicion and prompt further questioning. The absence of abnormal laboratory findings does not rule out chemical dependence.

Laboratory evaluation of suspected alcoholism or other drug dependence should include an SMA-12 panel, serum gamma-glutamyl transpeptidase (SGGT), electrolytes, complete blood count, urine analysis, and a urine or blood drug screen. Hepatitis profile, human immunodeficiency virus (HIV), prothrombin time, or blood cultures may be helpful if indicated. Chest X rays and EKGs are generally not helpful but should be done for patients over 40 years of age or for younger patients with a history of cardiac or pulmonary disease.[8]

Alcoholism

Elevated laboratory tests that may be associated with alcoholism include SGGT, alanine transferase (ALT; formerly known as SGPT), aspartate transferase (AST; formerly known as SGOT), lactic dehydrogenase (LDH), serum amylase, mean cell volume (MCV), serum cholesterol, serum triglyceride, alkaline phosphatase, total bilirubin, and uric acid.[20-23]

The SGGT is generally thought to be the most sensitive enzyme test of liver disease, yet it is abnormal in only between 31 and 70 percent of diagnosed alcoholics. The SGGT is a hepatic microsomal enzyme that is subject to induction; its elevation may, therefore, indicate either microsomal induction or hepatic injury. Alcoholism is the most common cause of its elevation; it is not elevated in social drinkers. (Anticonvulsants that induce hepatic enzymes may be a nonalcoholic cause of elevated SGGT.) It is normally higher in men than in women.[3,23-25] Unfortunately, the SGGT is not on the SMA-12 or most other screening panels. It should be ordered separately if it is not already being done so.

Excessive consumption of alcohol is also the most common cause of an elevated MCV. Patients may or may not have anemia. Other causes of an elevated MCV include reticulocytosis, folic acid deficiency, Vitamin B_{12} deficiency, and nonalcoholic liver disease. Prothrombin time (PT) may be prolonged by alcoholic liver disease, and patients occasionally have decreased platelet counts along with decreased white blood cell counts secondary to bone marrow depression by alcohol. Serum magnesium, calcium, phosphorus, potassium, and BUN may also be decreased.[21]

Alcoholics may have hypoglycemia or hyperglycemia. Alcohol impairs gluconeogenesis so that blood glucose levels may fall, especially in patients suffering from poor nutrition. Once the pancreas is damaged, it may not secrete enough insulin to respond to sugar loads, producing high blood sugar. Alcoholism should be considered in diabetic patients who have difficulty maintaining reasonable control of their diabetes.[17]

Combinations of abnormal laboratory values carry more weight in diagnosing alcoholism than do individual values. The combination of elevated SGGT, AST, and MCV, for example, is often found in alcoholics.

Laboratory measurements that may be abnormal in alcoholics are summarized in Table 2.8.

Other Drug Dependencies

Laboratory tests are not nearly as helpful for the diagnosis of dependence on other drugs as they are for alcoholism. For the most part, they represent non-specific findings or are the result of infections due to intravenous, subcutaneous, or intramuscular drug use. A urine drug screen may be helpful.

Inhalant use may initially cause leukocytosis and anemia, followed by pan-cytopenia or aplastic anemia. Myeloid leukemia has been reported. White blood cells, erythrocytes, and protein may be found in a patient's urine. Renal tubular necrosis may occur and lead to acute renal failure, with elevated BUN and creatinine. Liver toxicity may cause bilirubin, AST, ALT, LDH, and alkaline phosphatase to be elevated.[8]

Opioid use may produce a depressed testosterone level, a high resting glucose level, an abnormal glucose tolerance test, and, sometimes, eosinophilia. It may also cause false positive serological tests for pregnancy or syphilis. Acute myoglobinemia and myoglobinuria may occur with heroin use or phencyclidine overdose. Abnormal arterial blood gases (elevated Pco_2, depressed Po_2 and pH) may result from the pulmonary edema associated with heroin injection or from overdoses of drugs (depressants, opioids) that depress respiration.[8]

TABLE 2.6. Physical findings that may indicate other drug dependencies.

CNS depressants

Acute/chronic use—sedation, confusion, disorientation, slurred speech, ataxia, difficulty thinking, slowness of speech and comprehension, dizziness, impaired psychomotor performance, poor memory, faulty judgment, narrowed range of attention, emotional lability, irritability, quarrelsome, untidiness in personal habits, depression and suicidal gestures or attempts

Overdose—shallow breathing, respiratory depression, hypotension, aspiration pneumonia, respiratory arrest and circulatory collapse, depressed sensorium to coma, death

Withdrawal—insomnia, anxiety, panics attacks, tremor, nausea, vomiting, elevated blood pressure and pulse rate, irritability, agitation, sweating, hyperactive reflexes, pleading for drugs, grand mal seizures, confusion, delirium, psychosis

Opioids

Acute/chronic use—decreased pain, sleepiness, euphoria, nausea, vomiting, pupillary constriction, constipation, decreased libido and altered menstrual cycle, generalized itching, suppression of cough reflex, grand mal seizures

Overdose—drowsiness, hypothermia, pinpoint pupils (may be dilated with meperidine), aspiration pneumonia, hypotension, respiratory depression, pulmonary edema, respiratory arrest, coma, death

Withdrawal—lacrimation, rhinorrhea, yawning, irritability, sweating, restlessness, tremor, insomnia, piloerection, abdominal cramps, nausea, vomiting, diarrhea, muscle and bone pain, increased pulse and blood pressure, drug craving with drug seeking behavior

CNS stimulants

Acute/chronic use—euphoria with acute use/dysphoria with chronic use, increased energy with acute use/fatigue with chronic use, increased feelings of sexuality with acute use/decreased feelings of sexuality with chronic use, decreased appetite, insomnia, weight loss, excitement, tremor, pupillary dilation, increased blood pressure and pulse rate, indifference to pain, rhinitis, nasal bleeding, sinus problems, dull frontal headache, hyperemic nasal turbinates, nasal spray abuse, septal perforation, hoarseness, difficulty swallowing, personal neglect, delusions, suspiciousness, paranoid pychosis

Overdose—headache, flushed skin, tactile sensations (coke bugs), hallucinations, acute anxiety, agitation, confusion, malignant hyperthermia, tachycardia and hypertension, stereotypical repetitious behavior, bruxism and face picking, toxic psychosis, chest pain with cardiac arrythmias, myocardial infarction, grand mal seizures, cerebral hemorrhages, hypothermia, circulatory collapse, coma, death

Withdrawal—negativism, pessimism, lack of patience, irritability, depression, lack of energy, sleepiness, sleep disturbances, fear, paranoia, nervousness, diaphoresis, chills, hunger, drug craving

Cannabinoids

Acute/chronic use—euphoria, decreased psychomotor performance, increased pulse rate, decreased pulmonary function, exacerbation of asthma, conjunctival injection, uveitis, pharyngitis, bronchitis, stuffy nose, dry mouth, sinusitis, disruption of menstrual cycle, perceptual delusions, paranoid feelings, mood shifts (joy to sorrow, fear to elation), sleepiness, heightened sexual arousal, anxiety to panic, amotivational syndrome with chronic use, angina in those with preexisting heart trouble

Overdose—tachycardia, hypertension, delusions, hallucinations, seizures in epileptics, acute toxic psychosis

Withdrawal—irritability, restlessness, nervousness, insomnia, mild tremor, mild body temperature elevation

TABLE 2.6. (*Continued*).

Phencyclidines
Acute/chronic use—increased blood pressure and pulse rate, increased respiratory rate, dizziness, lack of coordination, ataxia, slurred speech, vertical and horizontal nystagmus, paranoid delusions, delusions of superhuman strength, agitation, unpredictable behavior, nudity in public
Overdose—vertigo, skin flushing, nausea, vomiting, auditory and visual hallucinations, hyperreflexia, rhabdomyolysis and acute renal failure, tremor, bilateral ptosis, tachycardia, decreased respiration, grand mal seizures, acute toxic psychosis, fever, body rigidity, coma-like state with eyes open and temporary periods of excitation, decreased pain perception, respiratory depression, hypertensive crisis, death
Withdrawal—Nervousness, anxiety, and depression may occur

Hallucinogens
Acute/chronic use—visual hallucinations, flushed face, pupillary dilation, fine tremor, increased blood pressure and pulse rate, increased body temperature, hyperreflexia, muscle weakness, tremor, dizziness, weakness, nausea, vomiting, parasthesia, labile mood, anxiety, panic attacks, depression, flashbacks
Overdose—toxic psychosis, tachycardia, hypertension, cardiac arrythmias, hyperpyrexia, shock, convulsions
Withdrawal—none known

Inhalants
Acute/chronic use—central nervous system effects (headache, euphoria, excitement, slurred speech, drowsiness, irritability, mental dullness, tremors, emotional lability, nystagmus, ataxia, polyneuropathies, permanent encephalopathies), intestinal effects (mucus membrane irritation, unpleasant breath odor, nausea, vomiting, gastric pain, anorexia, dyspepsia, chronic gastritis, hepatomegally, weight loss), urinary dysfunction (renal tubular necrosis, renal failure), cardiovascular (irregular heart beat, increased pulse rate), other (eye irritation, rash around mouth or nose, cough, chemical pneumonia, muscle weakness and atrophy)
Overdose—confusion, disorientation, cardiac arrythmias, respiratory depression, decreased sensorium, loss of consciousness, sudden death
Withdrawal—probably none

Vomiting caused by drug use or withdrawal may produce electrolyte abnormalities (elevated HCO_3^- and pH, decreased K^+ and Cl^-).[8]

Abnormal laboratory findings associated with infection include an increased white blood cell count and positive blood cultures. The most common offending organisms with acute infective endocarditis are *Staphylococcus aureus*, enterococci, gram negative bacteria, and *Candida albicans*. The hemoglobin and hematocrit may be depressed with infective endocarditis secondary to hemolysis; an echocardiogram may be diagnostic. Laboratory findings with hepatitis B include elevated bilirubin, AST, ALT, LDH, and alkaline phosphatase. X rays or a bone scan may be helpful for making the diagnosis of osteomyelitis. An elevated white blood cell count or positive culture on aspirated joint fluid may be helpful for diagnosing septic arthritis. Infection with the human immunodeficiency virus may produce a depressed lymphocyte count as well as a variety of abnormal tests resulting from infection with opportunistic organisms.[8]

Laboratory values that may be abnormal in other drug dependencies are given in Table 2.9.

TABLE 2.7. Physical findings related to drug injection.

skin tracks and related scars on neck, axilla, forearm, wrist, foot, ankle, under the tongue, and penile
    veins; new lesions may be inflamed
needle puncture marks located over veins
pock mark–like scars from subcutaneous injections (especially in the deltoid, gluteal areas, abdomen,
    thigh, and shoulder)
wheals or hives at injection site
abscesses, infections or ulcerations on the arm, thigh, shoulder, abdomen, chest, hand, or finger
necrosis of the skin (spaceloderma)
edema of the hand or irreducible finger flexion (camptodactylia); this occurs when drugs are injected
    into the veins of the fingers or the hands
thrombophlebitis at possible injection sites
accidental "tattoos" at injection sites; these result from carbon produced by heating needles to steri-
    lize them
dermatitis at injection sites
allergic reactions (purpura, urticaria, pruritis)
tourniquet pigmentation; this is a poorly defined linear mark above the antecubital space
signs of hepatitis B (fever, jaundice, hepatomegaly, nausea, vomiting)
signs of acute infective endocarditis (fever, mitral regurgitation murmur, septic pulmonary emboli,
    Roth's spots, Janeway lesions, Osler's nodes)
signs of septic arthritis or osteomyelitis (fever, local joint, limb, or back pain)
signs of AIDS (fatigue, anorexia, weight loss, fever, diarrhea, lymphademopathy, *Pneumocystis
    carinii* pneumonia, pulmonary aspergillosis, candida esophogitis, tuberculosis, histoplasmosis,
    cryptococcal meningitis)

TABLE 2.8. Laboratory values that may be abnormal in alcoholics.

Measurement	Normal range	Alcoholic change
gamma-glutamyltransferase	Male: 15–85 µ/L	increased
	Female: 5–55 µ/L	
alanine aminotransferase	6–36 µ/L	increased
aspartate aminotransferase	10–40 µ/L	increased
alkaline phosphatase	13–39 µ/L	increased
lactate dehydrogenase	60–120 µ/L	increased
bilirubin (total)	0.3–1.0 mg/dL	increased
amylase	4.0–25 µ/L	increased
uric acid	3.0–7.0 mg/dL	increased
triglyceride	40–150 mg/dL	increased
cholesterol	120–220 mg/dL	increased
mean corpuscular volume	80–94 cu microns	increased
blood alcohol level	zero	increased
prothrombin time	11.0–12.5 seconds	prolonged
calcium	8.0–10.5 mg/dL	decreased
phosphorus	3.0–4.5 mg/dL	decreased
magnesium	1.5–2.0 mEq/L	decreased
potassium	3.5–5.0 mEq/L	decreased
blood urea nitrogen	8–25 mg/dL	decreased
white blood cell count	4,300–10,800/mm³	decreased
platelet count	150,000–300,000/mm³	decreased
hematocrit	Male: 45–52%	decreased
	Female: 37–48%	
glucose	70–110 mg/dL	decreased or increased

From H.T. Milhorn, Jr., The diagnosis of alcoholism, *American Family Physician* 37:175–183, 1988.
Published by the American Academy of Physicians.

TABLE 2.9. Laboratory values that may be abnormal in other drug dependencies.

Measurement	Normal range	Drug-related change
gamma-glutamyltransferase	Male: 15–85 µ/L	increased
	Female: 5–55 µ/L	
alanine aminotransferase	6–36 µ/L	increased
aspartate aminotransferase	10–40 µ/L	increased
lactate dehydrogenase	60–120 µ/L	increased
bilirubin (total)	0.3–1.0 mg/dL	increased
prothrombin time	11.0–12.5 seconds	prolonged
glucose	70–110 mg/dL	increased
blood urea nitrogen	8–25 mg/dL	increased
creatinine	0.6–1.5 mg/100 ml	increased
bicarbonate	24–30 mEq/L	increased
potassium	3.5–5.0 mEq/L	decreased
chloride	100–106 mEq/L	decreased
platelet count	150,000–300,000/mm^3	decreased
white blood cell count	4,300–10,800/mm^3	increased or decreased
hematocrit	Male: 45–52%	decreased
	Female: 37–48%	
eosinophil count	0–5 percent	increased
lymphocyte count	12–50 percent	decreased
Pco$_2$	35–45 torr	increased
Po$_2$	75–100 torr (age dependent)	decreased
pH	7.35–7.45	increased or decreased
blood cultures	negative	positive
drug screen	negative	positive
serological tests (syphilis, pregnancy)	negative	positive
serum or urine myoglobin	zero	increased
urine white blood cell count	zero	increased
urine red blood cell count	zero	increased
urine protein	zero	increased

Drug Screening

General Principles

Laboratory procedures for detecting drugs are divided into screening tests and confirmatory tests. Screening tests offer high sensitivity but sacrifice specificity; therefore, in screening it is important to use tests that yield few false negative results. Most screens detect drugs in 99 percent or more of specimens in which they are present at concentrations greater than a predetermined cutoff level. The number of false positive results may be high. Confirmatory tests, on the other hand, are very specific and separate true positives from false positives with great accuracy.[26]

Although a number of body fluids can be used for drug testing, the most commonly used is urine. It is easy to collect, collecting it is noninvasive, it is easier to analyze than blood or other fluids, and it can be refrigerated and stored. Drugs and their metabolites are usually found in higher concentrations in urine than in other body fluids because of the concentrating functions of the kidney.[26]

Lab results do not give any indication of patients' patterns of drug use (how they administer drugs, how frequently they take them, when they last took them, the amount they used), whether patients are one-time users or are chemically dependent, and they do not tell whether patients are impaired physically or mentally by use of a drug.[26-28]

Routine urine screening tests usually do not detect hallucinogens, many designer drugs, or alcohol. Specific requests must be made for tests of these substances, and such tests are usually fairly expensive. Alcohol is better tested for in a blood sample.[26]

False negative screens occur for several reasons. A mix up of samples is an obvious cause, and it occasionally happens. A chain of custody should prevent this. False negative screens may occur when patients have taken drugs so recently that they have not undergone sufficient renal excretion to be detectable in urine. Also, renal impairment may delay excretion. Patients afraid of testing positive for drug use may adulterate their urine samples with a variety of substances (salt, vinegar, bleach, lemon juice, water) or substitute a urine sample from drug-free individuals. Patients should be directly observed while collecting urine samples.

Also, drug users often ingest one drug, believing it to be another one. For example, a patient may use PCP thinking it is cocaine. A test for cocaine would, therefore, be negative.[26,28]

The larger the dose, the longer a drug can be detected in the urine. If a patient is a chronic user, a drug may reach a steady state in the body, in which case the time needed to clear the drug from the body is longer than would be needed after an acute ingestion.[26,28]

The half-life, volume of distribution, lipophilicity, and dissociation constant (pKa) of a drug affect its rate of excretion. Drugs that are cleared by first-order kinetics (drugs for which the rate of clearance is proportional to serum concentration) are about 94 percent eliminated in four half-lives. Decreased cardiac output, as well as decreased liver or kidney function, can decrease the rate of excretion and, thereby, increase the half-life of a drug. Drugs with a small volume of distribution clear faster than those with a larger volume of distribution. Weak acids are excreted more rapidly in alkaline urine, and weak bases are excreted more rapidly in acidic urine.[26,28]

Because of their affinity for adipose tissue, cannabinoids can be detected in the urine for up to 25 days after patients stop heavy chronic marijuana use, for up to 8 days after patients stop moderate use, and for up to 2 days after patients stop occasional use. Long-acting barbiturates and methaqualone may be detected up to 7 days after use, and PCP for up to 8 days. Most other drugs are not detectable after between 1 to 3 days, depending on the drug.[26,28]

Screening Tests

Two screening tests are currently in use—thin-layer chromatography and immunoassays. Thin-layer chromatography is based on the principle that drugs of different solubilities migrate at different rates and, thus, occupy different positions on a strip after a specified period of time. Migration is allowed to occur under acidic and basic conditions. The strips are then examined under ultraviolet light and combined with iodine. Under each of these four conditions (acidic, basic, ultraviolet light, iodine), a given drug has a characteristic pattern of migration and color. By comparison to controls, individual drugs can be identified. This test is, therefore, not quantitative but is read merely as positive or negative.[26-27]

Immunoassays involve binding a drug (antigen) with an antibody, from a test kit, that has been generated to recognize and bind exclusively to it. Two immunoassays are in common use—enzyme immunoassay and radioimmunoassay. The two methods differ in the way they measure the concentration of the resulting complex. The enzyme immunoassay determines the concentration of the antigen-antibody complex by measuring the activity of an enzyme attached to the antigen. The Enzyme Multiplied Immunoassay Technique (EMIT) is the most widely used test of this type. The radioimmunoassay determines the concentration of antigen-antibody complex by measuring the activity of a radioisotopically labeled antigen. Immunoassays give quantitative results.[26,28]

False positive results in such tests sometimes occur because of a phenomenon known as cross-reactivity. Several drugs in the same chemical class may give positive tests on assays intended to detect a specific drug. For instance, phenylpropanolamine, ephedrine, or pseudophedrine may give positive results when physicians are testing for amphetamines. In such instances false positive tests can be identified by confirmatory tests.[26,28]

Confirmatory Tests

Confirmatory techniques include gas chromatography, gas chromatography/ mass spectrometry, and high-pressure liquid chromatography. All give highly specific results. Gas chromatology consists of a column, usually a glass tube, packed with an absorbent material and contained in a heated, ovenlike area. An inert gas continuously passes through the column. The mixture of drugs contained in an organic solvent is injected into one end of the column. The injected material is volatilized by the heat and carried through the column as a vapor. The components are separated as they pass through the column and pass out the other end one at a time. A drug's identity is determined by the amount of time required to traverse the column.[26,28]

Gas chromatography/mass spectrometry combines the separating power of the gas chromatograph with the molecular identifying power of the mass spectrometer. The gas chromatograph separates the compounds, and the mass spectrometer identifies them.[26,28]

High-pressure liquid chromatography in principle works much like gas chromatography. A solvent mixture is pumped under high pressure through an absorbent material packed into a column, usually made of stainless steel. The mixture of drugs contained in an organic solvent is injected into one end of the column. Individual drugs are identified by their ultraviolet spectrum as they exit the other end.[26,28]

National Council on Alcoholism and Drug Dependence Criteria

The National Council on Alcoholism and Drug Dependence (NCADD) considers individuals to be alcoholic who are physically dependent on alcohol, develop significant tolerance to it, have a major alcohol-related disease, or continue to drink in spite of a strong indication to quit (Table 2.10). The determination of any one of these findings is sufficient to make a diagnosis. It should be noted that the NCADD criteria define an advanced state of alcoholism.[7]

Mixed Drug Dependencies

Few addicts use only one drug. However, virtually all can identify the drug they most prefer. Often, but not always, this drug produces the predominant signs and symptoms in the face of mixed drug use, which complicates making a diagnosis. Urine or serum drug screens can be of considerable help if they can be obtained rapidly.

Two depressant drugs used simultaneously (alcohol and a barbiturate, for example) act synergistically to depress the central nervous system and can lead to respiratory depression, coma, and death. The simultaneous use of a depressant and an opioid acts much in the same manner.

Stimulants and depressants are often used together (alcohol to take the edge off cocaine or amphetamines to reduce the sleepiness from alcohol). Although some antagonism occurs at lower doses, at higher doses the depressant tends to dominate. Stimulants and the chronic use of alcohol act synergistically to increase blood pressure.

TABLE 2.10. National Council on Alcoholism and Drug Dependence's diagnostic criteria for alcoholism.

Physiological dependence (withdrawal signs/symptoms)
   gross tremor (alcohol-related)
   hallucinosis (hallucinations with a clear sensorium)
   withdrawal seizures
   delirium tremens
Alcohol tolerance
   blood alcohol concentration (BAC) greater than 0.1 gm % during any office visit
   BAC greater than 0.15 gm % without obvious signs of intoxication
   BAC greater than 0.30 gm % at any time
   consumption of one-fifth gallon of whiskey or an equivalent amount of wine or beer daily for more
     than one day by a 180-pound individual
Major alcohol-related illness
   alcoholic hepatitis
   alcoholic cerebellar degeneration
Drinking in spite of strong indication known to patient
   medical contraindication (pregnancy, alcohol-related medical problems)
   social contraindication (divorce, separation, loss of job, arrest, or driving under the influence)
   blatant indiscriminate use of alcohol (skid row behavior)

Based on A.J. Mooney, Alcohol abuse and dependence. In *Family Medicine*, R.B. Taylor, ed., Springer-Verlag, New York, 1983.

Hallucinogens and stimulants act together to produce stimulatory side effects such as increased pulse rate and blood pressure.

Marijuana may increase the depressant effect of alcohol and other CNS depressants on the central nervous system. Patients showing signs of alcohol intoxication that do not correspond to their blood alcohol levels may have used other drugs as well, such as marijuana, other depressants, or opioids. When used together, marijuana and stimulants synergistically increase pulse rate and blood pressure. Marijuana and alcohol or other depressant use decreases motor performance.

Presenting the Diagnosis

Discussing the diagnosis of chemical dependence with a patient is never easy. The major barrier is the patient's denial, which physicians should view as a symptom of the disease in the same way that thirst is a symptom of diabetes. By realizing that denial is primarily the result of unconscious psychological mechanisms and not of willful misrepresentation, physicians can maintain a sympathetic, nonjudgmental therapeutic stance. They should present the diagnosis as an expression of concern for a patient's health or safety. Moralization or threatening a patient is counterproductive.[29]

Many drug users are unaware of the basic facts about drugs and chemical dependence. Educating patients about these facts in a nonthreatening manner is appropriate. Discussing chemical dependence as a disease legitimizes seeking care for the dependence itself, not just for the medical consequences of the drug use. Comparing chemical dependence to other chronic diseases that require behavioral changes, such as hypertension or diabetes, reinforces the fact that abstinence from drugs is therapy, not punishment. Understanding chemical dependence as a disease allows patients to address the problem with less guilt. Although recovery from chemical dependence can take place only after patients accept the diagnosis, their refusal to call themselves drug addicts or alcoholics at this point need not stand in the way of treatment. Getting patients into treatment is much more important than agreeing on a diagnostic label.[29]

Final Comments

Alcoholism and other drug dependencies are commonplace in medical practice. Diagnosing dependencies primarily involves finding significant impairment from physiological, psychological, or social dysfunction caused by persistent and excessive use of a chemical substance. A variety of diagnostic tools are available to help physicians make a diagnosis. As with many diseases, awareness of the possibility of alcoholism or other drug dependence is the key to diagnosis.

References

1. Mulry, J. T., M. L. Brewer, and D. L. Spencer. The effect of an inpatient chemical dependency rotation on residents' clinical behavior. *Family Medicine*, July/August: 276–280, 1987.

2. Schuckit, M. A. *Drug and Alcohol Abuse.* Plenum Press, New York, 1984.

3. Sherin, K. M., S. H. Piotrowski, S. M. Panek, and M. C. Doot. Screening for alcoholism in a community hospital. *Journal of Family Practice,* 15:1091–1095, 1982.

4. Milhorn, H. T., Jr., L. C. Gardner, and R. D. Blondell. Effect of a chemical dependency rotation on residents' attitudes. *Family Practice Research Journal,* submitted.

5. Milhorn, H. T., Jr. Chemical dependency: Is medical education falling short? *Mississippi State Impaired Physicians Newsletter,* April, 1989.

6. Spickard, A., Jr. Alcoholism: The missed diagnosis. *Southern Medical Journal,* 79:1489–1492, 1986.

7. Mooney, A. J. Alcohol abuse and dependence. In *Family Medicine,* Ed. by R. B. Taylor. Springer-Verlag, New York, 1983, pp. 1632–1661.

8. Milhorn, H. T., Jr. The diagnosis of alcoholism and other drug dependencies. In *Review Course Syllabus,* American Medical Society on Alcoholism and Other Drug Dependencies, New York, in press.

9. Selzer, M. L. The Michigan Alcohol Screening Test: The quest for a new diagnostic instrument. *American Journal of Psychiatry,* 127:1653–1658, 1971.

10. Selzer, M. L., A. Vinokur, and L. Van Rooijen. A self-administered short Michigan Alcohol Screening Test (SMAST). *Journal of Studies on Alcohol,* 36:117–126, 1975.

11. Creek, L. V., R. L. Zachrick, and W. E. Scheger. The use of standardized screening tests in family practice. *Family Practice Research Journal,* 2:11–17, 1982.

12. Bernadt, M. W., and Taylor, C. Comparison of questionnaire and laboratory tests in the detection of alcoholism. *Lancet,* 1:325–327, 1982.

13. Ewing, J. A. Detecting alcoholism: The CAGE questionnaire. *Journal of the American Medical Association,* 252:1905–1907, 1984.

14. Graham, K. Identifying and measuring alcohol abuse among the elderly: Serious problems with existing instrumentation. *Journal of Studies on Alcohol,* 47:322–326, 1986.

15. Van Cleave, S., W. Byrd, and K. Revell. *Counseling for Substance Abuse and Addiction.* Word Books, Waco, Texas, 1987.

16. Milhorn, H. T., Jr. The diagnosis of alcoholism. *American Family Physician,* 37:175–183, 1988.

17. Liepman, W. R., R. C. Anderson, and J. V. Fisher, (Eds.). *Family Medicine Curriculum Guide to Substance Abuse.* Society of Teachers of Family Medicine, Kansas City, Missouri, 1984.

18. Cloninger, C. R. Neurogenetic adaptive mechanics in alcoholism. *Science,* 236:410–416, 1987.

19. Wilford, B. B. (Ed.). Clinical complications of drug abuse. In *Drug Abuse: A Guide for the Primary Care Physician.* AMA, Chicago, 1981, pp. 177–202.

20. Gitlow, S. E., and H. S. Peyser. *Alcoholism: A Practical Treatment Guide.* Grune and Stratton, Orlando, Florida, 1980.

21. Wilford, B. B (Ed.). *Review Course Syllabus,* American Medical Society on Alcoholism and Other Drug Dependencies, New York, 1987.

22. Milhorn, H. T., Jr. Diagnosis and management of phencyclidine intoxication. *American Family Physician,* in press.

23. Gallant, D. S. *Alcohol and Drug Abuse Curriculum Guide for Psychiatry Faculty.* U.S. Department of Health and Human Services, Rockville, Maryland, 1982.

24. Hays, J. T., and W. A. Spickard, Jr. Alcoholism: Early diagnosis and intervention. *Journal of Internal Medicine,* 2:420–427, 1987.

25. Stamm, D., E. Hansert, and W. Feuerlein. Detection and exclusion of alcoholism in men on the basis of clinical laboratory findings. *Journal of Clinical Chemistry and Clinical Biochemistry*, 22:79–98, 1984.

26. Mullen, J., and H. S. Bracha. Toxicology screening: How to assure accurate results. *Postgraduate Medicine*, 84:141–148, 1988.

27. Gold, M., and C. A. Dackis. Role of the laboratory in suspected drug abuse. *Journal of Clinical Psychiatry*, 47:17–23, 1986.

28. Schonberg, S. K. (Ed.). *Substance Abuse: A Guide for Health Professionals*. American Academy of Pediatrics, Elk Grove Village, Illinois, 1988, pp. 48–66.

29. Barnes, H. N. Presenting the diagnosis: Working with denial. In *Alcoholism: A Guide for the Primary Care Physician*. Ed. by H. N. Barnes, M. D. Aronson, and T. L. Delbanco. Springer-Verlag, New York, 1987, pp. 59–65.

CHAPTER 3

Treatment

Treating a chemically dependent individual involves three steps — getting the person into treatment, the treatment itself, and aftercare.

Getting the Addict into Treatment

The first step in treating chemical dependence is to get an addict to agree to treatment. This is also the most difficult step. Until an addict experiences some major crisis that causes emotional pain, he or she is usually not willing to seek help. A crisis frequently occurs in one or more of the following areas.

1. *Legal problems*. Many chemically dependent people eventually reach a point where they have to steal, sell drugs, or prostitute themselves to support their addiction. These activities often lead to trouble with legal authorities. Addicts also tend to get arrested for driving under the influence, for possessing drugs, or for disorderly conduct. Many judges now mandate treatment in place of sending addicts to prison.[1]
2. *Family problems*. Spouses frequently leave drug users because of the effects of their behavior on the family. This is a crisis for addicts because spouses may be the only emotional support they have. Addicts often agree to treatment not to get well but in hopes of getting spouses back. At this point, this is a perfectly satisfactory reason for getting addicts into treatment and should not be discouraged.[1]
3. *Medical problems*. As their health deteriorates, addicts may realize that their drug use is killing them. They may become aware that their behavior is out of control, or it may take a life-threatening event, such as a violent injury from a shooting, a stabbing, or an automobile accident, to make them aware. Serious medical problems may prompt addicts to seek help. Addicted people suffer from depression, not only from the effects of drugs on their brains but also from the effects of drugs on their lives. Suicide attempts are common among the chemically dependent.[1]

4. *Work problems*. Chemically dependent people who are still drinking or using other drugs are poor employees because of their tardiness, absenteeism, and erratic job performance. They may eventually be threatened with loss of their jobs or may actually be fired. Many employers now require treatment as a condition for continued employment for drug users. This is particularly true of larger companies, many of which have established employee assistance programs to deal with such problems.[1]

5. *Intervention*. Intervention is designed to precipitate a crisis so as to get an addict into treatment earlier than he or she might go otherwise. It is a planned confrontation between the alcoholic or drug addict and family members and other significant people. The purpose of the intervention is to convince an addict of the effects of his or her destructive behavior and to get the person into treatment. Intervention is detailed further in Chapter 5.

6. *Court-ordered admission*. In some states, suspected addicts can be admitted to treatment centers for evaluation of chemical dependence by court order. Basically, a family member or close friend hires an attorney to present evidence to a chancery court judge. If the judge finds sufficient evidence to warrant further evaluation, he or she can order that the suspected addict be committed to a local treatment program for between three to seven days of evaluation. At the end of this period, a patient has a right to appeal the judge's decision. If necessary, a representative of the treatment center may present evidence the center has gathered.

Treatment Options

Once an addict agrees to treatment, a program suited to that particular person must be found. Generally, three options are available—inpatient treatment, outpatient treatment, and support groups such as Alcoholics Anonymous (AA), Narcotics Anonymous (NA), or Cocaine Anonymous (CA). Other types of treatment programs include therapeutic communities and halfway houses, sometimes referred to as residential treatments.

Treatment does not attempt to answer the question of why an addict drinks or uses drugs but instead takes a here-and-now approach—let's see what we have (assessment) and what needs to be done (treatment).

The goals for patients in treatment include learning factual information about alcohol and other drugs; accepting the disease of addiction; understanding what it means to be chemically dependent; learning to identify feelings and deal with them appropriately; learning to assume responsibility for their own behavior; learning to deal appropriately with stress, insomnia, and depression; eliminating maladaptive behaviors and substituting more adaptive ones; becoming physically active; becoming familiar with the twelve steps of Alcoholics Anonymous or various other support groups; learning risk factors for relapse; and learning how to prevent relapse.

Inpatient Treatment

Inpatient treatment takes place in a general medical-surgical hospital's chemical dependency unit or in a freestanding facility. It is often referred to as primary treatment. A good inpatient program uses a multifactorial approach to treatment. Elements of such a program include medical assessment, detoxification, treatment of medical problems, psychosocial assessment, treatment plan development, rehabilitation, aftercare planning, and family treatment. Other possible components of an inpatient program include occupational therapy, vocational rehabilitation, and social services. On admission, each patient is assigned a counselor who guides his or her treatment. Inpatient treatment usually takes about a month.[2]

Medical Assessment

Medical assessment consists of an initial drug history, a routine medical history, a physical examination, and laboratory studies. The initial drug history focuses on a patient's recent drug history rather than on that person's lifelong drug history. This is primarily for the purpose of planning detoxification.[3]

The routine medical history includes questions about medical problems that chemically dependent people commonly encounter. Physicians ask patients about a history of blackouts, seizures, hallucinations, and delirium tremens. Because of the current AIDS epidemic, physicians may also ask patients about sharing needles or about homosexuality. If patients reveal a history of either of these, they may be offered HIV testing. Physicians obtain information about family history of chemical dependence and question patients about previous treatment for chemical dependence or for psychiatric problems. Because many chemically dependent people are depressed, physicians should ask patients about recent suicide thoughts or attempts. If patients have suicidal ideation, physicians should take precautions to prevent suicide and should arrange for psychiatric consultations for patients.[3]

The physical examination focuses on physical abnormalities resulting from substance use, such as an enlarged liver, needle tracks, and abscesses formed from nonsterile injections.[3]

Laboratory studies may include an SMA-12, serum gamma glutamyl transferase (SGGT), electrolytes, complete blood count, urine analysis, and urine drug screen. If the patient is over 40 years old or has a history of a heart or pulmonary problem, an electrocardiogram and/or chest X ray may be obtained.[3]

Detoxification

Based on information obtained in the medical assessment, physicians formulate a detoxification plan. In general, detoxification is required only for drugs that produce central nervous system depression, such as alcohol, barbiturates, benzodiazepines, and opioids. The dosing and scheduling of detoxification medication depend on several factors, such as a patient's age, sex, weight, health, and level of drug intake. Many patients, including some on inadequate levels of depressant drugs or those on such drugs for too short a time to have become physically dependent, do not require detoxification. However, because addicts may not be totally truthful about their use, they should be observed for withdrawal symptoms for at least 24 hours. Nursing care is extremely important during this phase of treatment.

Treatment of Medical Problems

Chemically dependent people have more health problems than other people do. Although many health problems are drug-related, others are problems encountered in any general medical practice. Physicians address these early in treatment. Because drug abuse can produce some common medical problems (gastritis, hypertension, gout, depression, insomnia), physicians can decide at admission which medications to discontinue and which to continue. Again, nursing care plays a major role. Physicians should request records from a patient's personal physician when they are pertinent.

Psychosocial Assessment

Patients need to be extensively assessed psychologically and socially. Psychological assessment consists primarily of testing. Two commonly used tests are the Minnesota Multiphasic Personality Inventory (MMPI) and the Shipley Institute of Living Scale (SILS). The MMPI consists of 566 statements to which patients respond true or false. It is divided into two sets of scales. The first set, consisting of three scales, reflects a patient's degree of cooperation with the testing and indicates the extent to which the clinical profile should be considered valid. The second set, consisting of ten scales, reflects personality characteristics and possible delusional, disorganized, or psychotic thinking.[4]

The SILS is a brief test used to estimate verbal intelligence quotient (IQ). It also estimates cognitive quotient (CQ), which is an indication of a patient's ability to think and reason. The verbal IQ is usually minimally affected by drug abuse, but the CQ may be depressed, indicating an acute or chronic brain syndrome. The SILS, thus, indicates a patient's range of intellectual functioning. If test results indicate that additional testing is appropriate, a physician can refer a patient for neuropsychological testing. Both tests—the MMPI and SILS—are administered shortly after detoxification. The SILS may be repeated about three weeks later if initial results indicate the need.[4]

Social assessment involves collecting data from patients, members of their families, and employers on patients' social functioning. Information counselors gather includes educational level, employment history, leisure activities, marriage/divorce history, history of childhood abuse, legal history, and detailed drug history. In addition, counselors gather information about a patient's childhood role models and family life.

Treatment Plan Development

From medical and psychosocial assessments, physicians and counselors identify problems and list them on a master problem list. Individual problems may be dealt with in treatment, may be noted and merely monitored, may be dealt with after treatment, or may require no action. Problems to be dealt with in treatment might include such things as alcoholic gastritis, denial of chemical dependence, or poor coping skills. For each problem to be addressed in treatment, physicians and counselors develop a treatment plan that sets forth specific objectives for resolving the problem and states how each objective is to be achieved and in what period of time. Each patient is assigned a treatment team that meets weekly to discuss the patient's progress on each identified problem and to update the treatment plan.

Rehabilitation

This process involves putting the treatment plan into action. This is done using education, group therapy, individual therapy, peer assessment, recreational therapy, coping skills and relaxation training, support group participation, and spirituality.[5] A typical daily patient schedule is given in Table 3.1.

Education. Patients usually attend lectures or view films daily on such diverse subjects as the disease concept of chemical dependence; medical, psychological, and social aspects of addiction to specific drugs; cross-addiction; various steps of Alcoholics Anonymous; recovery; and preventing relapse. They may also be given specific reading assignments dealing with chemical dependence.

TABLE 3.1. Typical daily schedule for an inpatient program.

Morning	
7:00– 8:00	Breakfast
8:00– 8:30	Devotional
8:30–9:30	Lecture/film
9:30–10:00	Break
10:00–11:00	Group Therapy (combined male and female groups)
11:00–12:00	Group therapy (separate male and female groups)
Afternoon	
12:00– 1:00	Lunch
1:00– 2:00	Peer
2:00– 3:00	Coping skills/relaxation training
3:00– 4:00	Recreational therapy
4:00– 5:00	Free time/individual therapy
Evening	
5:00– 6:00	Dinner
6:00– 7:00	Free time
7:00– 8:00	Support group attendance
8:00–11:00	Free time
11:00	Lights out

Group therapy. Involving ten to fifteen patients and a group leader, who is usually a certified alcohol and drug counselor (CADC) and who moderates discussion, group therapy is an opportunity for patients to deal with a variety of issues, aided by other group members. Patients are more apt to accept insights or criticism when they come from fellow addicts. Group therapy helps patients see themselves with the psychological camouflage stripped away. Denial of chemical dependence and dishonesty are common problems patients deal with in group therapy. Many patients, if not all, develop low-self esteem because of their drug use and its effects. As a result, over the years they build up a wall of defenses against anything that might threaten their self-esteem. They simply do not want to deal with such issues. Group therapy helps them to do this. Many times, their first group assignment will be to report their life story, focusing on their drug use and the effects it has had on their health, family, friends, and job. This helps them be honest with themselves and to let other group members get to know them. Patients can also use group time to report family conferences and to deal with feelings, which are often intense, about what transpired in such conferences. Ideally, group therapy helps patients identify feelings, see how their addiction has hurt themselves and others, and begin to see the need for change.

Many treatment centers have specialized groups designed for specific patient categories—groups for men, women, adolescents, the elderly, and for patients prone to relapse. Some centers have recently started groups for cocaine addicts. This is probably unwise, because having their own groups sets them apart from other patients. Many cocaine addicts already feel that they are members of an elite group because of the drug they use; having their own therapy groups only perpetuates this feeling.

Individual therapy. Problems inappropriate for group discussion or problems better dealt with in one-on-one situations can be addressed in individual therapy. Initially, therapy time is used to assess a patient's needs and to begin to plan treatment. The concept of addiction as a disease is reinforced, specific character defects (self-centeredness, intolerance, procrastination, self-pity, impatience) are dealt with, and patients' undesirable behaviors in the treatment center are related to behaviors that have caused them problems in the past. Poor relationships with spouses, parents, or significant others are discussed and plans made for improving them. Individual problems, such as irresponsibility and lack of trust, are addressed. Written assignments are made and discussed when completed. Reading assignments, important to patient treatment, are made and later discussed in relation to how the material applies to a patient.

Peer assessment. A special type of group, peer assessment allows patients an opportunity to contribute constructively to the treatment of another patient who is having difficulty understanding his or her behavior. Areas dealt with include dishonesty, defense mechanisms, and character defects. A patient's behavior in the treatment center may also be addressed, as may not participating in treatment, isolating, inappropriate behavior with the opposite sex, and playing counselor. A patient is not allowed to respond defensively to these discussions.

Recreational therapy. Chemically dependent individuals, as a rule, do not regularly exercise. Under supervision, patients are encouraged to participate in various physical activities, usually three times a week. These activities may include basketball, volleyball, racketball, walking or running, or swimming. Exercise decreases depression, gives a person a sense of well-being, and promotes a good night's sleep without alcohol or sleeping pills.

Coping skills and relaxation therapy. Many chemically dependent people have for years used drugs to cope with stress, to get to sleep, or to relax. Without drugs, they have to learn new ways of doing these things. Role-playing specific situations that have led to stress and taking drugs in the past teaches patients appropriate ways of dealing with such situations. Learning communication skills is also a major part of treatment. Instead of reaching for a bottle or a pill, patients with anxiety or insomnia learn to listen to tapes or to use other techniques to relax or to get to sleep.

Support group attendance. Attendance and participation in support groups, such as Alcoholics Anonymous, Narcotics Anonymous, or Cocaine Anonymous, are important parts of virtually all treatment programs. Initially, these meetings are held among patients in the treatment center. Later, as patients progress in treatment, they attend outside, local community meetings. Attendance at these meetings while in treatment is important because it introduces patients to support groups and familiarizes them with their function. After discharge from treatment, patients are expected to continue attending support groups in their hometowns for the rest of their lives.

Spirituality. An elusive concept, spirituality is a term that is commonly associated with religion. However, in the treatment of chemical dependence it is used in a broader sense. Spirituality has been defined as being in harmony with yourself, with those around you, and with a power greater than you. Alcoholics Anonymous, for example, is a deeply spiritual program, yet it has no religious orientation. It is embraced by people of all faiths and by some with no religious preference or background. Working the AA program one day at a time is a spiritual experience.[6]

Discharge Planning

Assessing the needs that individual patients will have following discharge from treatment is called discharge planning. From these needs, the patient and treatment staff jointly develop a personalized aftercare plan. If a treatment center has its own aftercare program, patients may be required to attend it. Patients are generally introduced to the aftercare program a week or so before discharge. They are also expected to attend local support groups once back at home. They may be given the names of contact people in support groups in their local areas and are referred back to their local physicians for specific care for individual needs, such as marriage counseling. Patients who need further treatment for their chemical dependence may be referred to halfway houses. A patient and an aftercare coordinator usually sign an aftercare contract.

Family Treatment

Chemical dependence is an illness that dramatically affects all members of a family. For successful recovery of an addict and other members of the family, treatment must include the family. Family treatment primarily involves education, group therapy, and support group participation. It is discussed in Chapter 5.

Outpatient Treatment

Typically about ten weeks in length, outpatient programs take place for two to three hours in the evening, three days a week. They have fewer components than inpatient programs. Common components include psychosocial assessment, developing treatment plans, rehabilitation, discharge planning, and family treatment. Rehabilitation consists of group therapy, individual therapy, peer assessment, support group attendance, and spirituality. In addition, because addicts have more access to drugs in outpatient programs, frequent random urine drug screening is important.

Day programs have recently become popular. These programs are very similar to inpatient treatment except that patients live at home and attend treatment during the day, usually all day every day, Monday through Friday. The intensity of treatment is virtually the same as inpatient treatment. Day programs are sometimes referred to as partial hospitalization.

Support Groups

A support group consists of recovering addicts who voluntarily meet regularly to help one another maintain sobriety. Alcoholics Anonymous is the oldest, largest, and best known of these organizations; others—for instance Cocaine Anonymous and Narcotics Anonymous—have based their programs on AA concepts. We will discuss AA.

History of AA

Alcoholics Anonymous was established in Akron, Ohio, in 1935 by two alcoholics, Bill Wilson (a stockbroker) and Dr. Bob Smith (a surgeon), who are affectionately referred to by AA members as Bill W and Doctor Bob. Unable to stay sober by themselves, they achieved sobriety through mutual support. They then directed their energies toward helping other alcoholics. They formulated their experiences into the Twelve Steps of AA in 1938. These steps provide guidelines for the personal growth necessary to achieve a stable recovery. The book *Alcoholics Anonymous*, known as the Big Book, was published in 1939.[7-8]

As the organization grew, it developed, for its own preservation, a set of guidelines—the Twelve Traditions (Table 3.2). These traditions assured that AA would not affiliate with organizations, would espouse no cause other than helping individuals achieve sobriety, and would never accept outside funding or charge fees. Anonymity was insisted on at all levels of the organization to prevent

TABLE 3.2. The twelve traditions of AA.

1. Our common welfare should come first; personal recovery depends upon AA unity.
2. For our group purpose, there is but one ultimate authority—a loving God as he may express himself in our group conscious. Our leaders are trusted servants—they do not govern.
3. The only requirement for AA membership is a desire to stop drinking.
4. Each group should be autonomous, except in matters affecting other groups or AA as a whole.
5. Each group has but one primary purpose—to carry its message to the alcoholic who still suffers.
6. An AA group ought never to endorse, finance, or lend the AA name to any related facility or outside enterprise lest problems of money, property, and prestige direct us from our primary purpose.
7. Every AA group ought to be fully self-supporting, declining outside contributions.
8. AA should remain forever nonprofessional, but our service centers may employ special workers.
9. AA, as such, ought never to be organized; but we may create service boards or committees directly responsible to those they serve.
10. AA has no opinion on outside issues; hence the AA name ought never to be drawn into public controversy.
11. Our public relations policy is based on attraction rather than promotion; we need always maintain personal anonymity at the level of press, radio, and films.
12. Anonymity is the spiritual foundation of all our traditions, ever reminding us to place principle above personalities.

individuals from using AA for personal gain. With the exception of some paid secretarial help, AA is staffed entirely by recovering members who volunteer their time.[7-9]

Each autonomous AA group sponsors meetings that take place on a regular schedule one or more times a week.[10] There are now over 48,000 groups in at least 92 countries. AA has more than 1 million members in the United States alone.[5,7-8]

Philosophy of AA

The single focus of AA is on staying sober, not analyzing why a person drank. Total abstinence is a basic tenet, which AA believes is the only way to stay sober. Sobriety is more than just abstinence; it involves a healthy, happy way of living without alcohol. The term dry drunk is used in AA to describe abstinent alcoholics who are living and behaving as if they were still drinking. AA considers alcoholism to be a disease, sort of an allergy to alcohol. It has no requirement for membership except a desire to stop drinking. There are no membership cards—people are members if they say so. It is free, supported only by voluntary contributions from members. Being anonymous, there are no membership lists.[8]

AA slogans for newly sober alcoholic members are purposefully simple, direct, and catchy, designed to be comprehended by the recently detoxified brain. Such slogans include "Don't drink—go to meetings" (immerse yourself in a network of recovering alcoholics), "Easy does it" (avoid stress), and "One day at a time" (focus on not drinking today).[7]

AA does not solicit members, promote any religion, provide social services, run hospitals or treatment services, follow up on its members, claim to be a help with any problem other than alcoholism, accept outside money for services or contributions, make medical or psychological diagnoses, prescribe or pay for treatment, or claim to be the only successful approach to alcoholism.[8]

The Twelve Suggested Steps of AA

The Twelve Steps of AA are a suggested model for the process of change and growth (Table 3.3). The fact that the word *alcohol* appears in only the first step underscores AA's contention that the main work of sobriety is restructuring of an alcoholic's personality. Step 1 is admitting that one is an alcoholic and has lost control of his or her life. This sounds like an obvious and simple step to take, but because of the tremendous denial systems most alcoholics have built up, it is usually the most difficult one. Having admitted powerlessness, Steps 2 and 3 give hope – that is, the recognition that something can lead the alcoholic on a path of sobriety. The phrase "God as we understood him" is little less than a stroke of genius. It was an attempt to diffuse the religious language of the Twelve Steps. AA members usually refer to this "God as we understood him" as their "higher power." For agnostic members of AA, their higher power may be AA itself or whatever they choose.

Steps 4 and 5 involve self-examination. The purpose of this self-examination is not to dwell on the past but to prevent relapse. Steps 6 and 7 allow God to change the alcoholic. Steps 8, 9, and 10 have to do with accepting responsibility and being accountable, two traits lacking in the alcoholic lifestyle. Step 11 is for continued spiritual growth, and Step 12 is the keystone of the program, for it

TABLE 3.3. The twelve suggested steps of AA.

1. We admitted we were powerless over alcohol – that our lives had become unmanageable.
2. We came to believe that a power greater than ourselves could restore us to sanity.
3. We made a decision to turn our will and our lives over to the care of God as we understood him.
4. We made a searching and fearless moral inventory of ourselves.
5. We admitted to God, to ourselves, and to another human being the exact nature of our wrongs.
6. We were entirely ready to have God remove all these defects of character.
7. We humbly asked Him to remove our shortcomings.
8. We made a list of all persons we had harmed, and became willing to make amends to them all.
9. We made direct amends to such people whenever possible, except when to do so would injure them or others.
10. We continued to take personal inventory and when we were wrong promptly admitted it.
11. We sought through prayer and meditation to improve our conscious contact with God, as we understood him, praying only for knowledge of his will and the power to carry that out.
12. Having had a spiritual awakening as the result of these steps, we tried to carry this message to alcoholics, and to practice these principles in all our affairs.

reinforces the work of the previous eleven steps. It involves helping drinking alcoholics in positive ways, such as accompanying them to meetings or helping them get medical care. By doing this work, recovering alcoholics not only help alcoholics who are still drinking but help develop an improved sense of their own self-worth.[1,7-10]

The Sponsor

Veteran AA members with at least one year of sobriety can serve as sponsors to offer guidance and support, including confrontation if a newcomer's behavior indicates he or she is ready to drink again. The most powerful influence sponsors exert may be as role models of people who have successfully achieved sobriety. Veteran AA members become a newcomer's sponsor by mutual agreement. Traditionally, to avoid development of intimate relationships, sponsors are of the same sex as their assigned newcomers.[7]

The AA Meeting

There are two basic types of AA meetings—open and closed. Anyone can attend open meetings, whether or not he or she has problems with alcohol. Only AA members and those wishing to stop drinking can attend closed meetings. Those who do not admit to having a problem with alcohol may be asked to leave. Unfortunately, at some meetings this includes those who have problems with drugs other than alcohol. In general, however, AA is becoming more lenient and accepting of these nonalcoholic addicts. Closed meetings usually have a stable core of members and function more or less as leaderless support groups.[7]

Although they vary somewhat, AA meetings generally follow similar formats (Table 3.4). A meeting begins with a moment of silence. Members may use this time to say a personal prayer, reflect on the happenings of the day, or just to feel gratitude for being sober. Next, the group, in unison, recites the serenity prayer:

TABLE 3.4. Typical agenda for an AA meeting.

Moment of silence
Recital of the Serenity Prayer
Reading of "What AA Is and Is Not"
Reading of "How It Works" (*Alcoholics Anonymous*, Chapter 5)
Program:
  Big Book study
  Step study
  Topic discussion
  Group discussion
  Speaker meeting
  Combination of these
Recital of the Lord's Prayer
Adjourn

God, grant me the serenity to accept the things I cannot change, the courage to change the things I can, and the wisdom to know the difference.

Someone is then asked to read a statement about what AA is and what it is not:

Alcoholics Anonymous is a fellowship of men and women who share their experience, strength, and hope with each other that they may solve their common problem and help others to recover from alcoholism.

The only requirement for membership is a desire to stop drinking. There are no dues or fees for AA membership; we are self-supporting through our own contributions. AA is not allied with any sect, denomination, politics, organization, or institution; does not wish to engage in any controversy; neither endorses nor opposes any causes. Our primary purpose is to stay sober and help other alcoholics to achieve sobriety.

Next, someone is asked to read the first part of Chapter 5, "How It Works," from *Alcoholics Anonymous*.

Our stories disclose in a general way what we used to be like, what happened, and what we are like now. If you have decided you want what we have and are willing to go to any length to get it—then you are ready to take certain steps.

At some of these we balked. We thought we could find an easier, softer way. But we could not. With all the earnestness at our command, we beg of you to be fearless and thorough from the very start. Some of us have tried to hold on to our old ideas and the result was nil until we let go absolutely.

Remember that we deal with alcohol—cunning, baffling, powerful! Without help it is too much for us. But there is One who has all power—that One is God. May you find Him now!

Half measures availed us nothing. We stood at the turning point. We asked His protection and care with complete abandon.

Here are the steps we took, which are suggested as a program of recovery.[11]

The Twelve Suggested Steps of AA are then read. Afterwards, the reading continues from Chapter 5 of the Big Book.

Many of us exclaimed, "What an order! I can't go through with it." Do not be discouraged. No one among us has been able to maintain anything like perfect adherence to these principles. We are not saints. The point is that we are willing to grow along spiritual lines. The principles we have set down are guides to progress. We claim spiritual progress rather than spiritual perfection.

Our description of the alcoholic, the chapter to the agnostic, and our personal adventures before and after make clear three pertinent ideas:
(a) That we were alcoholic and could not manage our own lives.
(b) That probably no human power could have relieved our alcoholism.
(c) That God could and would if He were sought.[11]

Next, the major portion of the meeting takes place—the program. It may take one of several forms. For instance, in a Big Book program members read sections of *Alcoholics Anonymous*. After each section, members discuss how the particular passage relates to their experiences. In a step program, members discuss the various steps of AA. In a topic program, members discuss a topic such as gratitude, acceptance, honesty, or resentment. Each member relates what the topic means to him or her. A topic is usually selected by the chairperson prior to the meeting. Some meetings are used to discuss personal problems related to the maintenance of sobriety, and in speaker meetings recovering alcoholics, usually from different AA groups, tell their stories, which are called "drunkalogues." These are accounts of alcoholics' troubles with drinking and their recovery through AA. Many times they are humorous. In larger meetings, members may separate into smaller groups so that several of these types of programs may go on at the same time.

Finally, the meeting ends with a group recital of the Lord's Prayer, usually with members holding hands:

Our Father, which art in heaven, hallowed be Thy name. Thy kingdom come. Thy will be done, on earth as it is in heaven. Give us this day our daily bread, and forgive us our debts, as we forgive our debtors. And lead us not into temptation, but deliver us from evil: For thine is the kingdom, and the power, and the glory, for ever. Amen.

The meeting is then adjourned.

In addition to meetings, many local AA organizations operate clubhouses. These are open during the day and sometimes in the evening, and alcoholics can spend time there chatting with other recovering alcoholics. This setting provides a variety of benefits: It replaces the drinking environment and provides alcoholics a new social group and a supportive environment.[4]

Residential Treatment

Two other forms of treatment that should be mentioned are therapeutic communities and halfway houses, commonly referred to as residential treatment.

Therapeutic Communities

Usually three months to two years in length, therapeutic community programs share a number of common components with short-term programs. One feature that distinguishes therapeutic communities from short-term treatment, however, is their emphasis on a patient's resocialization. Some therapeutic community programs require that participants be forcibly separated from the outside world. Therapy is strongly confrontive. Other therapeutic community programs are similar to short-term programs but extend treatment over a longer period of time and involve less confrontation and less separation from the outside world. Therapeutic communities usually have dormitory-style living, daily chores, family-style meals, and require members to help maintain the facility. They may offer educational and vocational training. Therapeutic community treatment is best suited for adolescents.[1,8]

Halfway Houses

Basically a structured transitional living situation between inpatient treatment and returning home, halfway houses are frequently referred to as secondary treatment or extended treatment. They are best suited for those who have not made satisfactory progress in primary treatment or who should not return home because of an unresolved family situation (as in the case of a female patient with an abusive spouse at home). In halfway house programs, ten to twenty patients live together, sharing responsibility for maintaining the house. They do their own grocery shopping, cook their own meals, do housework, and wash their own clothes. They are employed outside the house, which provides a supportive living environment, a low level of treatment, and a place to hold AA meetings. Patients also attend other AA meetings in the local community. The level of intensity in halfway house programs varies considerably. Some are little more than a group living situation, while others function almost as an inpatient treatment program. Halfway house treatment usually lasts two to six months.[12]

Choosing a Treatment Program

Having made the diagnosis and gotten the addict to agree to treatment, a physician must now make a decision about which program is best for that particular patient. This consists of two steps — evaluating a patient to see which type of treatment (inpatient, outpatient, AA) is best suited for him or her and evaluating the type and quality of the various available treatment programs.

Patient Evaluation

Particular characteristics and situations may make a patient more suitable for one type of treatment program than another (these are outlined in Table 3.5). Characteristics that may make a patient more suitable for inpatient treatment include significant denial of chemical dependence, physical dependence on CNS depressant drugs or opioids, significant medical problems or debility because of advanced age, failed outpatient treatment, adolescence, refusal to enter an outpatient program, and dual diagnosis.

TABLE 3.5. Guidelines for inpatient treatment.

Patient characteristics
    significant denial of chemical dependence
    physical addiction to CNS depressants or opioids
    significant medical problems or debility due to advanced age
    failed outpatient treatment
    adolescents who are chemically dependent; those diagnosed as using or abusing drugs may be suit-
      able for outpatient treatment
    refusal to enter outpatient program
    dual diagnosis

Patient situations
    poor family support
    drug-using spouse or significant other at home
    distance greater than 40 miles from nearest outpatient program or lack of transportation
    court-ordered inpatient treatment

Situations that may make a patient more suitable for inpatient treatment include poor family support, a drug-using spouse or significant other at home, living further than 40 miles from the nearest outpatient program or not having transportation to get to that program, and court order to attend inpatient treatment. Most patients who do not meet these guidelines are probably best suited for outpatient treatment.

Alcoholics Anonymous is used as a primary treatment only when patients will not accept inpatient or outpatient treatment under any conditions or when public programs or funds for private programs are not available. Many times, patients who will not agree to formal treatment will agree to attend AA. When this is the case, they should agree to attend a fixed number of meetings in a given time period. Traditionally, 90 meetings in 90 days, followed by less intensive but regular attendance, have been recommended. Patients should sign written contracts agreeing to enter treatment if they are not able to maintain sobriety by this method; physicians also sign the contracts.[13]

Program Evaluation

Both inpatient and outpatient treatments have advantages and disadvantages, some of which are listed in Table 3.6. Advantages of inpatient treatment include a structured environment, lack of access to drugs, more intense treatment, an impression on patients of the gravity of their situation, and more integrated healthcare services. Disadvantages include the fact that inpatient treatment is considerably more expensive than outpatient treatment, patients must be away from home, and patients must take time off from work.[12]

Advantages of outpatient treatment are that it is considerably less expensive than inpatient treatment, patients can continue to live at home, and they can

TABLE 3.6. Inpatient versus outpatient treatment.

Inpatient treatment	
Advantages	*Disadvantages*
structured environment	higher costs
no access to drugs	away from home
more intense treatment	absence from work
impression on patient of gravity of situation	
more integrated healthcare	

Outpatient treatment	
Advantages	*Disadvantages*
less expensive	lack of structured environment
can live at home	more access to drugs
can continue to work	less intense treatment
	less impression on patient of gravity of situation
	less integrated healthcare

continue to go to work. Disadvantages are the lack of a structured environment, more access to drugs, less intensive treatment than inpatient treatment, less of an impression is made on patients of the gravity of their situation, and healthcare services are less integrated.[12-13]

A good inpatient treatment program should consist of medical assessment, detoxification, treatment of medical problems, psychosocial assessment, the development of a treatment plan, rehabilitation, discharge planning, and family treatment. Rehabilitation in such a program should, at a minimum, include education, group therapy, individual therapy, peer assessment, recreational therapy, coping skills and relaxation training, support group attendance, and spirituality (these components are listed in Table 3.7). In addition, good medical and nursing care is extremely important, and a program's medical director should be certified in addiction medicine.[1]

Components of a good outpatient program include psychosocial assessment, the development of a treatment plan, rehabilitation, frequent urine drug screens, discharge planning, and family treatment. Rehabilitation in such a program should include group therapy, individual therapy, peer assessment, support group attendance, and spirituality (these components are listed in Table 3.7).

Counselors in both inpatient and outpatient treatment programs should be certified in chemical dependence. Programs should teach the disease concept of addiction, emphasize the twelve-step process, and have a strong commitment to aftercare.[1]

TABLE 3.7. Components of a good treatment program.

Inpatient	Outpatient
medical assessment	psychosocial assessment
recent drug history	treatment plan development
medical history	rehabilitation
physical examination	group therapy
laboratory studies	individual therapy
detoxification	peer assessment
treatment of medical problems	support group attendance
psychosocial assessment	spirituality
psychological testing	frequent urine drug screens
social assessment	discharge planning
treatment plan development	family treatment
rehabilitation	
education	
group therapy	
individual therapy	
peer assessment	
recreational therapy	
coping skills/relaxation training	
support group attendance	
spirituality	
discharge planning	
family treatment	

Aftercare

Each treatment program, inpatient and outpatient, should have its own aftercare program. Most commonly, facilities conduct aftercare programs two evenings a week. Aftercare usually lasts for one to three months; however, some programs extend it to as long as two years. It should not be viewed as another kind of treatment but as a continuation of the initial treatment. It differs from outpatient treatment in that its goals are very limited, dealing with the problems of reentry while simultaneously attempting to consolidate the gains made during treatment.[12] Each patient is assisted in making the transition from treatment to family, job, and community. The recovering addict is also expected to attend two to three support group meetings a week. Because chemical dependence, like any chronic disease, requires lifelong care, recovering patients are expected to continue to attend support groups long after aftercare has ended.[8]

Confidentiality

A federal statute mandates confidentiality in the treatment of chemical dependence. Specifically, the law applies to records of a patient's identity, diagnosis, prognosis, or treatment and records that are maintained for the purposes of education, training, treatment, rehabilitation, or research. The statute is applicable if the treatment facility receives any federal assistance, including registration to dispense a controlled substance (if it is used to treat chemical dependence), tax-free exemptions, or Medicare. When not in use, written records must be maintained in a secure room, in a locked file cabinet, safe, or other similar container.[14]

Information in a patient's record can be disclosed only with that patient's written consent. In general, records cannot be used in making criminal charges or in investigating a patient.[14]

The federal regulations do not apply to the Veterans' Administration or the Armed Forces. They also do not apply to communication within a treatment program or between a program and an agency with administrative control of the program. The statute also exempts crimes on program premises or against program personnel, situations involving serious risk of bodily harm to a third party, and reports of suspected child abuse and neglect. Information identifying patients may be disclosed to medical personnel in medical emergencies. Immediately following it, such a disclosure must be documented in a patient's records. The statute is not considered by most healthcare workers to prevent them from reporting venereal diseases to local health authorities. Identifying information can also be disclosed to qualified individuals for research purposes if the information will not be redisclosed and if the research has been approved by an independent group of three or more individuals who find that patient rights would be adequately protected and that the benefits of the research outweigh risks to patients' confidentiality.[14]

A treatment center's acknowledgment of a patient's presence in its program also requires the patient's written consent. Insurance information that a patient furnishes for admission constitutes permission for the treatment center to disclose information to the insurance company or its representative. Additionally, observations of patients by former patients attending support groups in the center or by visiting family members of other patients do not violate the statute. If the treatment facility is a unit of a general hospital, the acknowledgment that a person is a patient in the general hospital is not considered a breech of confidentiality.[14]

In the case of an adult patient who has been judged to lack the capacity to manage his or her own affairs, consent may be given by a guardian or other person authorized under state law to act in the patient's behalf.[14] The statute also addresses confidentiality of patients who have not yet reached the age of majority as specified in state law or, in the absence of a state law, are not yet 18 years of age. If the minor patient acting alone has the legal capacity under state law to apply for and obtain alcohol or drug-abuse treatment, only that patient may give written consent for disclosure. Where state law requires consent of a parent or guardian, both the minor patient and his or her parent or guardian must give authorization for disclosure. When a minor patient is judged to lack the capacity for rational choice (because of extreme youth or a mental or physical condition), a parent or guardian may act in the minor's behalf.[14]

A patient must be informed in writing at the time of admission, or as soon thereafter as the patient is capable of rational communication, of the confidentiality requirement.[14]

The statute provides for criminal penalties for those who violate its provisions.[14]

The Role of the Referring Physician

Having made the diagnosis of chemical dependence, a physician should evaluate factors in a patient's life that might be used as leverage to get him or her to agree to treatment (legal problems, family problems, medical problems, work problems). If this does not prompt the addict to seek treatment, the family may wish to intervene (intervention is discussed in Chapter 5). The patient's physician can guide the family on intervention and may even wish to be a member of the intervention team. If the intervention fails or if the family does not want to use this approach, physicians can instruct family members on how to get a court order mandating treatment (depending on the law in the patient's state). Physicians should be aware that federal statute mandates confidentiality of patient records in a treatment facility.

Should patients agree to treatment, physicians must be able to decide which type of treatment is best suited for particular patients (inpatient, outpatient, support group). They should also have a good understanding of AA and other support groups and be familiar with treatment, both inpatient and outpatient. They should be able to evaluate the quality of various local treatment programs.

Finally, when treatment is completed, physicians should be involved in the long-term recovery of patients. They should discuss attending support groups with patients at each office visit, be aware of prescribed medication that may lead to relapse, be alert for signs of relapse, and help patients get back into treatment should relapse occur.

Comment

Treatment of chemically dependent individuals is rapidly undergoing change as we learn more about which techniques are useful and which are not. Also, criteria for inpatient versus outpatient treatment will undoubtedly undergo change, as will the length and structure of the various types of treatment programs.

References

1. Van Cleave, S., W. Byrd, and K. Revell. What really works in treatment. In *Counseling for Substance Abuse and Addiction*. Word Book, Waco, Texas, 1987, pp. 133–143.
2. Cook, C. C. H. The Minnesota model in the management of drug and alcohol dependency: Miracle, method or myth? Part I. The Philosophy and the Programme. *British Journal of Addiction*, 83:625–634, 1988.
3. Milhorn, H. T., Jr. Diagnosis of alcoholism and other drug dependencies. In *Review Course Syllabus*, American Medical Society on Alcoholism and Other Drug Dependencies, in press.
4. Alford, G. S. Psychoactive substance use disorders. In *Recent Developments in Adolescent Psychiatry*. Ed. by L. K. G. Hsu and M. Hersen. Wiley, New York, 1988, pp. 309–331.
5. Anderson, R. C., J. V. Fisher, C. L. Whitfield, and M. R. Liepman. Substance abuse rehabilitation. In *Family Medicine Guide to Substance Abuse*. STFM, Kansas City, Missouri, 1984, pp. 6-1 through 6-18.
6. King, P. Spirituality. *Adolescent Counselor*, April/May, 1989, p. 16.
7. O'Neill, S. F., and H. N. Barnes. Alcoholics Anonymous. In *Alcoholism: A Guide for the Primary Care Physician*. Ed. by H. N. Barnes, M. D. Aronson, and T. L. Delbanco. Springer-Verlag, New York, 1987, pp. 93–101.
8. Royce, J. E. Alcoholic Anonymous. In *Alcohol Problems and Alcoholism*. Free Press, New York, 1981, pp. 242–255.
9. *The Twelve Steps and Twelve Traditions*. Alcoholics Anonymous World Services, Inc., New York, 1976.
10. Van Cleave, S., W. Byrd, and K. Revell. The road to recovery: What it takes to get out of addiction. In *Counseling for Substance Abuse and Addiction*, Word Books, Waco, Texas, 1987, pp. 101–117.

11. How it works. In *Alcoholics Anonymous*. Alcoholics Anonymous World Services, Inc., New York, 1976, pp. 58–71.

12. Shulman, G. D., and R. D. O'Connor. The rehabilitation of the alcoholic. In *Alcoholism: A Practical Treatment Guide*. Ed. by S. E. Gittow and H. S. Peyser. Grune and Stratton, Orlando, Florida, 1980, pp. 103–129.

13. Spickard, A., and B. R. Thompson. Paths to sobriety. In *Dying for a Drink: What You Should Know About Alcoholism*. Word Books, Waco, Texas, 1985, pp. 136–144.

14. Weger, C. D., and R. J. Diehl. *The Counselor's Guide to Confidentiality*. Program Information Associates, Honolulu, Hawaii, 1987.

CHAPTER 4

Recovery and Relapse

Recovery

Abstinence is not using addictive chemicals. It allows recovery to begin. Learning to live normally without the use of addictive chemicals requires more than abstinence. *Recovery* is a process in which the physiological, psychological, and social damage caused by chemical dependence is healed. Addicts learn to live healthy and productive lives without the need for alcohol or other drugs. Recovery is an individual process; no two people recover at exactly the same rate.[1]

Recovery has no time limit. It is a lifetime program. Physicians must be prepared to enter into a lifelong relationship with recovering individuals and their families. Many crises — including relapse — may occur, especially in the first two years of recovery. By developing an open relationship with patients and their families, physicians will be more likely to be consulted when such crises occur.[2]

Tasks of Recovery

The first task of recovery is for addicts to recognize that they have a debilitating, life-threatening disease. Once they recognize this, the second task of recovery is total abstinence from psychoactive substances. The third task is to recognize the need for a program to give support and assistance in staying sober one day at a time.[1]

The Recovery Process

The recovery process moves from basic to more complex tasks. The progression is from abstinence (learning to live without drugs) to sobriety (learning to cope with life without drugs), to comfortable living (learning how to live comfortably while abstinent), to productive living (learning how to build a meaningful sober life). Gorski and Miller divide the recovery process into six developmental periods: (1) pretreatment, (2) stabilization, (3) early recovery, (4) middle recovery, (5) late recovery, and (6) maintenance.[1]

1. *Pretreatment.* In pretreatment, addicts learn from the consequences of drug use that they cannot safely use psychoactive substances. As the consequences become more and more severe, addicts attempt to control their drug use. When this fails, they attempt periods of abstinence. Finally, they admit defeat and realize that they cannot control their drug use. Addicts are often forced into treatment before they recognize that chemical dependence is a problem. The recognition of addiction that comes as a result of treatment is part of the pretreatment experience.[1]

2. *Stabilization.* Stabilization is regaining control of thought processes, emotions, judgment, and behavior. It involves recovery from acute withdrawal and physical health problems. The major motivational life crisis that caused an addict to enter this period is stabilized.[1]

3. *Early recovery.* Early recovery involves accepting the disease of addiction and learning to function without psychoactive substances. Addicts begin to recuperate from serious physiological, psychological, and social damage caused by chemical dependence. This period relies heavily on structured recovery programs, which are often developed for addicts in treatment programs and later as aftercare plans. It creates an environment that educates addicts and their families about chemical dependence and recovery. This period may be difficult for some because of the postacute withdrawal syndrome.[1]

4. *Middle recovery.* In the middle recovery period, the primary goal is to change lifestyles. Addicts work at developing normal, balanced lifestyles that are based on sobriety-centered values and activities. This involves living a recovery program that is active but less intense than that of early recovery. It includes work activities, family activities, social activities, self-development, recreation, exercise, and proper diet. Resisting the temptation to substitute another addiction, such as gambling, is an important issue in middle recovery. Sobriety can be maintained in this period with a less restrictive recovery program than in the early recovery period.[1]

5. *Late recovery.* The primary goal of the late recovery period is to develop self-esteem, the capacity for healthy intimacy, and the ability to live happily and productively. Personal beliefs, beliefs about self and others, self-defeating patterns of living, intimacy, and relationship skills are evaluated and, if necessary, restructured. For some recovering people—usually addicts who come from relatively functional families—the late recovery period poses no serious problems. From childhood they learned healthy beliefs and values, but their chemical use interfered with their ability to live productively. For these people, recovery means rehabilitation— that is, returning to a previous level of health and well-being. Other recovering individuals are not as fortunate. They have a great deal of work to do in the late recovery period, either because they grew up in dysfunctional families or because they began using alcohol or other drugs at such a young age that their emotional growth and development were arrested. They never learned normal, healthy beliefs and attitudes. Participating in Adult Children of Alcoholics (ACOA) support groups may be helpful to

those who grew up in dysfunctional families. Those whose arrested emotional growth and development resulted from early use of psychoactive substances must undergo a long course of habilitation—that is, developing healthy beliefs and attitudes for the first time.[1]

6. *Maintenance.*   The primary goal of the maintenance period is for addicts to stay sober and live productively. This involves maintaining themselves on effective recovery programs, identifying warning signs of relapse, daily problem solving, maintaining honesty, and living productively. Addicts continue to avoid addictive chemicals. Recovery from chemical dependence is a lifelong process; the disease of addiction never goes away.[1]

Partial Recovery

Recovery does not follow a progressive, straight line. Addicts reach and overcome plateaus, slip backwards occasionally, but usually move on. Many recovering people eventually achieve long-term and comfortable sobriety. Others, however, do not make it all the way through the recovery process. *Partial recovery* begins when they confront a recovery task that they believe to be unmanageable or insurmountable. They get stuck at this level of recovery and only achieve a low-quality sobriety. Instead of taking productive steps to overcome their failure to progress, many deny that something is wrong. With help, many of these people overcome their denial and again begin to make progress. Unfortunately, in others, failure to progress causes relapse. Even then, some will become aware of what is happening to them and prevent the relapse episode before it actually occurs. Others go on to relapse. The Big Book of AA calls the failure to take the necessary steps to progress in recovery half measures. These individuals tend to believe that attendance at AA meetings alone will keep them sober.[1]

Controlled Drinking

The controversy over whether alcoholics can learn to drink socially reached its peak with the publication of the Rand report in 1976. This study found that successful social drinking among men treated 18 months previously for alcoholism was not uncommon.[3] Since that time, most studies have been less optimistic. In general, the longer the interval studied, the fewer alcoholics were found to be able to sustain moderate problem-free drinking. Thus far, the only factors identified as common to alcoholics who are able to drink moderately are that they have milder cases of alcoholism (fewer lifetime alcohol-related problems) and greater social support. In a review of the literature, Taylor, Helzer, and Robins found that data from the majority of studies indicate that successful moderate drinking among treated alcoholics is uncommon.[4] Even if a small percentage of alcoholics are able to drink socially, there is currently no way to identify them. Therefore, an alcoholic attempting to drink moderately plays a form of Russian roulette. A realistic goal for the treatment of alcoholism is still abstinence.

Drugs That May Be Hazardous to Recovery

The Drugs

Numerous drugs (legal, prescription, over-the-counter, illicit) may be hazardous to recovery; some of these are listed in Table 4.1. This concept is based on what is known in the treatment field as *cross-addiction*. The basic tenet of cross-addiction is that if a person has ever been addicted to a psychoactive substance, he or she can never again use any psychoactive substance without increasing the risk of relapse. It is not wise for a cocaine addict, for example, to begin drinking alcohol after treatment. The individual may become addicted to alcohol, or the alcohol may lead back to addiction to cocaine. The drugs listed in Table 4.1 are often referred to as mood-altering drugs (MAD).

Recovering individuals are at particular risk for relapse when taking prescription drugs prescribed by well-meaning physicians who are not knowledgeable about chemical dependence. It is not unusual for these physicians to get angry

TABLE 4.1. Drugs that may be hazardous to recovery.

Alcoholic beverages
  all

Prescription drugs
  barbiturates
  barbiturate-like drugs (ethchlorvynol, ethinamate,
    glutethimide, methyprylone)
  benzodiazepines
  meprobamate
  chloral hydrate
  amphetamines
  methylphenidate, pemoline
  diet pills
  narcotics and narcotic combination drugs
  muscle relaxants
  antihistamines
  decongestants
  antitussives
  antidepressants
  phenothiazines and similar drugs
  all prescription drugs containing alcohol

Over-the-counter drugs
  antihistamines
  decongestants
  antitussives
  diet pills
  sleeping pills
  all over-the-counter drugs containing alcohol

Illicit drugs
  all

when recovering patients tell them that they cannot take a medication because it may be hazardous to their sobriety. Over-the-counter cough and cold preparations are particularly dangerous to recovering people; some have 30 to 40 proof alcohol concentrations.

Treatment personnel usually tell recovering patients to avoid nonaddicting drugs that tend to cause sedation, such as classic antihistamines. There is little evidence to indicate that the use of these drugs leads to relapse. However, many recovering addicts will tell you that if they use them they will abuse them. Since we now have newer nonsedating antihistamines, it is probably better to continue to tell recovering patients to avoid classic antihistamines. Other nonaddicting but sedating drugs (muscle relaxants, antidepressants) should be used only when absolutely necessary and then under the care of a knowledgeable physician.

Rational Use of Medications in Recovery

Recovering patients who must undergo surgery can have narcotics for postsurgical pain and can in fact have just as much of it as anyone else. However, some special rules apply. When possible, patients should be maintained in a hospital an extra few days if it means they can go home narcotic-free. Use of some of the nonsteroidal drugs such as ibuprofen (Motrin) for mild to moderate pain, rather than narcotic preparations, has been very helpful. When an addict's pain is such that postdischarge narcotic medication is absolutely necessary, someone in his or her family or a close friend should keep the narcotic and dispense it as prescribed. The patient should never have direct access to it. It should be prescribed as short a time as possible. As soon as they are physically able, addictive patients should temporarily increase their attendance at support groups. The same rules apply for dental procedures requiring pain medication or other medical procedures requiring psychoactive substances.

Patients with severe primary psychiatric disorders (unipolar or bipolar affective disorders, schizophrenia) and chemical dependence may require drugs (antidepressants, lithium, phenothiazines) to control the psychiatric symptoms before their chemical dependence can be treated. For lesser psychiatric illnesses, such as anxiety disorders, nonpharmacological approaches should be used first, followed by drugs with the least possible potential for abuse. Some patients with psychiatric disorders will require medication indefinitely. This sometimes presents a problem in AA meetings.

Pharmacological Approaches

Two pharmacological approaches to help support recovery are the use of disulfiram (Antabuse) for alcoholism and naltrexone (Trexan) for opioid addiction.

Disulfiram

A chemical barrier to support abstinence, disulfiram is especially useful in the first year or two of sobriety. It is a safe medication with relatively few side effects. Disulfiram, by interfering with the action of aldehyde dehydrogenase, causes rapid accumulation of a toxic catabolite, acetaldehyde, after ethanol ingestion. Within 15 minutes after they consume alcohol, alcoholics' faces turn beet red and they sweat and suffer palpitations, dyspnea, tachycardia, hypotension, syncope, chest pain, nausea, and vomiting. EKG changes of ST depression, T-wave flattening, and QT prolongation may occur. Disulfiram should always be prescribed with a patient's full knowledge and consent.

Although any substances that contain alcohol, including mouthwashes, aftershave lotions, food sauces, and cough medicine, can produce a reaction, the likelihood of them doing so has been exaggerated. When reactions occur, it usually means that alcoholics have deliberately consumed alcohol. However, patients should be given lists of common products containing alcohol and be advised to avoid them. They should wear bracelets or carry cards to alert medical personnel that they are taking disulfiram.[2]

Treating alcohol-induced reactions to disulfiram mainly involves restoring normal blood pressure and controlling shock if it should occur. Most reactions are mild and last 30 minutes to several hours. Intravenous diphenhydramine (50 to 100 mg) and ascorbic acid (1000 mg) may be beneficial.[2]

Addicts daily take a 500-mg tablet of disulfiram at bedtime for five days and take 250 mg daily thereafter. They should have consumed no alcohol for at least 12 hours before they begin taking disulfiram. The drug is slowly excreted. Therefore, reactions to alcohol usually continue to occur up to 5 to 7 days after patients stop taking the drug.[2]

Side effects of disulfiram are usually mild and consist of fatigue, somnolence, headache, dizziness, skin rash, gastrointestinal distress, and a garliclike taste and odor from the mouth. These side effects usually disappear in a week or two. If they are particularly troublesome, physicians can lower the drug's dosage for two weeks then return it to its previous level. A rare, idiosyncratic disulfiram-induced hepatitis, which is potentially fatal, has been reported. As a result, some doctors recommend that patients undergo tests of their liver function before they begin treatment and that these tests be repeated at two-week intervals for the first two months of treatment and at three- to six-month intervals after that. If a patient's liver function tests become abnormal, the drug should be discontinued. Alcoholics can take disulfiram indefinitely, but they usually only need it early in their recovery.[2,6-7]

There are few contraindications to the use of disulfiram. Alcoholics with cardiac or other serious medical problems should not take the drug. Likewise, mentally impaired alcoholics should not take it because they tend to forget whether or not they *have* taken it. Psychotic patients are also poor candidates for disulfiram treatment. Disulfiram may intensify the effects of anesthetics, sedative-hypnotics, phenytoin, and coumadin. When used by patients taking izoniozid, disulfiram occasionally causes confusion, changes in mental status, or unstable gait. Many drugs have been reported to produce a disulfiramlike reaction if patients ingest alcohol while taking them. These include oral hypoglycemic agents (chlorpropamide, tolbutamide), antibiotics (metronitazole, quinacrine, sulfonamides, chloramphenicol), some anti-inflammatory drugs (phenylbutazone, phenacetin), ethacryinic acid, and trinitroglycerin.[2,5,8]

At AA meetings, some members who reject all drugs as crutches may criticize patients taking disulfiram. Fortunately, most AA groups accept disulfiram today, and such criticism is declining.[2]

Patients who do well on disulfiram are older, well-motivated people with long drinking histories; their social lives are stable, and they tend to be binge drinkers. Disulfiram therapy by itself is ineffective and should be coupled with appropriate counseling and attendance at AA meetings.[5,8] Its use is controversial. A major Veteran's Administration study found no difference in sobriety between a group of patients treated with disulfiram and counseling and a control group treated with placebo and counseling.[9]

Naltrexone

Occasionally a useful adjunctive treatment for maintaining abstinence in detoxi-fied opioid addicts, naltrexone is a potent, long-acting opioid antagonist that reduces or eliminates the euphoria and drug-seeking behavior opioids produce. Physicians should not attempt to treat patients with naltrexone until they have stopped taking opioids for seven to ten days. If in doubt, physicians can perform a Narcan challenge test. If patients do not show withdrawal symptoms, physi-cians can start them on naltrexone therapy.

Naltrexone's side effects consist mainly of mild gastrointestinal disturbances (nausea, vomiting), anxiety, and insomnia, all of which tend to disappear over a few days. The usual oral dose is 100 mg on Mondays and Wednesdays and 150 mg on Fridays. In doses higher than 300 mg per day, some patients show hepatic toxicity. Many patients drop out of treatment and stop taking the drug. When it is combined with family support and counseling, patients are more apt to remain opioid-free.[10-12]

Relapse

The Relapse Syndrome

Just as it is important for addicts to understand that recovery is more than absti-nence, they need to recognize that relapse is not simply the act of taking a drink or using a drug. It, too, is a process. Addicts who believe that abstinence is syn-onymous with recovery also believe that not using alcohol or other drugs is their main task in recovery. As a result, when their behavior is dysfunctional, they become confused because their mistaken belief keeps them from identifying the real problem—their failure to progress in recovery. They believe that when they are abstinent the only way to lose control is to use alcohol or other drugs.[1]

A common mistaken belief about relapse is that it just suddenly occurs without warning. The truth is that many warning signs precede a relapse. Addicts who believe that relapse just suddenly occurs are unable to identify warning signs.

They also forget that denial carries over into sobriety and can block their recognition of warning signs, which occur very late in the relapse process. By the time they develop, many addicts have already lost control of their judgment and behavior. As a result, they are unable to act to reverse the relapse process.[1]

In the early days of AA, alcoholics were considered to relapse only when they began drinking again. As alcoholics started substituting other sedative drugs (such as tranquilizers and sleeping pills) for alcohol, it became obvious that they could not safely use any sedative. So relapse came to mean the use of any sedative, including alcohol. In the 1960s physicians found that relapse was also associated with other drugs, such as marijuana, cocaine, amphetamines, and narcotics. As a result, relapse came to mean the use of any psychoactive substance.[1]

The relapse process includes becoming dysfunctional in recovery. The dysfunction begins as a mental process that in AA is called stinking thinking. This thinking leads to a change in behavior that AA calls a setup for relapse. The dysfunctional behavior in AA is called a dry drunk, which is sometimes thought of as an alcoholic's thinking and acting as if he or she were drinking despite being abstinent.[1]

The Relapse Process

Although it has no definite timetable and may last from one to several months, relapse has been divided by Gorski and Miller into the following ten phases (these are also listed in Table 4.2).[1]

1. *Return of denial.* During this phase, individuals in the relapse process become unable to recognize and honestly tell others what they are thinking or feeling. The most common symptoms of this phase are a concern about well-being (addicts feel uneasy, afraid, and anxious, but the uneasiness comes and goes, usually only lasting a short time) and denial of the concern (to tolerate these periods of worry, fear, and anxiety, addicts ignore or deny these feelings in the same way they at one time denied addiction).
2. *Avoidance and defensive behavior.* During this phase, addicts begin to avoid anything or anybody that would force them to look at themselves. When asked questions about their well-being, they tend to become defensive. They believe that they will never drink or take drugs again, so that a daily recovery program seems unnecessary to them. They tend to worry about others instead of themselves, judging others' recovery programs rather than their own. In AA this is called working the other guy's program. Addicts in this phase also become defensive, defending themselves even when they do not need to. They become compulsive, or rigid, in the way they think and behave, tending to do the same things over and over again without good reasons. They also tend to control conversations either by talking too much or by not talking at all. They tend to work more than they need to, become involved in many activities, and may appear to be models of recovery because of their heavy work on AA's twelfth step and their chairing of AA

TABLE 4.2. Phases of relapse.

Phase 1. Return of denial
  concern about well-being
  denial of the concern
Phase 2. Avoidance and defensive behavior
  belief they will never drink or use again
  worrying about others instead of themselves
  defensiveness
  compulsive behavior
  impulsive behavior
  loneliness
Phase 3. Crisis building
  tunnel vision
  minor depression
  loss of constructive planning
  plans begin to fail
Phase 4. Immobilization
  daydreaming and wishful thinking
  feeling that nothing can be solved
  immature wish to be happy
Phase 5. Confusion and overreaction
  periods of confusion
  irritation with friends
  easily angered
Phase 6. Depression
  irregular eating habits
  lack of desire to take action
  irregular sleep habits
  loss of daily structure
  periods of deep depression

Phase 7. Behavioral loss of control
  irregular attendance of support group
    meetings
  development of an "I don't care" attitude
  open rejection of help
  dissatisfaction with life
  feelings of powerlessness and helplessness
Phase 8. Recognition of loss of control
  self-pity
  thoughts of social drinking or using
  conscious lying
  complete loss of self-confidence
Phase 9. Option reduction
  unreasonable resentment
  discontinuance of all support group meetings
  overwhelming loneliness, frustration, anger,
    and tension
  loss of behavioral control
Phase 10. The relapse episode
  initial use
  shame and guilt
  helplessness and hopelessness
  complete loss of control
  biopsychosocial damage
  complete collapse

meetings. They are well-known by counselors for playing counselor. They avoid casual or informal involvement with people, however. They are impulsive, acting without thought or self-control, usually during times of high stress. As a result, they may make decisions that seriously damage their recovery program. Lastly, addicts in this phase are lonely—they begin to spend more time alone and usually have good reasons and excuses for staying away from other people.

3. *Crisis building.* During this phase, addicts have problems that result from denying personal feelings, isolating themselves, and neglecting their recovery programs. They commonly suffer tunnel vision—seeing only one small

part of life rather than the big picture, which sometimes creates the illusion that everything is secure and going well. They blow small problems way out of proportion and come to believe that they are being treated unfairly and are powerless to do anything about it. Addicts also often suffer minor depressions, the symptoms of which begin to appear and to persist. They are usually able to distract themselves from these moods by getting busy with other things, and they do not talk about depression. Addicts stop planning, often mistaking the AA slogan "one day at a time" to mean that people shouldn't plan or think about what they are going to do. They pay less and less attention to details and make plans more on wishful thinking than on reality. Finally, their plans begin to fail because they are unrealistic. As a result, addicts develop problems in their lives.

4. *Immobilization.* During this phase, addicts are unable to initiate action and merely go through the motions of living. Common symptoms of this phase include daydreaming and wishful thinking. Addicts have difficulty concentrating, and they frequently use the expression "If only" in conversation. They begin to have fantasies of escape and of being rescued by events that are unlikely to happen. Addicts also begin to develop a sense of failure, which may be real or imagined. They blow small failures out of proportion. They also harbor an immature wish to be happy, without identifying what they need to be happy. They want things to get better without doing anything to make them better.

5. *Confusion and overreaction.* During this phase, addicts cannot think clearly. They become upset with themselves and those around them and are irritable, overreacting to small things. Symptoms of this phase include periods of confusion, which steadily become more frequent, last longer, and cause more problems. Addicts often are angry with themselves because they cannot figure things out. They become irritable with friends, straining relationships with friends, family, and support group members. The conflicts continue to increase in spite of their efforts to resolve them. And addicts are easily angered, becoming frustrated, resentful, and irritable for no reason. They frequently overreact to small things and become increasingly stressed and anxious.

6. *Depression.* During this phase, addicts become so depressed that they have difficulty sticking to normal routines. At times they think of suicide, drinking, or using drugs. Their depression is severe and persistent. The most common symptoms are irregular sleeping habits, inability to take action, irregular eating habits, loss of daily structure, and periods of deep depression.

7. *Behavioral loss of control.* During this phase, addicts are unable to control their behavior and their daily schedules, but they deny being out of control. Their lives become chaotic. Their attendance at support group meetings becomes irregular, as they find excuses for missing meetings and don't recognize the importance of attendance. Other things seem more important to

them. They develop an "I don't care" attitude, trying to act as if they are unconcerned about their problems. They use this attitude to hide feelings of helplessness and a growing lack of self-respect and self-confidence. They reject help, cutting themselves off from those who could help with fits of anger, by criticizing or putting others down, or by quietly withdrawing from others. They become dissatisfied with life, which seems to them to have become unmanageable since they stopped drinking or using drugs. They begin to feel that they might as well start drinking or using drugs again. Finally, they feel powerless and helpless. They have trouble getting started, thinking clearly, concentrating, and thinking abstractly. They begin to feel there is no way out.

8. *Recognition of loss of control.* During this phase, addicts' denial breaks and they realize how severe their problems really are, how unmanageable their lives have become, and how little power they have to solve any of their problems. By this time, they are so isolated that they have no one to turn to for help. They commonly begin to feel sorry for themselves and often use self-pity to get attention from family members and from support group members. They think about social drinking, imagining that alcohol or other drugs would make them feel better and they begin to think that they can control use. They recognize their lying, denial, and the excuses they make but are unable to do anything about them. They lose self-confidence, feel trapped and overwhelmed by the inability to think clearly and take action. This feeling of powerlessness leads them to believe that they are useless and incompetent.

9. *Option reduction.* During this phase, addicts feel trapped, with only three ways out—insanity, suicide, or drug use. They no longer believe that anyone or anything can help them. They feel an unreasonable resentment and anger because they cannot behave the way they want to. They stop attending all support group meetings and feel overwhelming loneliness, frustration, anger, and tension. They have intense fears of insanity and feelings of help-lessness and desperation. Finally, they lose control over their behavior and have more and more difficulty controlling their thoughts, emotions, and judgment. They are unable to regain control.

10. *The relapse episode.* During this phase, addicts begin to use alcohol or other drugs again. Their failed struggle for abstinence leads to shame and guilt. Eventually, they lose all control and develop serious biopsychosocial problems. They begin using alcohol or other drugs in attempts to control their dysfunction, and their shame and guilt isolates them and makes them afraid their relapse will be discovered. They feel helpless and hopeless—that they can do nothing to stop the relapse. They stop attempting to control their use of alcohol or other drugs and begin using them often, heavily, and des-tructively. The progressive relapse damages their physical, psychological, and social health. They become so ill that they cannot function. They either seek treatment, have a physical or emotional collapse, commit suicide, or die from medical complications.[1]

Factors Contributing to Relapse

Talbott has identified 13 factors that contribute to relapse (these are listed in Table 4.3).[13]

1. *Failure to understand and accept chemical dependence as a disease.* This is the fundamental factor that can precipitate relapse. Addicts who do not believe addiction to be a disease tend to think that by willpower alone they can control their drinking and using.
2. *Denial of loss of control.* Addicts who don't believe in loss of control feel that they can drink or use as long as they do so carefully. They do not connect their abuse of psychoactive substances and the problems that follow. They continue with the same behavior but expect different results.
3. *Dishonesty.* For addicts, dishonesty usually means distorting reality and concealing emotions. It may include extensive rationalizations. Addicts may have extramarital affairs, which are likely to contribute to relapse.
4. *The dysfunctional family.* A family can contribute immeasurably to an addict's recovery. In the same way that the dysfunctional family contributed to the progression of the disease, however, it can also contribute to relapse.
5. *The lack of a spiritual program.* The lack of a spiritual program leads addicts to believe that no source of strength, other than themselves, is available to them. The concept of a higher power ceases to be important in their recovery.
6. *Stress.* The old way addicts handled stress was to take chemicals to get high. In recovery, they have to learn nonchemical coping skills. Emotional and physical traps that often are said to lead to relapse include getting too hungry, angry, lonely, or tired (HALT), as well as self-pity. Recognizing these traps, and getting out of them is essential.

TABLE 4.3. Factors that contribute to relapse.

1. Failure to understand and accept the disease of chemical dependence
2. Denial of loss of control
3. Dishonesty
4. The dysfunctional family
5. The lack of a spiritual program
6. Stress and the inability to cope with it
7. Isolation and failure to become an active member of a support group
8. Cross-addiction
9. Holiday syndrome
10. Withdrawal
11. Overconfidence
12. A return to friends who drink and use drugs and to old habits
13. Guilt over the past

Based on G.D. Talbott, Elements of the impaired physician's program, *Journal of the Medical Association of Georgia*, 73:749–751, 1984.

7. *Isolation.* Withdrawal from relationships to avoid conflict can also lead to relapse. Isolation in recovery can lead addicts to feel hopelessly different and worthless; addicts must combat it with the tools of recovery.
8. *Cross-addiction.* Recovering individuals may take over-the-counter or prescription medications without being aware of their mood-altering or addictive qualities. Addicts have relapsed while taking legitimately prescribed medication for pain, for anxiety, or for surgical procedures.
9. *Holiday syndrome.* The risk of relapse is high at special times of the year, such as Thanksgiving, Christmas, birthdays, or anniversaries, when memories of the past surface and increase the pain of the present. During such periods addicts must go to more support group meetings, call their sponsors, and work the steps of the support group.
10. *Withdrawal.* Many people consider withdrawal from chemical dependence to consist of the obvious acute physical signs—tremors, seizures, delirium—that occur when addicts stop taking drugs. However, the physical and emotional effects of addiction may last up to a year or longer after addicts stop taking drugs. This is sometimes referred to as the postacute withdrawal syndrome.
11. *Overconfidence.* When in recovery, life's problems at last seem manageable to addicts. They can easily believe that things will continue to go well and can easily discard a sense of humility and dependence on a higher power. Such an attitude sets up an addict for relapse.
12. *Returning to drinking or drug-taking friends and to old habits.* When recovering individuals come to believe that they can handle the temptations they experience in such settings, the next step is for them to believe that they, too, can drink or use drugs. The AA wisdom of avoiding old faces and old places is good advice.
13. *Guilt over the past.* To achieve sobriety with a measure of serenity, addicts must take a moral inventory (AA Step 4) and make amends for their past actions and attitudes (AA Step 9), thus acknowledging the past and making peace with it.[13]

Preventing Relapse

Many addicts relapse because they do not understand relapse and what to do to prevent it. Gorski and Miller identify nine steps in preventing relapse (these are also listed in Table 4.4).[1]

1. *Stabilization.* Before addicts in recovery can prevent relapse, they must be in control of themselves. Stabilization involves gaining control of thoughts, emotions, memories, judgment, and behavior. Addicts may need professional help.
2. *Assessment.* The past is the best teacher. Addicts should review previous relapses and learn from them. The information they gain should be included in their relapse prevention plans.
3. *Education.* To prevent relapse, addicts must understand it. The more information they have about addiction, recovery, and relapse the more tools they

TABLE 4.4. The steps of relapse prevention.

1. Stabilization
2. Self-assessment
3. Relapse education
4. Identifying warning signs
5. Managing warning signs
6. Inventory training
7. Reviewing the recovery program
8. Involvement of significant others
9. Follow-up and Reinforcement

Based on T.L. Gorski and M. Miller, *Staying Sober: A Guide for Relapse Prevention*, Independence Press, Independence, Missouri, 1986, pp. 157–170. This material is copyrighted and propriety information of the CENAPS Corporation. It is reproduced here with the permission of the CENAPS Corporation. Any further reproduction is specifically prohibited without written permission of the CENAPS Corporation, P.O. Box 84, Hazel Crest, IL 60429, 708-334-3606.

have to maintain recovery. They should be familiar with the warning signs of relapse, as well as factors that contribute to it.

4. *Identifying warning signs.* Every addict has a unique set of personal warning signs that indicate he or she is relapsing. These may be health problems, thinking problems, emotional problems, memory problems, or problems with judgment and appropriate behavior. Each addict should develop a list of personal warning signs.

5. *Managing warning signs.* For each warning sign that an addict identifies, he or she should develop a plan for coping with it. Listing several alternatives may be helpful.

6. *Inventory training.* A successful recovery program involves a daily inventory (AA Step 10), which helps identify warning signs of relapse. Two daily inventory rituals are recommended. First, each morning addicts should read the daily entry in the 24-Hour-a-Day Book and briefly outline plans for the day. Each evening, they should review the day's tasks, identifying what they handled well and what they need to improve.

7. *Review of the recovery program.* When addicts are not recovering, they are in danger of relapsing. They should periodically review their personal recovery program to identify strengths and weaknesses and correct the weaknesses.

8. *Involvement of significant others.* Recovery cannot take place in isolation. It involves the help and support of others. Since relapse is often totally unconscious, family members, coworkers, and fellow support group members can be extremely helpful in recognizing warning signs. For them to help, they must know an addict's personal warning signs, information the addict should share with significant individuals in his or her life.

9. *Follow-up and reinforcement.* Like recovery, preventing relapse should be a way of life. Addicts should practice it until it becomes a habit. Addicts should periodically revise and update the relapse prevention plan as they grow and change in recovery.[1]

TABLE 4.5. What to do when relapse occurs.

When relapse occurs, addicts should:

1. Call their sponsors
2. Go to support group meetings
3. Call support group friends
4. Discuss the relapse with their physicians
5. Pick up white chips
6. Talk with their spouses, families, or significant others

Based on G.D. Talbott, Elements of the impaired physicians' program, *Journal of the Medical Association of Georgia*, 73:749–751, 1984.

What to Do When Relapse Occurs

It is not uncommon for people who have had a period of recovery to relapse. The relapse should be interrupted as soon as possible so that minimum damage is done to recovery. The experience should be used to build a stronger recovery. When relapse occurs, addicts should be instructed to do the following (these steps are also listed in Table 4.5).[13]

1. *Call their sponsors.*   Recovering addicts should have sponsors in their support groups. This is especially important in the first few months of recovery. Addicts will then, it is hoped, call their sponsors before using psychoactive substances.
2. *Go to a support group meeting.*   Addicts should be instructed to go to a meeting immediately and at least daily thereafter to resolve the conflict that resulted in the relapse.
3. *Call support group friends.*   Addicts should share honestly with support group friends psychoactive substance use or the urge to drink or use drugs.
4. *Discuss the relapse with their physicians.*   Addicts should discuss their relapse with their primary care physicians. In many cases, addicts can talk to their treatment program physicians for advice.
5. *Pick up a white chip.*   In AA a white chip denotes the desire to become abstinent and to begin a recovery program. Addicts who have relapsed should be instructed to pick up white chips at support group meetings and to begin again with the first step of AA.
6. *Talk with their spouses, families, or significant others.*   Although it may be difficult for addicts' spouses, families, or significant others to accept their relapse, they should share the experience with these people.[13]

Methadone Maintenance

A form of outpatient treatment for heroin addiction, methadone maintenance involves giving patients methadone daily. Since methadone is an opioid, methadone maintenance obviously does not have abstinence as its goal.[14]

Methadone (Dolophine) is a synthetic opioid that in large doses produces a degree of euphoria comparable to that of heroin (see Chapter 11). It has the advantage of having a longer half-life than heroin and of being effective in an oral form. Methadone often produces side effects, including sedation, constipation, excessive sweating, urine retention, and reduced sex drive. Intoxicated patients should not be given methadone because its effect with alcohol is synergistic.[14]

The goals of methadone maintenance are to reduce illicit drug use, reduce criminal activity, increase productivity (as indicated by employment), increase self-esteem, and improve family and community functioning. In addition, because addicts take methadone orally, they reduce their risk of acquiring serious infectious complications of intravenous drug use, such as bacterial endocarditis, hepatitis B, and AIDS. Methadone maintenance helps a large number of people who are not motivated to become abstinent and who otherwise would return to criminal activity and illicit drug use.[12] Patients on methadone maintenance commonly use cocaine, alcohol, and benzodiazepines.[15,16]

Originally, physicians used large doses of methadone (100–200 mg/day) to block the effects of heroin. Currently, they disagree over the appropriate dosage for methadone. Daily doses in the range of 40 to 50 mg appear to achieve comparable results by reducing addicts' craving for opioids, indicating that the blocking ability of high doses is not as important as the relief of cravings for opioids.[12]

A typical methadone maintenance clinic provides addicts daily doses of oral methadone, plus ancillary services such as vocational, legal, and social counseling. They usually also provide group therapy. Methadone maintenance programs periodically analyze addicts' urine for heroin and other drugs. Addicts take the medication in the presence of nurses or other responsible employees. After a few months of satisfactory cooperation with the program, programs may allow patients to take home a day's supply of methadone. As they continue to act reliably and responsibly, programs may permit them to take home a three-day supply.[12,14,17]

Methadone maintenance programs are subject to stringent federal and state regulations. Some states do not allow this treatment. Federal regulations require that such programs be registered with the Drug Enforcement Administration (DEA) and comply with specific DEA reporting requirements. Further, regulations require detoxification, rather than maintenance, of patients who have been dependent on opioids for less than one year.[14,17]

The Role of the Physician

Physicians, in the long-term management of chemically dependent individuals and their families, should follow a few simple rules. They should not assume responsibility for keeping patients sober. That is the responsibility of their patients. They should be careful with their prescription pads, and they should not try to treat patients alone. In times of crisis, such as relapse, they should get help from appropriate professionals. Physicians should monitor patients' recovery by watching for warning signs of relapse, inquiring about their families, jobs, friends, and support group attendance, and by giving them general support.[2]

References

1. Gorski, T. L., and M. Miller. *Staying Sober: A Guide for Relapse Prevention*. Independence Press, Independence, Missouri, 1986.
2. Zuska, J. J., and J. A. Pursch. Long-term management. In *Alcoholism: A Practical Treatment Guide*. Ed. by S. E. Gitlow and H. S. Peyser. Grune and Stratton, Orlando, Florida, 1980, pp. 131–164.
3. Armor, D. J., J. M. Polich, and H. B. Stambul. Alcoholism and treatment. Prepared for the National Institute on Alcohol Abuse and Alcoholism, Rand Corporation, Santa Monica, California, 1976.
4. Taylor, J. R., J. E. Helzer, and N. Robins. Moderate drinking in ex-alcoholics: Recent studies. *Journal of Studies on Alcohol*, 47:115–121, 1986.
5. Barnes, H. N. The use of disulfiram. In *Alcoholism: A Guide for the Primary Care Physician*. Ed. by H. N. Barnes, M. D. Aronson, and T. L. Delbanco. Springer-Verlag, New York, 1987, pp. 73–77.
6. Wright C. IV, J. A. Vafier, and C. R. Lake. Disulfiram-induced fulminating hepatitis: Guidelines for liver-panel monitoring. *Journal of Clinical Psychiatry*, 49:430–434, 1988.
7. Cereda, J., J. Bernuau, C. Degott, B. Rueff, and J. Benhamou. Fatal liver failure due to disulfiram. *Journal of Clinical Gastroenterology*, 11:98–100, 1989.
8. Forest, G. G. Antabuse treatment. In *Alcoholism and Substance Abuse*. Ed. by T. E. Bratter and G. G. Forest. The Free Press, New York, 1985, pp. 451–460.
9. Fuller, R. K., L. Branchey, D. R. Brightwell, et al. Disulfiram treatment of alcoholism: A Veteran's Administration cooperative study. *Journal of the American Medical Association*, 250:1449–1455, 1986.
10. Gonzalez, J. P., and R. N. Brogden. Naltrexone: A review of its pharmacodynamic properties and therapeutic efficacy in the management of opioid dependence. *Drugs*, 35:192–213, 1988.
11. Santos, E. F. Naltrexone: Useful tool in the treatment of heroin users: A review of the literature. *Henry Ford Hospital Medical Journal*, 35:95–100, 1988.
12. Wilford, B. B. (Ed.). *Review Course Syllabus*, American Medical Society on Alcoholism and Other Drug Dependencies, New York, 1987, pp. 279–363.
13. Talbott, G. D. Elements of the impaired physician's program. *Journal of the Medical Association of Georgia*, 73:749–751, 1984.
14. Wilford, B. B. (Ed.). *Drug Abuse: A Guide for the Primary Care Physician*. American Medical Association, Chicago, 1981, pp. 203–247.
15. Methadone maintenance and patients in alcoholism treatment. In *Alcohol Alert*, Department of Health and Human Services, Rockville, Maryland, August, 1988.
16. Hanbury, R., V. Sturiano, M. Cohen, B. Stimmel, and C. Aguillaume. Cocaine use in persons on methadone maintenance. *Advances in Alcohol and Substance Abuse*, 6:97–106, 1986.
17. Cohen, S. Methadone maintenance. In *The Substance Abuse Problems: Volume One*. Haworth Press, New York, 1981, pp. 251–256.

CHAPTER 5

The Family

Introduction

The effects of substance abuse on the family are profound. If one accepts 10 million as the number of adult alcoholics in the United States, probably 40 million people are codependent for alcoholism. How many people are addicted to other drugs or codependent with those who are is not known, but it is thought to be a substantial number. A *codependent* is a person who lets another person's behavior (the addict) adversely affect him or her and who is obsessed with controlling that person's behavior.[1-2]

Although we will discuss alcohol in this chapter, the principles outlined apply to any family that has a chemically dependent member, regardless of the drug that person abuses.

The Healthy Family

Most families are basically healthy, and family members are usually happy, working, contributing members of society. A healthy family, however, is not necessarily perfect. Members go through the illnesses, career crises, accidents, and losses that are part of normal living. Their lives are disrupted, and they suffer stress as children grow up. Healthy families remain intact because they adjust to changes in a healthy manner. Curran has identified 15 traits of a healthy family; these are listed in Table 5.1.[3]

The Alcoholic Family

Alcoholism exacts a tremendous emotional toll on a family and its individual members. As a result, a family develops a denial system and specific rules, and members tend to assume specific roles.

TABLE 5.1. Traits of the healthy family.

The healthy family:

1. Communicates and listens
2. Has members that affirm and support one another
3. Teaches respect for others
4. Develops a sense of trust
5. Has a sense of play and humor
6. Shares responsibility
7. Teaches a sense of right and wrong
8. Has rituals and traditions
9. Has a balance of interaction
10. Has a shared religious core
11. Has members who respect one another's privacy
12. Values service to others
13. Values shared meals and conversation
14. Shares leisure time
15. Admits to and seeks help with problems

Based on D. Curran, *Traits of a Healthy Family,* Winston Press, Minneapolis, 1983.

A Family Disease

Everyone whose life touches the alcoholic's is, in one way or another, affected by the disease, but its most direct consequences fall on family members. A boss can dismiss him or her, employees can quit, and friends can drift away. Family members, however, can not so easily turn their backs on the addict and that person's problem. To do so would mean totally disrupting their own lives as well as deserting someone they love. So they often choose to stay and adapt to the addict's illness. Unfortunately, there is no healthy way to adapt to alcoholism.[4] It is in the family environment, therefore, that alcoholics find their greatest allies. Here, the people who suffer the most from the addict's behavior become the people who nurture that addiction. The enabling relationships that develop follow a predictable pattern and cause alcoholism to be accurately labeled "a family disease."[5]

Family Denial

One of the most baffling aspects of alcoholism is the inability of the people closest to an alcoholic to recognize the reality of the addiction. Even more puzzling, many family members continue to deny the alcoholic's addiction long after he or she has died from an alcohol-related disease or accident.[4] Several important factors contribute to the family's distorted perception of reality.

1. *Isolation.* It is rare to find a family that talks together about an alcoholic in its midst. Shame and embarrassment build a wall of silence around each individual member and gradually cut off all but superficial communication. Family members increase their isolation by gradually separating themselves from outside friends and interests. The world of the family gradually narrows until it includes only those essential for its survival.[5]

2. *Emotional turmoil.*   Family members eventually become trapped in much the same emotional turmoil that afflicts an alcoholic. They wrongfully feel guilty for causing the alcoholic to drink and for hating or resenting someone they know they should love. They are ashamed and embarrassed by the alcoholic's actions, and they are angry at their own helplessness. They seldom share their emotions with one another. Instead, they suppress them and allow them to fester into despair and self-hatred. The alcoholic's unpredictable behavior leads to fear and anxiety about the future; increasing isolation leads to loneliness and depression.[5]
3. *Alcoholic centricity.*   In a healthy family, no one person is always the center of attention. However, in a family with an alcoholic, that person is the primary focus of everyone's attention. The family is always on guard, trying to predict the unpredictable and hoping to keep a bad situation from becoming worse. Because of the stresses on individual family members, they often internalize the rationalizations and projections of the alcoholic, and like the alcoholic, they deny the addiction, even while they pay an extraordinarily high price for it.[5]

As alcoholics gradually lose control over their own lives and behavior, they wield more and more power over those close to them. Although they are increasingly dependent on those people for emotional, social, and financial support, they play dictator to get them. Addicts control what family members say, what they do, and even what they think. Soon everyone displays the psychological symptoms of the disease.[4]

Rules in the Alcoholic Family

The person who holds the power in the family—the alcoholic—makes the rules. Thus, the most powerful person in terms of rule making is also the most dysfunctional. These rules are never openly stated, but everyone in the family understands them and lives by them. Wegscheider-Cruse has identified six such rules, which are listed in Table 5.2.[4]

Rule 1: An alcoholic's use of alcohol is the most important thing in a family's life.
   The alcoholic is obsessed with maintaining a supply of alcohol, and the rest of the family is obsessed with cutting it off. The family plans its day around the

TABLE 5.2. Rules in the alcoholic family.

1. The use of alcohol is the most important thing in the family's life.
2. Someone or something else caused the alcoholic dependency; the alcoholic is not to blame.
3. The status quo must be maintained at all costs.
4. Everyone in the family must be an enabler.
5. No one may discuss what is really going on in the family, either with one another or outsiders.
6. No one may say what he or she is really thinking.

Based on S. Wegscheider-Cruse, The family disease. In *Another Chance*, Behavioral Books, Inc., Palo Alto, California, 1981, pp. 76–103.

alcoholic's drinking hours. The alcoholic's drinking is the concern everything else in the family revolves around.

Rule 2: Someone or something else caused the alcoholic dependency. The alcoholic is not to blame, and that person's increasing tendency to blame something or someone else for his or her situation develops into a rule that is imposed on the rest of the family.

Rule 3: The status quo must be maintained at all costs. Alcoholics are afraid to quit drinking, for without alcohol they are afraid they cannot survive. So, as the rule makers, they make sure that their families remain rigid enough to protect them from change.

Rule 4: Everyone in the family must be an enabler. Family members, if asked, will very quickly say that they would do anything to get an alcoholic to quit drinking. But all the while they unconsciously help, or *enable* that person to keep drinking. They make up alibis for the person, cover up, take over that person's responsibilities, and accept that person's rules. They defend these actions on the basis of love, loyalty, or family honor, but the actions effectively preserve the status quo.

Rule 5: No one may discuss what is really going on in the family, either with one another or with outsiders. Feeling threatened, the rule maker tries to avoid letting people outside know about family affairs, specifically his or her degree of dependence and the magnitude of its impact on the rest of the family. An alcoholic also avoids letting family members have access to new information and advice from outside that might undermine their willingness to enable.

Rule 6: No one may say what he or she is really feeling. The rule maker is in so much emotional pain that he or she cannot handle the painful feelings of the family. So that person requires everyone to hide his or her feelings. As a result, communication among family members is severely hampered.[4]

Roles in the Alcoholic Family

In addition to the alcoholic, Wegscheider-Cruse has identified five roles dysfunctional family members tend to assume in attempts to adapt to the stresses in their lives: (1) the Chief Enabler, (2) the Hero, (3) the Scapegoat, (4) the Lost Child, and (5) the Mascot (these are listed in Table 5.3).[4] Each role grows out of its own kind of pain, has its own symptoms, offers its own payoffs for both the individual and the family, and ultimately exacts its own price.[1] A spouse is usually the Chief Enabler, but a parent or a close friend may assume the role. An oldest child usually becomes the Hero, the second child the Scapegoat, the next child the Lost Child, and the youngest the Mascot. Roles may change over time, especially as children grow older and leave home. When a family has fewer than four children, the children may take on parts of more than one role. Pain and confusion may be particularly overwhelming for an only child.[4,6]

TABLE 5.3. Roles in the alcoholic family.

	Alcoholic	Chief Enabler	Hero	Scapegoat	Lost Child	Mascot
Feeling	shame, inadequacy, guilt	anger and helplessness	guilt	inferiority	loneliness	fear of catastrophe
Behavior	addiction	worry and over-protection, lashing out in anger	overachievement	delinquent, rebellious	passivity	joking, clowning, overactivity
Defense mechanism	denial	avoidance of crisis situations	obsessive-compulsive and rigid behavior	substitution	withdrawal or retreat	diversion
Payoff	relief of emotional pain	temporary peace (at any cost) and increased self-esteem	positive attention and praise	attention (negative)	escape from chaos	relief of fear
Price	personal destruction	self-deception, perpetuation of the addiction	workaholism, possible burnout	rejection and alienation	social isolation	psychological immaturity

Based on S. Van Cleave, W. Byrd, and K. Revell, *Counseling for Substance Abuse and Addiction*, Word Books, Waco, Texas, 1987.

Alcoholic

The alcoholic's life is motivated largely by shame, inadequacy, and guilt—shame over using a chemical crutch, inadequacy in not finding another way to cope with the pressures of life and the world, and guilt about the effects of his or her drinking on the family.[4,6] Alcoholics are protected from the painful results of their drinking by the chemical effect of alcohol on their judgment and memory, their sophisticated denial systems, and the well-intentioned efforts of the people closest to them.[5]

Alcoholics' behavior is addiction, and their defense mechanism is denial of their alcoholism. Their payoff from addiction is temporary relief from emotional pain. The price they pay is personal destruction.[4,6]

Chief Enabler

Usually some key person in the alcoholic's immediate family—a spouse, parent, or close friend—undertakes the role of Chief Enabler. That person suffers depression, anxiety, and physical symptoms, resulting in more frequent visits to physicians than other people make.[7] The Chief Enabler feels compelled to try, at all costs, to decrease the chaos the alcoholism produces. However, in doing so that person only helps perpetuate the addiction. Without the Chief Enabler it would be difficult for the alcoholic to continue drinking. In the early years the Chief Enabler tries to control the alcoholic's drinking by cutting off that person's supply of alcohol, searching the house for hidden bottles, pouring liquor down the drain, and diluting the alcoholic's drinks. The Chief Enabler becomes irritated at friends who drink and thereby tempt the alcoholic and stops accepting invitations to parties where alcohol is served. Despite such efforts, the alcoholic continues to drink.[4-6]

Chief Enablers pick up the responsibilities that alcoholics give up or simply take responsibilities away from them. Chief Enablers pay bills, fix the plumbing, and discipline the children. They lie to alcoholics' bosses about their absences from work, bail alcoholics out of jail, take their side in drunk driving accidents, and drive them to work when they lose their license. Chief Enablers continually try to rescue alcoholics and will not let them suffer the consequences of their addiction. They make excuses to the children about alcoholics' behavior and thus take the heat off them. This only adds to the children's confusion.[5-6]

The good intentions of Chief Enablers create for alcoholics an increasingly comfortable environment in which to drink. Alcoholics' meals are cooked, their laundry is done, and their transportation is provided. And just when Chief Enablers have had enough, alcoholics sober up temporarily, only to begin drinking again at some time in the future. These periods of abstinence keep Chief Enablers hanging on for years, hoping that sooner or later they will find the solution to their spouses' drinking problem.[5]

The primary feeling Chief Enablers develop is anger, although they often mask it with a veneer of concern and unselfishness. They may also feel helpless. They primarily worry and overprotect alcoholics, their principle defense mechanism being avoidance of crises. Their payoff is temporary peace at any cost and increased self-esteem for doing right. The price they pay is self-deception and perpetuation of the addiction. The Chief Enabler's parental message is that what the alcoholic did was terrible, but that person was not responsible because he or she was drunk.[4,7]

Hero

The Hero is the individual who feels somehow responsible for the alcoholic's addiction. This responsible, adultlike child takes on the duties of a missing or overburdened parent—preparing meals, worrying about finances, looking out for the welfare of younger brothers or sisters, and trying to keep the family functioning as normally as possible. At school, the Hero makes better than average grades, runs for class office, or is an athlete, always working hard to accomplish difficult goals and win the approval of teachers and authority figures.[4-6]

The Hero's characteristic behavior is overachievement. By achieving, he or she believes that maybe the alcoholic can be made to feel better and stop drinking. The personality defense mechanism the Hero most often uses is obsessive, compulsive behavior. The Hero bases his or her self-worth on performance and by excelling shows the world that all is right with the family. The Hero's payoff is positive attention and praise, resulting in temporary boosts to self-worth. The price the Hero pays is eventual workaholism and possible burnout. A Hero often grows up to marry an alcoholic or goes into one of the helping professions, such as medicine. The parental message to the Hero is "It's your successes that make my life bearable."[4,6]

Scapegoat

The Scapegoat in the family feels inferior, often like a victim. For this person, attention for being bad is better than no attention at all. Delinquent and rebellious behavior is common in a Scapegoat, behavior that may progress to criminal activity. A Scapegoat's defense against emotional pain is substitution—substituting anything for relief of emotional pain. For example, a Scapegoat may withdraw from the family and totally substitute peers as a source of approval. A Scapegoat may drop out of school and is an easy prey for cults, the wrong crowd, the latest fad in dress or music, or drug addiction itself. He or she clamors incessantly for attention and a sense of belonging, commonly using anger to cover up fear, sadness, or hurt. The payoff for this person is attention, even if it is negative; the price he or she pays is rejection and alienation from normal living. The parental message to the Scapegoat is "If you would stop causing trouble, everything would be OK."[4,6]

Lost Child

This person withdraws from the family in a quiet way, not in the openly defiant way of the Scapegoat. He or she is an adaptor, accepting with a shrug the arbitrarily canceled vacation, the sudden fight, or the unexpected slap. Lost Children often separate themselves from the rest of the family and spend a great deal of time in their room, creating a fantasy world. They are often seen by outsiders as model children.[4-6]

The Lost Child most commonly feels lonely and uses emotional withdrawal and physical retreat as a defense against the painful events occurring in the home. The Lost Child's payoff is escape from chaos in the family; the price he or she pays is social isolation. The Lost Child is at high risk for suicide. The parental message to him or her is "I love you. Now go away."[4,6]

Mascot

The Mascot is the family clown or joker, the one who feels that the chaos at home will suddenly reach a boiling point and explode. The Mascot uses humor and superficiality as a diversion to cheer up the depressing atmosphere and relieve tension. He or she tries to smooth over conflicts before they develop and attempts to heal the hurts of others by giving of himself or herself. The main defense the Mascot uses is laughter, tending to laugh or smile when dealing with painful emotions. His or her payoff is relief of fear; the price he or she pays is often psychological emotional immaturity in adulthood. The parental message to the Mascot is "You are cute and entertaining, but not important."[4-6]

The Grief Process

Families with a member who is addicted to alcohol or other drugs often grieve the loss. They may go through the five stages of grief—denial, anger, bargaining, depression, and acceptance. Denial of the problem is often the longest of these stages and may prevent the chemically dependent member from receiving help for years.[7]

Getting the Alcoholic Sober

Pain—emotional, physical, spiritual—is the dominant feeling in the alcoholic's life. This pain may result from loss of a job, being arrested, severe illness, self-disgust, shame, separation from spouse and children, or rejection by family and friends. Addicts can temporarily cover up the pain with more alcohol, but sooner or later they will hit bottom and have to come to grips with it. This process can be speeded up by the use of two concepts: tough love and intervention by confrontation.

Tough Love

The application of tough love consists of five steps: open acceptance, education, joining support groups, assigning responsibility, and allowing the consequences.

1. *Open acceptance.*   Open acceptance is based on an alcoholic's need for a relationship with a significant other—a relationship he or she values and does not want to lose. This person is usually the Chief Enabler, and that person's objective is to openly accept the alcoholic as a person worthy of love. This love is based on the alcoholic's needs, not on his or her behavior, which the Chief Enabler should not condone.[6]
2. *Education.*   Family members should learn as much as they can about alcoholism and codependency. As they learn the hard facts of addiction, they will acquire the emotional detachment necessary to overcome their fear and their dependence on the alcoholic. This objectivity will allow them to think and behave rationally enough to implement the remaining steps of tough love.[5]
3. *Support groups.*   Families should find local support groups, such as Al-Anon and Alateen, and should attend their meetings. Alcoholics are threatened by anything that undermines their ability to control the people around them and will go to great lengths to prevent their families from attending these meetings. Family members should attend regardless of addicts' resistance. They should inform alcoholics that they are attending the meetings for themselves to learn more about the disease that is making their entire family ill.[5]
4. *Assigning responsibility.*   In this step, the family quits making excuses for an alcoholic's behavior and actions and no longer accept that person's rationalizations and excuses. The alcoholic is expected to take responsibility for and to be accountable for his or her behavior.[6]
5. *Allowing the consequences.*   As an alcoholic's pain increases from being forced to face the consequences of his or her actions, he or she may plead to be rescued. The family must take a loving but firm stand. As a result, the alcoholic may eventually reach a point where he or she is ready for treatment. If not, the family may need to intervene and confront the addict.[6]

Intervention by Confrontation

Intervention by confrontation consists of two steps: preparing for the confrontation and the actual event itself.

Preparing for the Confrontation

The purpose of direct confrontation is to convince alcoholics of the effects of their destructive behavior and insist that they get treatment. During confrontations, alcoholics are told the harmful effects of their behavior on themselves and on the people close to them; are told the consequences of continuing an alcoholic life-style; and are offered a way to avoid the consequences—treatment.[6]

A family prepares for a confrontation by taking six steps: consulting a professional, choosing members of the team, choosing the confrontation date, choosing its time, holding a practice confrontation, and investigating treatment options.

Step 1: Consult a professional.   The first step in preparing for the confrontation is for the family to consult a professional. Every intervention team should have a drug abuse counselor or a physician familiar with the process to supervise the preparation and direct the actual confrontation. Families can usually find such a person by calling a local treatment center[5]

Step 2: Choose members of the team.   Families should select members of the intervention team on the basis of their close relationships with the alcoholic and their willingness to participate in a confrontation. Not all family members will be appropriate for the team. The most strategically important members of the intervention team are the Chief Enabler, an employer, and the alcoholic's physician, if he or she is knowledgeable about addiction. Individuals that should be excluded include those whose psychological state is too fragile to withstand the emotional impact of the confrontation, anyone likely to berate the alcoholic or preach moralistically, and family members too angry or full of hate to perceive the alcoholic as a sick person in need of help[5]

Step 3: Choose the data.   With the help of the professional, each team member selects three or four examples of the alcoholic's inappropriate behavior. These should be as detailed and as current as possible. Team members should focus on facts and observations rather than feelings and judgments. They should not use the data to humiliate the alcoholic but to help him or her see the seriousness of addictive behavior. Angry, hostile remarks will only activate the alcoholic's defense mechanisms[5]

Step 4: Choose the time.   A team should confront the alcoholic when he or she is sober, or at least as sober as possible. If the alcoholic is drunk at the scheduled confrontation time, the meeting should be postponed. It may be necessary to schedule the meeting early in the morning before the alcoholic has had time to do much drinking[5]

Step 5: Hold a practice confrontation.   Members of the intervention team need to meet at least once, and preferably twice, to rehearse the confrontation. During these meetings, the professional plays the role of the alcoholic, and team members practice giving their evidence in a detached, nonjudgmental manner. They also practice how they will respond to the alcoholic's manipulation, evasion, or anger[5]

Step 6: Investigate treatment options.   The last step is for team members to investigate local treatment options for types of programs offered, the costs of each, and their appropriateness for the particular alcoholic. Members should take care of financial matters, such as insurance clearance so that, should the intervention be successful, there will be no delay in getting the alcoholic into treatment[5]

The Confrontation

Family members, the professional, and significant others assemble at the planned time. Once the alcoholic arrives, the facilitator speaks first, explaining to the alcoholic why they have gathered and asking him or her to listen without speaking for a while. When everyone else is finished speaking, the alcoholic will have a turn. As rehearsed, each person then speaks directly to the alcoholic, sharing facts, events, and personal reactions to that person's behavior, telling how it has adversely affected him or her. Members then share options for help. The group should be prepared for the alcoholic's tearful acceptance, anger, hostility, counteraccusations, or bolting from the room. If the alcoholic agrees to enter treatment, he or she should not be allowed to bargain with the group or postpone it, which only gives the alcoholic time to develop new excuses and rationalizations for his or her behavior, allowing him or her to deny the facts members present in the intervention. Once the group makes a decision, the alcoholic should enter treatment without delay.[6]

If the intervention is unsuccessful, the family has three options. They can secure the alcoholic's word to stop drinking, having him or her sign a contract agreeing to enter treatment if he or she drinks again. They can continue to live with the actively drinking alcoholic, in which case they should continue to work on their own recovery by attending Al-Anon and Alateen meetings. And, in many states, the family can obtain a court order to commit the alcoholic to treatment against his or her will.

Getting the Family Well

Once the alcoholic enters treatment, all too often family members believe their problems are over. In reality they are not, and in some cases when the alcoholic gets better, without treatment, the family gets worse. Therefore, it is imperative that the entire family go through a treatment process just as the alcoholic does.[6]

Importance of Family Treatment

Treatment of the family is important for several reasons. Most family members do not realize the extent to which their responses to the alcoholic — isolation, enabling, depression, anxiety, physical illness — have resulted in dysfunctional behavior. Also, without a better understanding of alcoholism and its effects on the family, spouses of alcoholics commonly remarry alcoholics and their sons and daughters often marry alcoholics. Treatment of the family helps to set the groundwork for leading a normal family life during the alcoholic's recovery. A couple facing a sober marriage after many years of alcoholism may have unrealistic expectations. Recovering alcoholics may throw themselves so heavily in Alcoholics Anonymous that their spouses may sense competition from new partners. Recovering alcoholics must be given responsibility for roles that they relinquished due to their drinking; spouses may find it difficult to relinquish such roles. And, finally, the children of alcoholic parents are more likely to be healthy in the long run if the whole family participates in treatment.[8-9]

Family Treatment Resources

Three useful treatment resources are available for the family: family therapy, codependent treatment, and self-help groups.

Family Therapy Programs

Approaches to family therapy include individual treatment of couples or group treatment with several couples. In some programs, families join alcoholics for up to a week at a treatment center, with follow-up group therapy for couples after alcoholics return home. A typical family week at a treatment center would include interviews with all family members to assess their understanding of alcoholism. Presentations on the pharmacology of alcohol, its medical complications, and the concept of alcoholism as a disease follow.[10-11]

Group sessions with members of several families are helpful for sharing experiences, for recognizing that an alcoholic's problem is truly a family problem, and for breaking down defenses family members have developed. Properly supervised confrontations between an alcoholic and family members are helpful in releasing long-standing anger and resentment. They help reestablish communication and lead both parties to better insights into each other's needs. Commonly, weekly group sessions involving several couples are conducted for up to six months after an alcoholic has returned home from a treatment center.[10-11]

Codependent Treatment

Treatment for family members and close friends who have been adversely affected by an alcoholic's drinking (codependents) is available in many programs. The majority are outpatient, although more inpatient programs are becoming available. A typical outpatient program lasts about a month and meets for two to three hours, usually in the evening, three days a week. Treatment is directed at breaking through codependents' denial about their role in the disease of alcoholism, educating them about codependency, and giving them an opportunity to express and deal with feelings in a group setting. They are introduced to a twelve-step program adapted from that of Alcoholics Anonymous, and they are encouraged to join support groups such as Al-Anon and Alateen. The treatment's premise is that codependents can get well whether an alcoholic does or not.[2,12]

Support Groups

Al-Anon is a fellowship of men and women whose lives have been adversely affected by an alcoholic family member or close friend. It developed as an outgrowth of AA in the 1940s because family members of early AA groups learned from experience that they needed to apply the AA principles to their own affairs. As a result, they began to work together in their own groups. Today Al-Anon groups are found virtually everywhere, generally meeting at the same time that AA meetings take place. So closely did the twelve steps of AA meet their needs that they changed only one word. The word "alcoholics" was changed to "others" in step 12: "Having had a spiritual awakening as a result of these steps, we tried to carry this message to others, and to practice these principles in all our affairs." In essence, they admit they cannot control the excessive drinking of their spouse, parent, or close friend. They learn that an alcoholic is sick, not weak-willed or malicious. This shifts their focus from the alcoholic to learning how to manage their own lives more effectively. No longer can they blame an alcoholic's drinking for their shortcomings. They learn that shielding an alcoholic by lying to his or her boss, paying bail, and all other such behavior only helps an alcoholic keep drinking. Members learn to detach from the problem, not the person. Denial plays a big role in the family as it does in an alcoholic's thinking. The group helps to penetrate this denial by sharing insights.[13-15]

Like AA, Al-Anon is compatible with all religions and offends none. It is a spiritual program that lets members conceive of God in their own way. The fellowship of Al-Anon lets people know they are not alone, that others have the same fears and frustrations and have made the same mistakes. It also gives them the opportunity to help others, a source of great personal satisfaction for them.[15]

Al-Anon's primary purpose is not to try to stop alcoholics from drinking but to help those who have been affected by that drinking lead saner, happier, and more productive lives. Among Al-Anon members are the relatives and close friends of AA members who are leading sober lives, alcoholics who are still drinking sporadically but who are trying to overcome their compulsion, alcoholics who continue to drink and refuse help from any source, and alcoholics who are divorced or separated from their families or have died.[13]

In 1957, a teenager whose parents were in AA and Al-Anon began a group for people his own age. It was called Alateen. Alateen meetings, too, are widely available.[9]

The Family in Recovery

In recovering families, individuals develop flexible roles, and they depend on one another, which they acknowledge and respond to. Families develop a sense of purpose and grow over time toward their optimal level of functioning. Recovering members should gauge their progress by their sense of stability, adaptability, and flexibility in relationships rather than by comparing their evolving families with an idealistic normal family. Families should begin to feel free to talk about anything, to think any thoughts, to ask for what each member wants, to express any emotion, to pursue any goal. Indicators of family recovery are clear communication; cooperation; empowerment rather than subjugation; enhancement of individual uniqueness; using authority to guide rather than forcing compliance; love, valuing, and respect among members; personal and social responsibility; and an ability to use problems as challenges. Families begin to take on many of the traits of the healthy family discussed earlier in this chapter. Support groups such as Al-Anon and Alateen continue to play important roles in recovery.[16]

Adult Children of Alcoholics (ACOAs)

Between 20 and 34 million adults in the United States grew up in alcoholic homes and around 7 million children currently live in such environments.[6,11]

Consequences of Growing Up in an Alcoholic Home

The tremendous emotional scars inflicted on children growing up in alcoholic families lead directly to marital discord, emotional depression, vocational insta-bility, and job dissatisfaction when they become adults.[4] Being a child of an alco-holic increases your likelihood of growing up to be an alcoholic, marrying an alcoholic, or both, thereby perpetuating the cycle.[15]

Dysfunctional Characteristics of ACOAs

Children of alcoholics may carry into adult life certain dysfunctional characteris-tics, ones not only ACOAs possess but many adults who grew up in dysfunctional families, regardless of the cause of their dysfunction.[16-17] Woititz has identified 12 characteristics of ACOAs (these are listed in Table 5.4).[17]

1. *ACOAs guess what normal is.*   ACOAs grew up in homes that, because of alcoholism, were not normal. They simply have no experience with what is normal. They often bring a fantasized concept of the perfect family into a marriage, thus, making life very difficult.

TABLE 5.4. Characteristics of adult children of alcoholics (ACOAs).

ACOAs
1. Guess what normal is
2. Have difficulty following a project through from beginning to end
3. Lie when it would be just as easy to tell the truth
4. Judge themselves without mercy
5. Have difficulty having fun; they take themselves very seriously
6. Have difficulty with intimate relations
7. Overreact to changes they have no control over
8. Constantly seek approval and confirmation
9. Usually feel different from other people
10. Are superresponsible or superirresponsible
11. Are extremely loyal, even in the face of evidence that the loyalty is undeserved
12. Are impulsive, tending to lock themselves into courses of action without giving consideration to alternative behaviors or possible consequences

Based on J.G. Woititz, *Adult Children of Alcoholics,* Health Communications, Inc., Pompano Beach, Florida, 1983.

2. *ACOAs have trouble following a project through from beginning to end.*   In the typical alcoholic family, there are a lot of promises. The great job was always just around the corner; the big deal was almost always about to be made; the work that needed to be done around the house would be done. But these things never happened. Thus, ACOAs had role models for their procrastination. Not only that, they really never had anyone to show them how to carry a project through from beginning to end, which they then have difficulty doing in later life.

3. *ACOAs lie when it would be just as easy to tell the truth.*   Lying is basic to an alcoholic family. The first and most basic lie is the family's denial of the problem, so the pretense that everything at home is in order is a lie. The nonalcoholic parent lies to cover up for the alcoholic and makes excuses for that person's not fulfilling an obligation, not being on time, or not showing up for an appointment. Alcoholics make a lot of promises that turn out to be lies. Because lying is a habit in an alcoholic's household, it is not surprising that children carry this habit over into adulthood.

4. *ACOAs judge themselves without mercy.*   When they were children, ACOAs never felt they were good enough. They were constantly criticized. Because they were never able to meet the standards of perfection expected of them in childhood, they carry the feeling into adulthood that, what ever they do, it is not quite good enough. They have trouble accepting compliments, and they do not judge others nearly as harshly as they judge themselves.

5. *ACOAs have difficulty having fun.*   The childhoods of ACOAs were probably not much fun. They seldom heard their parents laughing and joking. Life was a very serious business, and they grew up with the same attitude. They tend not to join in games because they are afraid of looking foolish or making mistakes (that is, they are afraid of not playing the game perfectly). They have difficulty having fun and take themselves very seriously.

6. *ACOAs have difficulty with intimate relationships.*   ACOAs have trouble developing healthy, intimate relationships because they do not have a frame of reference for such relationships because they did not grow up in one. They grew up with inconsistent parent-child relationships—were loved one day and rejected the next. They have developed a fear of being close, yet have a need for it, and develop a fear of abandonment that causes them to lack confidence in relationships.

7. *ACOAs overreact to changes they have no control over.*   Growing up, ACOAs were not in charge of their lives. Alcoholics inflicted their lives on them. As a result, they fear that when a change is made without them participating in it, they will lose control of their lives. Therefore, they tend to overreact—they simply don't adjust to change well. They are often accused of being controlling, rigid, and unspontaneous.

8. *ACOAs constantly seek approval and confirmation.*   Children begin to believe who they are from the messages they get from their parents. As they get older, they internalize these messages, which then contribute significantly to their self-images. These messages were confusing to them, so that they grew up lacking self-confidence. They feel that anyone who would care

about them must not be worth very much and constantly seek approval and confirmation of their self-worth.

9. *ACOAs usually feel different from other people.* ACOAs assume that in any group of people, everyone else feels comfortable and they are the only ones who feel awkward. They feel different from other people. When growing up, they became isolated and so did not develop the social skills necessary to feel comfortable as part of a group. It is difficult for ACOAs to believe that they can be accepted because of who they are and that they do not have to earn the acceptance.

10. *ACOAs are superresponsible or superirresponsible.* ACOAs tried unsuccessfully as children to please their parents by doing more and more. Some continue this characteristic into adulthood, while others reach the point where they realize it doesn't really matter and begin doing as little as they can. Those that continue to strive feel that if they are not perfect they will be rejected, so they tend to be superresponsible. They subject themselves to enormous pressure trying to be perfect spouses, perfect parents, perfect friends, and perfect employees. Those who are superirresponsible tend to procrastinate and have trouble getting started.

11. *ACOAs are extremely loyal.* Family members of alcoholics are extremely loyal and remain in bad situations long after reason dictates they should leave. They do not walk away just because the going gets tough. This leads ACOAs to remain in relationships that they would be better off leaving. Because making friends or developing relationships is so difficult for them, the relationships and friendships they make tend to be permanent. The fact that they may be treated poorly doesn't matter; they can rationalize that.

12. *ACOAs are impulsive.* ACOAs grew up in homes in which impulsive behavior by alcoholics was the norm. The alcoholic never seriously considered what happened the last time or what the consequences would be this time. The reality in the alcoholic home was that if something were not done immediately, it never got done. ACOAs tend to be impulsive, which leads them to be confused, to loathe themselves, and to lose control over their environment. They spend an excessive amount of time cleaning up the mess.[17]

Support Groups for ACOAs

Because of the needs of ACOAs, much like the needs of alcoholics for AA, a support organization for ACOAs evolved, which adapted the twelve steps of AA. In addition to the change in step 12 made by Al-Anon, the word "alcohol" was changed to "the past" in step 1: "We admitted we were powerless over the past. Our lives had become unmanageable." The other steps remain the same.[16]

The Role of the Physician

Physicians who uncover underlying alcoholism by recognizing roles (Chief Enabler, Hero, Scapegoat, Lost Child, Mascot) that develop in a family are in a position to provide valuable assistance to the family and the alcoholic. Those who do not recognize these roles will unwittingly enable an alcoholic to continue drinking and cause the family to continue to suffer. An informed physician will (1) understand that alcoholism is a family illness, (2) detect alcoholism through its impact on family members, (3) be aware of the stresses on the family at the time of intervention and early recovery, (4) participate in an intervention if he or she feels comfortable in that role, (5) recognize the value of family therapy, codependent treatment, and support groups for the recovery of family members, (6) refer family members to Al-Anon or Alateen when appropriate, (7) understand the dynamics of the recovering family, and (8) be aware of the dysfunctional characteristics of adult children of alcoholics and their need for help. Physicians should refer those people to ACOA support groups when such groups are available.[9,16-17]

References

1. Mulry, J. T. Codependency: A family addiction. *American Family Physician*, 35:215–219, 1987.
2. Beattie, M. *Codependent No More.* Hazelden Press, Minnesota, 1987.
3. Curran, D. *Traits of a Healthy Family.* Winston Press, Minneapolis, 1983.
4. Wegscheider, S. The family disease. In *Another Chance.* Science and Behavioral Books, Inc., Palo Alto, California, 1981, pp. 76–103.
5. Spickard, A., and B. R. Thompson. The family trap. In *Dying for a Drink: What You Should Know About Alcoholism.* Word Book, Waco, Texas, 1985, pp. 68–75.
6. Van Cleave, S., W. Byrd, and K. Revell. Addiction is a family affair. In *Counseling for Substance Abuse and Addiction.* Word Books, Waco, Texas, 1987, pp. 76–88.
7. Lamping, R. A., and V. McAdams-Mahoud. Families in recovery. *Insight*, 10:28–31, 1989.
8. Kaufman, E. The family of the alcoholic patient. *Psychosomatics*, 27:347–360, 1986.
9. Griner, M. E., and P. F. Griner. Alcoholism and the family. In *Alcoholism: A Guide for the Primary Care Physician.* Edited by H. N. Barnes, M. D. Aronson, and T. L. Debanco. Springer-Verlag, New York, 1987, pp. 159–166.
10. Usher, M. L., J. Jay, and D. R. Glass. Family therapy as a treatment modality for alcoholism. *Journal of Studies of Alcoholism*, 43:927–938, 1989.
11. Anderson, R. C., and M. R. Liepman. Chemical dependency in the family. In *Family Medicine Curriculum Guide to Substance Abuse.* Ed. by M. R. Liepman, R. C. Anderson, and J. V. Fisher. Society of Teachers of Family Medicine, Kansas City, Missouri, 1984, pp. 8-1 to 8-34.
12. Cermak, T. L. *Diagnosing and Treating Co-dependence.* Johnson Institute Books, Minneapolis, 1986.
13. *Al-Anon Family Groups.* Al-Anon Family Groups Headquarters, Inc., New York, 1987.
14. *Al-Anon's Twelve Steps and Twelve Traditions.* Al-Anon Family Group Headquarters, Inc., New York, 1988.
15. Royce, J. E. Alcoholics Anonymous. In *Alcohol Problems and Alcoholism.* Free Press, London, 1981, pp. 242–255.
16. Friel, J., and L. Friel. *Adult Children: The Secrets of Dysfunctional Families.* Health Communications, Inc., Deerfield Beach, Florida, 1988.
17. Woititz, J. G. *Adult Children of Alcoholics.* Health Communications, Inc., Pompano Beach, Florida, 1983.

CHAPTER 6

Prevention

Introduction

Preventing substance abuse is a complex and difficult activity in our society, but one that is critically needed. Use, misuse, and attempts to control the use of drugs are apparently as old as civilization.[1] Prevention is customarily divided into primary, secondary, and tertiary types. Primary prevention involves keeping individuals from beginning to use drugs. Secondary prevention is aimed at getting individuals who are already using drugs, but who are not yet chemically dependent, to stop. Early detection is the key to secondary prevention. Employee assistance programs, physician screening, court ordered referral (especially family and traffic court), teachers, and counselors can play important roles.[2-3] Techniques used for primary prevention may be effective in some individuals, but others will require outpatient treatment. Tertiary prevention seeks to treat chemically dependent individuals and return them to society to lead lives of recovery. Outpatient treatment is effective for some individuals, but others, especially most adolescents, require inpatient treatment.

The first part of this chapter deals with primary prevention. The second part deals with preventing prescription drug abuse.

Primary Prevention

For practical purposes, primary prevention programs are directed at adolescents and preadolescent children. They attempt to reduce social influences that promote or support substance use; to increase resistance to social influences by teaching refusal skills and media resistance skills; to decrease susceptibility to social influences by increasing personal characteristics that make people less susceptible to them, such as high self-esteem, high sense of personal control, high self-efficacy, and low anxiety; and to foster the acquisition of adaptive coping skills that make substance use as a coping response unnecessary.[4]

Adolescent Development

As children approach adolescence, their moral orientation shifts from a rigid and inflexible notion of right and wrong to one that takes into account a myriad of situational factors. With this new orientation, adolescents can accept deviations from established rules and norms and come to believe that a behavior that might be considered wrong in one situation might be right in another. They also become less likely to accept authority.[4]

During adolescence, individuals characteristically experiment with a variety of behaviors and life-style patterns as part of the natural process of separating from parents, developing a sense of autonomy and independence, establishing an identity, and acquiring the skills necessary to function in an adult world. As individuals approach adolescence, they are less influenced by parents and more influenced by peers. Much of the experimentation young people do, including substance use, they do in peer groups. Increased dependence on peer groups typically accompanies a corresponding rise in conformity. Dependent, anxious individuals with low self-esteem and high social sensitivity tend to conform more.[4-5]

One of the major developmental tasks of adolescence is the formation of an identity separate and distinct from parents and other family members. This leads adolescents to be overconcerned about their public images and about how others perceive them. They focus on appearance, personal qualities, and abilities. This may lead them to be uncomfortable or anxious in social situations. Adolescents may be motivated to smoke, drink, or use drugs because of the positive social image those activities are given in the media.[4]

The decline in parental influence, the increased reliance on peer groups, the increased tendency to conform to peer group norms, and the positive media portrayal of drugs increase the risk for adolescents of yielding to the influence to smoke, drink, or use other drugs.[4]

History of Prevention Efforts

The modern history of drug use prevention began in the 1960s in response to increasing numbers of American youth who were "turning on, tuning in, and dropping out." The earliest prevention programs relied on promoting overblown and inaccurate risks of drug use—that is, they relied on scare tactics. They did little more than impair their credibility. Another early approach involved presenting factual physiological, psychological, and social information in an attempt to encourage rational decisions about drug use.[3]

In the early 1970s, programs began to focus on improving traits that appeared to distinguish drug users from nonusers. Studies suggested a relationship between drug use and variables such as low self-esteem, poor decision-making skills, and poor communication skills. It was not clear which came first—the traits or the drug use. About the same time, programs developed that provided young people with a variety of alternatives to drug use, ranging from wilderness challenges to community service to drug-free rock concerts.[5]

In the late 1970s four new trends in prevention evolved. The first trend was the involvement of parents and communities in prevention efforts. The second trend was the idea that some drugs, particularly marijuana, were not harmful when used responsibly. The goal was to encourage youth to make responsible decisions about drug use. By the 1980s, this concept, for the most part, had disappeared. The third trend grew out of the recognition of the importance of peer pressure. The fourth trend was based on the concept of approaching prevention from many levels.[5]

Program Focus

Modern prevention programs focus on one or more aspects of life: individuals, families, peer groups, schools and communities, and the larger social environment (these are outlined in Table 6.1).[5]

Individual Focus

Programs that focus on the individual generally believe that chemical dependence arises out of the following six factors.

1. *Biological vulnerabilities.* This concept is based on the belief that some individuals are biologically more susceptible to becoming addicted than others and that biological markers will eventually be found to identify those people.
2. *Affective regulation.* This concept is based on the belief that individuals use drugs to self-medicate a variety of affective problems (depression, anxiety, boredom, loneliness) or that drug abuse is a symptom of a primary personality disorder. Affective programs are based on identifying individuals at risk and providing nonpharmacological treatment of their underlying problems.
3. *Knowledge deficits.* This concept is based on the belief that individuals use drugs because they do not know about the detrimental effects of drugs. Programs with this focus attempt to make young people more aware of the adverse health, social, and legal consequences of drug abuse. They assume that if young people are aware of the negative consequences they will make rational decisions not to smoke, drink, or use other drugs.[4] These programs may consist of simple, one-shot efforts, such as the use of pamphlets or films, or they may be larger, more complex efforts such as school drug curricula.[5]
4. *Life skills deficits.* This concept seeks to correct life skills deficits, such as low self-esteem, poor decision-making skills, and poor communication skills.
5. *Invulnerability.* This concept is based on the belief that, although young people recognize the risks of drug use, they do not believe that the risks apply to them. Some programs focus on short-term risks that are salient to young people, rather than on long-term risks that young people may consider irrelevant. A drinking prevention program, for instance, may focus on loss of driving privileges rather than on accident statistics.

TABLE 6.1. Prevention programs.

Individual focus
    biological vulnerabilities
    affective regulation
    knowledge deficits
    life skills deficits
    invulnerability
    sensation seeking

Family focus
    family dynamics
    socialization deficit
    parental modeling
    social control

Peer group focus
    conformity
    peer modeling
    peer influence

School and community focus
    deterrence
    availability
    social climate
    social bonding

Larger social environment focus
    advertising
    portrayal of drug use

Based on S.K. Schonberg (Ed.), Prevention programs, adapted with permission from *Substance Abuse: A Guide for Health Professionals,* Copyright © 1988 The American Academy of Pediatrics, Elk Grove, Illinois, pp. 77–99.

6. *Sensation seeking.* This concept is based on the theory that young people have a natural tendency to seek new, exciting, and sometimes risky experiences. Programs with this focus seek to provide alternative highs such as wilderness programs.[5]

Family Focus

Early family experience with substance use can have a profound impact on whether adolescents will become substance users. If any family member uses a drug, that substance will be present in the home, increasing the likelihood that children will experiment with it.

The family provides the first opportunity for individuals to learn basic social skills. It provides a supportive environment in which children can develop a sense of self-esteem, self-confidence, and autonomy. A high-quality parent-child relationship can offset or attenuate negative influences that come from peer groups.[5]

Since the goals of family-oriented prevention strategies are to strengthen families in a number of ways, family oriented prevention programs use a variety of approaches and techniques. Some work on improving parent-parent interactions, while others target parent-child interactions. Some target communication and effective skill building, while others focus on child management principles and parenting styles.[6] Prevention programs focused on the family view drug use in terms of one or more of the following four factors.[5]

1. *Family dynamics.* This concept considers the risk of drug abuse to be associated with factors such as parental permissiveness or inconsistency, loose family structure, harsh physical punishment, and poor family communication. Programs with this focus seek to improve parenting skills and, thereby, prevent substance abuse.
2. *Socialization deficit.* This concept considers that the family is the major socialization agent and that many families fail to teach children such values as self-control, self-motivation, and self-discipline. Programs with this focus teach parents ways of structuring the home environment to increase the likelihood that children will develop these skills.
3. *Parental modeling.* This concept is based on the belief that children's early notions about drug use are learned by observing how parents behave with tobacco, alcohol, over-the-counter medications, prescription medications, and illicit drugs (such as marijuana and cocaine). The goal of programs with this focus is to change parental behavior as a method for preventing drug use.
4. *Social control.* This concept is based on the assumption that many parents have abdicated their responsibilities for their children's drug use. Programs with this focus seek to get parents to reinstate social controls.[5]

Peer Group Focus

Prevention programs that focus on peer groups consider drug abuse to be the result of the following three factors.

1. *Conformity.* This concept is based on the assumption that a desire to fit in with the crowd is a major concern for adolescents. It attempts to inoculate young people against peer conformity by programs such as the "Just say no" campaign. Programs with this focus also attempt to teach young people that drug use is not the norm.
2. *Peer modeling.* This concept is based on the assumption that drug abuse is learned through peer modeling. It attempts to counteract negative peer models by exposing young people to attractive, positive models who communicate an antidrug message.
3. *Peer influence.* This concept is based on the assumption that young people use drugs because peers pressured them to. It teaches peer-pressure resistance skills.[5]

School and Community Focus

A variety of prevention activities have been implemented in schools throughout the country. Programs that focus on school and community address one or more of the following four factors.

1. *Deterrence.* Deterrence-based programs emphasize the importance of consistently enforcing school drug policies. They advocate a no-drug campus policy.[5,7]
2. *Availability.* Most community-based programs attempt to reduce the availability of drugs. Raising the legal drinking age to 21 years is one application of this principle.
3. *Social climate.* The social climate concept of prevention is based on a wide spectrum of efforts to alter the environment in which young people live. These include increased law enforcement efforts, strong school prevention programs, concerned parents groups, and antidrug editorials in local newspapers.
4. *Social bonding.* This concept is based on the assumption that drug abuse results from some young people's failure to bond to social institutions and their norms. Programs with this focus provide young people with opportunities to make positive contributions to the community and to develop positive social bonds as a result. They involve young people in community service programs such as historical restorations, programs for the elderly, and youth job services.[5]

In addition, school programs focus on increasing students' knowledge of the physical and social hazards of substance abuse. They attempt to mold attitudes and beliefs that do not support substance abuse.[7]

School-based programs are limited by a number of factors. The majority of a young person's day is spent outside of school, and most opportunities to use drugs occur outside of school. Adolescents spend most of their time at home, much of it watching television. The influences of family and mass media on them are enormous. They spend a considerable amount of time in predictable out-of-school locations, such as movie theaters, video arcades, and other recreation sites. These could become sources of positive influence. Young people at highest risk of drug abuse are least likely to attend school regularly and, thereby, benefit from drug prevention programs. Therefore, an optimal drug abuse prevention program would utilize not only school systems but also families, mass media, and community organizations.[8]

Larger Social Environment Focus

These programs are directed at the larger social environment in which young people live. They include advertising. For years, young people have been exposed, often during broadcasts of athletic events, to famous athletes advertising beers. Full pages of color in magazines advertise alcoholic beverages and cigarettes, associating them with adventure, sexual attractiveness, or sophistication. Attempts have been made to limit, reduce, or eliminate cigarette and alcohol advertising, to use advertisements that counteract cigarette and alcohol advertisements by lampooning popular advertisements, and to teach young people about advertising techniques to aid them in critiquing the persuasive messages in advertisements.

The mass communication system comprises an important part of the environment in which children develop, and television plays a major role in childrens' lives. On average they watch about 20 hours a week. It is a significant source of socialization.[9] Television messages are clear: If you can't sleep, take a sleeping pill; if you have a headache, take a pain pill. A pill is available to solve every problem. In addition, the average child sees alcohol consumed on television 75,000 times before he or she is of legal drinking age.[10] Thus, mass media contribute to the problem, but they may also be part of the solution. Unfortunately, many more messages in the media model the use of cigarettes, alcohol, and other drugs than discourage it.[9] Programs aimed at the portrayal of drug abuse in the mass media attempt to educate writers, producers, and directors about the drug messages their productions convey and to help these individuals present a more realistic picture of substance abuse.[5]

Prevention of Prescription Drug Abuse

Factors Contributing to Prescription Drug Abuse

Prescription drug abuse often results from overprescribing by physicians, which they do in response to two main influences—lack of knowledge and patient pressure. Some physicians are not as knowledgeable as they should be about the adverse consequences of excessive drug use, and some patients demand specific drugs almost as a right. It is often easier for physicians to give in to pressure from patients than to resist it.[11]

Other factors that contribute to prescription drug abuse include:

1. *Excessive use of prescribed drugs.* Patients may abuse prescription drugs to become intoxicated or intentionally increase the dose as they develop tolerance.
2. *Patients with complex problems.* Patients with long histories of physical and emotional disorders are highly susceptible to chemical dependence because of drug availability, the symptomatic relief obtained, and personality factors.
3. *Diversion of leftover drugs.* Leftover prescription drugs in the family medicine cabinet can be a source of supply for initiating or maintaining drug dependence in family members other than those for whom the drugs were prescribed.
4. *Patients with several physicians.* Some patients with many complaints visit several physicians and receive prescriptions from all of them.
5. *Careless prescription writing.* Many prescriptions can be easily altered (10 changed to 100 for example).
6. *Poor prescription security.* Addicts can use a stolen blank prescription pad to obtain thousands of doses of prescription drugs for illicit purpose.
7. *Poor safeguarding of supplies.* Repeated office break-ins occur when drug abusers discover that physicians keep large quantities of drugs and syringes in their offices or that security is poor.

TABLE 6.2. Factors contributing to prescription drug abuse.

Lack of knowledge by physicians
Patient pressure
Excessive use of prescribed drugs
Complex physical and emotional problems
Diversion of leftover drugs
Multiple physicians
Careless prescription writing
Poor prescription security
Poor safeguarding of supplies
Deception of physicians
The impaired physician
The script doc
Reimbursement regulations

Based on B.B. Wilford (Ed.), Prescribing practices and drug abuse, in *Drug Abuse: A Guide for the Primary Care Physician,* American Medical Association, Chicago, 1981, pp. 263–284.

8. *Deception of physicians.* The drug abuser's ability to deceive is often greater than the physician's ability to cope with deception.
9. *The script doc.* The script doc is a physician who deliberately overprescribes or misprescribes psychoactive substances for profit, or one who is so easily duped that he or she gains a reputation for gullibility.
10. *The impaired physician.* Drug-dependent physicians can become sources of illicit drugs by prescribing larger than necessary amounts as a reflection of their own addiction, in response to blackmail, or by becoming script docs to generate sufficient income to maintain their own dependence.
11. *Reimbursement regulations.* Regulations third-party payers impose can contribute to the drug abuse problem. For example, if a reimbursement policy allows a patient only one office visit a month, a patient suffering from chronic pain, anxiety, or depression may receive larger amounts of drugs at one time than he or she would ordinarily be prescribed. Factors that contribute to prescription drug abuse are summarized in Table 6.2.[11]

Guidelines for Prescribing Psychoactive Substances

The federal Drug Enforcement Administration has issued guidelines to counteract overprescribing or overutilization of psychoactive substance by physicians. The general guidelines state that:

1. Controlled substances have legitimate clinical usefulness; physicians should not hesitate to prescribe them when they are indicated for a patient's comfort and well-being.
2. Prescribing controlled substances for legitimate medical use requires special caution because of those drugs' potential for abuse and dependence.

3. Physicians should exercise good judgment in administering and prescribing controlled substances so that they are not diverted to illicit uses and so that patients do not develop drug dependence.
4. Physicians should guard against contributing to drug abuse through injudicious prescription writing practices or by acquiescing to unwarranted demands by some patients.
5. Physicians should examine their individual prescribing practices to ensure that they cautiously write all prescription orders for controlled substances.
6. Physicians should make a specific effort to ensure that patients are not obtaining several prescriptions from different prescribers.[12]

Specific guidelines issued by the Drug Enforcement Administration for writing prescription orders for controlled substances state that:

1. The prescription order must be signed by the physician when it is written. The physician's name, address, and DEA registration number, as well as the patient's full name and address, must be shown on prescriptions for controlled substances.
2. The written prescription order should be precise and distinctly legible to enhance exact and effective communication between physician and pharmacist.
3. The prescription order should indicate whether or not it may be renewed and, if so, the number of times or duration for which renewal is authorized. Prescription orders in Schedules III, IV, and V may be issued either orally or in writing and may be renewed on the prescription order for up to five times within a six-month period following the date of issue. A written prescription order is required for drugs in Schedule II. The renewing of Schedule II orders is prohibited. A pharmacist may accept a verbal order for Schedule II drugs only in an emergency, and this must be followed up by a written order within 72 hours.
4. Physicians should prescribe no greater quantity of a controlled substance than is needed until a patient's next office visit.
5. Prescription orders should be made alteration-proof. When prescribing a controlled substance, the actual number should be written out as well as given in Arabic numbers.
6. A separate prescription blank should be used for each controlled substance prescribed.
7. Physicians should avoid using prescription blanks that are preprinted with the name of the drug.
8. When they use institutional prescription blanks, physicians should print their name, address, and DEA registration number on them.[12]

Identifying the Patient Hustler

Almost all physicians will encounter patients who deliberately set out to deceive them to obtain psychoactive substances. Types of manipulative approaches patient hustlers use include feigning physical problems; feigning psychological problems; deception such as prescription theft, alteration, or forgery; and pressuring physicians (See Chapter 2). Physicians, in the face of such tactics, should maintain control of the doctor-patient relationship, remain professional, and regard drug seekers as patients with a serious illness.[13]

The Role of the Physician

Physicians should be familiar with primary prevention programs for several reasons. First, knowledge of these programs provides insight into a patient's and his or her parents' knowledge, attitudes, and beliefs about drug use and abuse. Physicians are in an excellent position to provide primary education and counseling about drug abuse. Second, knowledge of program content allows physicians to reinforce the positive messages that they convey. And third, as community experts in health issues, physicians may be asked to participate in the development of such programs.[5]

Through conscious awareness and screening programs, physicians are in a position to detect substance abuse or chemical dependence and assist families in getting treatment for patients. They have an opportunity to prevent drug abuse by closely monitoring their patients' use of psychoactive medications.[13]

References

1. Kumpfer, K. L., J. Moskowitz, H. W. Whiteside, and M. Klitzner. Future issues and promising directions in the prevention of substance abuse among youth. In *Childhood and Chemical Abuse*. Ed. by S. Griswold-Ezekoye, K. L. Kumpfer, and W. J. Bukoski. Haworth Press, New York, 1986, pp. 249–278.

2. Wilford, B. B. (Ed.). *Drug Abuse: A Guide for the Primary Care Physician*. AMA, Chicago, 1981, pp. 299–315.

3. Royce, J. E. *Alcohol Problems and Alcoholism*. The Free Press, New York, 1981, pp. 179–196.

4. Botvin, G. J., and S. Tortu. Peer relationships, social competence, and substance abuse prevention: Implications for the family. In *The Family Context of Adolescent Drug Abuse*. Ed. by R. H. Coombs. Haworth Press, New York, 1988, pp. 245–773.

5. Schonberg, S. K. (Ed.). Prevention programs. In *Substance Abuse: A Guide for Health Professionals*. American Academy of Pediatrics, Elk Grove, Illinois, 1988, pp. 77–99.

6. DeMarsh, J., and K. L. Kumpfer. Family-oriented interventions for prevention of chemical dependency in children and adolescents. In *Childhood and Chemical Abuse*. Ed. by S. Griswold-Ezekoye, K. L. Kumpfer, and W. J. Bukoski. Haworth Press, New York, 1986, pp. 117–151.

7. Bukoski, W. J. School-based substance abuse prevention: A review of program research. In *Childhood and Chemical Abuse*. Ed. by S. Griswold-Ezekoye, K. L. Kumpfer, and W. J. Bukoski. Haworth Press, New York, 1986, pp. 95–115.

8. Johnson, C. A., W. B. Hanger, and M. A. Pentz. Comprehensive community programs for drug abuse prevention. In *Childhood and Chemical Abuse*. Ed. by S. Griswold-Ezekoye, K. L. Kumpfer, and W. J. Bukoski. Haworth Press, New York, 1986, pp. 181–199.

9. Wallack, L. Mass media, youth and the prevention of substance abuse: Towards an integral approach. In *Childhood and Chemical Abuse*. Ed. by S. Griswold-Ezekoye, K. L. Kumpfer, and W. J. Bukoski. Haworth Press, New York, 1986, pp. 153–180.

10. Barum, K., and P. Bashe. *How to Keep the Children You Love Off Drugs*. The Atlantic Monthly Press, New York, 1988.

11. Cohen, S. Drug abuse and the prescribing physician. In *Frequently Prescribed and Abused Drugs: Their Indications, Efficacy, and Rational Prescribing*. Ed. by C. Buchwald, S. Cohen, D. Katz, and J. Solomon. Medical Monograph Series, National Institute of Drug Abuse, Rockville, Maryland, 1980.

12. Guidelines for prescribers of controlled substances. U.S. Department of Justice, Drug Enforcement Administration, Washington, D.C., 1979.

13. Wilford, B. B. (Ed.). *Drug Abuse: A Guide for the Primary Care Physician*. American Medical Association, Chicago, 1981, pp. 263–284.

Part II Psychoactive Substances

CHAPTER 7

Basic Principles of Pharmacology

An understanding of the basic principles of pharmacology is essential to understanding how psychoactive substances exert their effects.

Pharmacokinetics

Four major processes determine both the intensity and duration of a drug's action: absorption, distribution, metabolism, and excretion. The branch of pharmacology concerned with these four processes is called *pharmacokinetics*.[1]

Absorption

Route of Administration

Drugs can be ingested orally, insufflated (snorted) via the nasal mucosa, inhaled, or injected. Ingested drugs must cross the intestinal mucosa to reach the bloodstream. Some drugs—alcohol, for example—may be partially absorbed in the stomach. Drugs that are insufflated, such as cocaine, must cross the nasal mucosa, and drugs whose vapors are inhaled (amyl nitrite, butyl nitrite) or that are combusted and then inhaled (nicotine, marijuana, cocaine, phencyclidine) must cross the alveolar-capillary membrane to reach the bloodstream. Many drugs can be injected (cocaine, methamphetamine, heroin) subcutaneously, intramuscularly, or intravenously.[2-3]

The site of absorption can markedly affect the rapidity of onset of a drug's effect as well as the degree of its effect. Cocaine in the form of chewed coca leaf, for example, is slowly absorbed in the buccal mucosa and small intestine. It is absorbed more rapidly and reaches a higher peak when smoked. In fact, smoking cocaine approximates the rapid delivery of intravenous cocaine because drugs that reach the alveoli have rapid access to the bloodstream through the large alveolar-capillary membrane. Because most of the cardiac output passes through the pulmonary capillaries, the delivery of a drug from the alveoli to the brain is further enhanced.[2-3]

Diffusion

Diffusion of most psychoactive substances through biological membranes is passive and depends on both the concentration of a drug and its ability to pass through the membrane. Drugs move across membranes from areas of higher concentrations to areas of lower concentrations. In addition, a drug must have certain chemical properties to pass through membranes easily: relatively small molecular size, adequate solubility in lipids, and lack of electric charge.[4]

Partition Coefficient

Biological membranes behave as if they are lipid solvents. As a result, how well a drug passes through them depends in part on the drug's lipid solubility. The *partition coefficient* is a measure of the relative solubility of a drug. It is defined as the ratio of the concentration of the drug dissolved in oil to its concentration dissolved in water. The higher its partition coefficient, the easier a drug passes through a membrane. The cellular barrier of the blood vessel endothelium has gaps between the cells so that even drugs with low partition coefficients pass with ease.[2-3]

Effects of pH

The degree of acidity or alkalinity of a solution (pH) markedly alters the degree of charge on drugs that ionize in solution as weak acids or bases. A weak acid will be least charged in an acidic fluid and most charged in an alkaline fluid. On the other hand, a weak base will be most charged in an acidic fluid and least charged in an alkaline fluid. The greater a drug's charge, the less lipid soluble—and the more water soluble—the drug is. The converse is also true. Therefore, a weak acid, such as phenobarbital, in an alkaline solution will tend to be trapped on one side of a membrane because of its charge. A weak base, such as methadone, will be least charged in an alkaline solution and, therefore, tend to be trapped on the acidic side of a membrane.[2-3]

In summary, drugs are absorbed through biological membranes by a system of passive movement that is characterized by a tendency to move from higher concentrations to lower concentrations, a tendency for more lipid-soluble drugs to cross membranes more readily, and a tendency for charged particles of weak acids or bases to be trapped on one side of a membrane.

Distribution

Volume of Distribution

The simplest compartments of distribution for drugs can be described in terms of extracellular and intracellular water, with a subdivision of extracellular water into plasma (intravascular) and interstitial (extravascular) fluids (Figure 7.1). Drugs that stay in the plasma distribute to 3 liters of body fluid. Charged drugs may distribute only through extracellular fluid (3 + 10 = 13 liters), because they

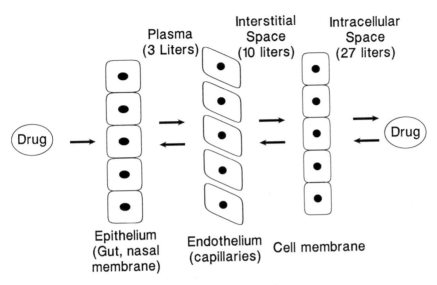

FIGURE 7.1. Drug distribution.

cannot readily cross cell membranes. Drugs that are water soluble and cross membranes readily, such as ethanol, may be distributed into all body water (3 + 10 + 27 = 40 liters).[4]

Some drugs in the plasma compartment are in solution, while others are combined with plasma proteins, most commonly albumin. A dynamic equilibrium exists between free drug and protein-bound drug. The binding constitutes a reservoir for the drug and may significantly affect the distribution of the drug to other sites in the body. Hence, both the drug's effect and its rate of elimination may be retarded. Methadone, for instance, has a relatively prolonged effect and a prolonged persistence in the body, in part because it is highly bound to plasma protein.[2-4]

The *volume of distribution* (Vd) of a drug is a ratio of the amount of drug in the body divided by the concentration of the drug in the plasma at that time. It is usually calculated by dividing the initial dose (Do) of drug by an extrapolated concentration at time zero (Co) as shown in Figure 7.2. The alpha phase is due to drug distribution; the beta phase is due to metabolism and excretion.[2-3,5]

Drug Accumulation in Adipose Tissue

Fatty (adipose) tissue can act as a depot for lipid-soluble drugs. Because blood flow through fat is rather slow, drugs that accumulate in fat, such as THC (the major psychoactive component of marijuana), tend to stay there for long periods of time and are usually released into the bloodstream slowly after use of the drug has stopped.[2-4]

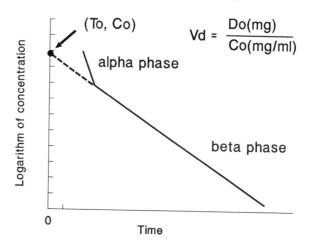

FIGURE 7.2. Decline of drug concentration in plasma over time.

The Blood-Brain Barrier

The capillary endothelial cells of the central nervous system (CNS) greatly reduce the ability of many drug molecules to diffuse across the membrane and reach effective concentrations in the brain. The blood-brain barrier probably evolved to protect the cells of the CNS against foreign substances. Only drugs that are very lipid-soluble can cross the blood-brain barrier well and produce achievable actions in the CNS. Such drugs include anesthetic gases, alcohol, sedatives, and hypnotics. Some portions of the CNS, such as the chemoreceptor trigger zone, which is responsible for nausea, are outside the barrier.[2-4]

The Placental Barrier

The capillary network of the placenta limits the ability of some drugs in the maternal circulation to reach the fetal circulation. The placental barrier serves as a means to protect the fetus against potentially harmful drug effects. Nevertheless, many drugs that enter the maternal circulation, including alcohol, nicotine, cocaine, and heroin, can cross the placental barrier and may cause fetal dependence, toxicity, and/or birth defects.[2-3]

Metabolism

Most drugs that enter the body are changed by a series of chemical reactions known as metabolism, or biotransformation. It is one of the two major processes for reducing the amount of active drug in the body. The other is excretion. The major site of drug metabolism is the liver.

Metabolites

Biotransformation transforms a drug to one or more other substances called *metabolites*, which are generally less active pharmacologically and, therefore, less toxic to the body. They are also more water-soluble so they can be excreted more readily. Some drugs are totally metabolized to other compounds before they are excreted. Others undergo no metabolism and are excreted unchanged. Most drugs, however, undergo both processes, with most of the drug being metabolized and the rest excreted without prior metabolism.[4,6]

Hepatic Drug Metabolism

Most liver cells (hepatocytes) contain many complex and active enzyme systems that metabolize drugs. Two of these are the microsomal and the nonmicrosomal enzyme systems. The microsomal enzymes are found primarily in the endoplasmic reticulum of the hepatocyte. They metabolize drugs with widely differing structures, such as phenobarbital, amphetamines, and meperidine (Demerol). Microsomal enzymes perform two basic types of chemical reactions on drugs — synthetic and nonsynthetic. Synthetic reactions involve chemically combining the parent or some of its metabolites with another compound such as an amino acid or a sugar. This is referred to as conjugation. Nonsynthetic reactions oxidize, reduce, or hydrolyze the parent drug or its metabolites.[2-3,6]

The nonmicrosomal enzyme system also metabolizes drugs nonspecifically. For example, alcohol dehydrogenase, the enzyme that metabolizes ethanol, also metabolizes ethylene glycol.[2-3]

Drugs administered orally pass through the liver, where many drugs that have just entered the body are transformed. Many orally administered drugs can be significantly inactivated the first time they pass through the liver, so that their concentrations in the blood are considerably less than they would otherwise be. This phenomenon is known as the *first-pass effect*.[2-4]

Several important factors can alter the liver's ability to metabolize a drug and therefore can dramatically influence a person's response to it. Such factors include a person's age, nutritional status, genetic makeup, and whether or not the person has liver disease.[4]

Types of Enzymatic Reactions

Two types of enzymatic reactions occur. In a *first-order reaction*, a drug's concentration is well below the level that would saturate the binding sites of the enzyme. The drug is, therefore, metabolized at a rate proportional to its concentration. Most drugs undergo first-order reactions. In a *zero-order reaction*, the binding sites on the enzymes are saturated. The rate of metabolism, therefore, is constant. Ethanol is an important example of a drug that undergoes a zero-order reaction. Some drugs, such as phenytoin (Dilantin), undergo first-order reactions at lower concentrations and zero-order reactions at higher concentrations.[2-3]

Enzyme Inhibition and Induction

Drug-metabolizing enzymes may be inhibited or induced (stimulated). Inhibition may be competitive or noncompetitive. *Competitive inhibition* occurs when another substance of similar structure combines reversibly with an enzyme's active sites. This type of inhibition may be overcome by increasing a drug's concentration. One example of competitive inhibition is the inhibition of acetaldehyde dehydrogenase by disulfiram (Antabuse). This results in a severe reaction when patients ingest ethanol, because the toxic acetaldehyde formed by the metabolism of the ethanol cannot be biotransformed. *Noncompetitive inhibition* occurs when an agent, unrelated in structure to the drug, binds in a distorted manner to prevent normal interaction between the drug and the enzyme. This form of inhibition cannot be overcome by increasing the drug's concentration.[2-3]

Microsomal enzymes undergo a quantitative increase in metabolizing ability (induction) when persistently exposed to a variety of drugs. Since most drugs that do this are lipid soluble, entering the liver cells is apparently necessary for drugs to cause enzyme induction. Phenobarbital is the most commonly known drug to do this. A few drugs, such as meprobamate (Equanil, Miltown) and gluthethamide (Doriden), may, by enzyme induction, hasten their own metabolism.[2-3]

Excretion

Renal Excretion

Drugs, or their metabolites, are excreted from the body primarily in the urine. Three processes affect the fate of a drug once it reaches the kidneys—glomerular filtration, tubular secretion, and tubular reabsorption. Glomerular filtration and tubular secretion increase the amount of a drug that is eliminated by the body, while tubular reabsorption reduces the amount of a drug that is eliminated. Water-soluble compounds remain in the urine after glomerular filtration or tubular secretion and are excreted from the body. Lipid-soluble compounds may passively diffuse across the renal tubular epithelium back into the bloodstream (tubular reabsorption) only to repeat the cycle over and over. If lipid-soluble drugs, such as phenobarbital, did not undergo metabolic conversion to water-soluble metabolites, they could remain in the body for months to years.[2-4]

By changing the pH of a patient's urine, it is possible to change the degree of charge of some compounds, rendering them less lipid-soluble and, hence, more readily excreted from the body in urine. Alkalinization of the urine, for example, may enhance the excretion of some weak acids, such as phenobarbital. Similarly, acidification of the urine may increase the excretion of some weak bases, such as amphetamines, methadone, and phencyclidine (PCP).[2-4]

Hepatic Excretion

The liver excretes some drugs via the bile into the duodenum. Probably the majority of these compounds are not excreted in significant amounts in the feces but instead are reabsorbed by the intestines to eventually be excreted by the kidneys. Glutethimide is thought to be intensively subjected to this *interhepatic circulation*, explaining why it persists in the body so long after an overdose.[2-4]

Other Sites of Excretion

An alternate but less important route of excretion is the lungs. The characteristic breath odor of an individual who has been drinking alcohol results from respiratory excretion of the drug. Alcohol concentrations in the breath are so closely related to blood alcohol levels that they are used to determine whether a person has a blood alcohol level above the legal limit for operating a motor vehicle. In addition, varying amounts of some drugs are excreted in sweat, breast milk, and saliva.[2-4]

Steady-State Relationships

The *half-life* of a drug is defined as the time required for the serum concentration of the drug to fall to 50 percent of its previous level. Only drugs that undergo first-order reactions can be described in terms of half-life. The time it takes drugs (such as alcohol) that undergo zero-order reactions to fall to 50 percent of their previous level depends on the dose—the greater the dose, the longer the time required for this to occur. The half-life of a drug is determined by the interaction between absorption, distribution, metabolism, and excretion.[7]

When a drug is administered at intervals less than, or equal to, its half-life, it will begin to accumulate in the serum because some of the previous dose is still in the blood when each subsequent dose is taken. Eventually a point of balance (a steady state) is reached in which the rate of excretion and metabolism is equal to the rate of administration. The dose markedly affects the steady-state level but does not effect the time required to reach it, which is a function only of the drug's half-life. The steady-state concentration, whatever it is going to be, will be reached in four or five half-lives of the drug, regardless of dose size.[2-3,7]

Pharmacodynamics

The study of how drugs exert their effects is called *pharmocodynamics*. It focuses on how the molecules of most drugs interact with specific receptors on target cells, how a biological response occurs, the relationship of the dose and the resultant response to a drug, and the way one drug can alter the response to another.[8-9]

Receptors

Many drugs produce their effects by interacting with specific macromolecules that are usually located on a cell's outer membrane. These specific interaction sites are called *receptors*. The shape, size, electrical charge, and other properties of the receptor surface are compatible with those of the specific drug molecules

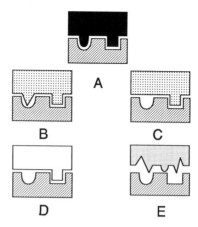

FIGURE 7.3. Lock-and-key analogy of drug-receptor interaction: (A) strong agonist, (B) and (C) weak agonist, (D) antagonist, (E) no interaction.

that interact with it. This interaction is often described by a lock and key analogy (Figure 7.3). *Agonists* interact with the receptor to form a drug-receptor complex and in doing so alter cell function to cause a response. Agonists whose characteristics exactly match those of the receptor cause a strong response (Figure 7.3a), while agonists that do not precisely match the receptor cause a weaker response (Figure 7.3b and c). Some drugs, called *antagonists*, have properties that allow them to bind to a receptor but produce no response (Figure 7.3d). By doing so, they prevent formation of an agonist-receptor complex and thereby block the response that would ordinarily occur. Naloxone (Narcan) and naltrexone (Trexan) are examples of opioid antagonists. They will actually displace drugs such as morphine and hydromorphone (Dilaudid) from receptors. Some analgesic drugs, such as pentazocine (Talwin) and nalbuphine (Nubain), have varying degrees of both agonist and antagonist activity. They will precipitate withdrawal symptoms in narcotic addicts. Finally, drugs that do not match receptor sites will not interact at all (Figure 7.3e).[8-10]

The binding of a drug molecule to its receptor is the first step leading to a response. In many cases this activates a second step. Drugs that cause muscle contraction, for example, do so by first forming a drug-receptor complex on the muscle cell. This activates adenyl cyclase, an enzyme that increases the formation of cyclic adenosine monophosphate (cAMP). In turn, cAMP increases the flow of calcium ions into the cell, activating the contractile proteins and causing muscle contraction.[8-10]

Dose-Response Curves

Dose-Response Plots

Drug-receptor interactions are usually discussed in terms of semi-logarithmic, dose-response plots of drug plasma concentration versus physiological response

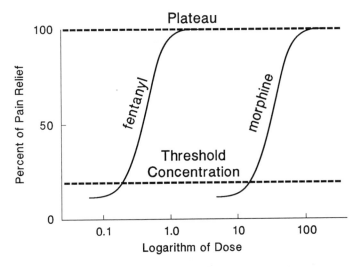

FIGURE 7.4. Dose-response curves of two opioid drugs.

(Figure 7.4). The semi-logarithmic plot has several advantages. It can display a wide range of doses, and its curves are usually S-shaped with linear middle segments. This implies that binding to the receptors is a first-order process within this linearity—that is, that the amount of a drug binding to the receptors is directly proportional to the drug's concentration. Drugs producing the same effects by the same mechanism produce dose-response curves whose linear segments parallel each other. When two drugs act individually by binding to the same receptors, they produce the same maximum response (plateau). The plateau means that all receptors have become saturated. In addition, a minimum plasma concentration of a drug is necessary to initiate a response. The amount of drug that produces this minimum concentration is called the *threshold* dose.[2-3,10]

Affinity, Potency, and Efficacy

The tendency of a drug to be bound at given receptor sites is known as its *affinity*. In Figure 7.4, fentanyl produces a response at a lower dose than morphine. Therefore, it has a greater affinity for the receptors, and is said to be more potent. *Potency* indicates the dose of a drug needed to produce a given response when compared to the dose of another drug required to produce the same response. Fentanyl and morphine reach the same plateau. They therefore have the same *efficacy* (response-producing ability) despite differing potencies. Drugs that plateau at lower maximum responses than other drugs are said to be less efficacious.[2-3,10]

Synaptic Transmission

The transmission of a nerve signal from one neuron to the next in the CNS requires the action of a chemical substance called a *neurotransmitter*. Neurotransmitters include catecholamines, choline esters, 5-hydroxytryptamine, amino acids, and neuropeptides.[11]

Synaptic Function

As the action potential moves down the *presynaptic neuron* (Figure 7.5), it reaches the nerve terminal where it causes the release of calcium ions. These, in turn, act on *storage vesicles* to initiate the release of neurotransmitter molecules. The neurotransmitter molecules then cross the *synaptic cleft*, where they momentarily interact with receptors on the *postsynaptic neuron*. Activation of the receptors causes the conversion of adenyl cyclase to cAMP which, in turn, initiates an action potential in the postsynaptic neuron. After brief interaction with the *postsynaptic receptors*, the neurotransmitter molecules tend to return to the presynaptic vesicles for storage and reuse. A portion of the neurotransmitter molecules is rendered inactive by a specific enzyme in the synaptic cleft. Synaptic transmission is very rapid, requiring only about 1/1000 of a second.[11]

Effects of Drugs on Synaptic Function

Drugs alter synaptic function by a variety of mechanisms. For example, the administration of neurotransmitter precursors may increase the availability of neurotransmitter in the presynaptic vesicles, such as when the amino acid tryptophan, which is a precursor of serotonin, is used. Other examples are monoamine oxidase inhibitors, such as phenelzine (Nardil), which decrease the activity of the metabolizing enzyme in the synaptic cleft, making more of the neurotransmitter available at the postsynaptic receptors. Antagonistic drugs may displace neurotransmitter molecules from the postsynaptic receptors; Atropine, for example, antagonizes the action of acetylcholine at muscarinic

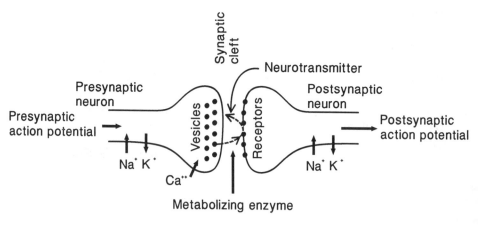

FIGURE 7.5. Synaptic transmission.

receptors. A drug may mimic the activity of the neurotransmitter to increase receptor activity. Bromocriptine (Parlodel), for example, activates the postsynaptic dopamine receptors. A drug may also block access to the receptor. Antipsychotic drugs, such as chlorpromazine (Thorazine), block access of dopamine to its receptors in the limbic system, producing their antipsychotic effects, and in the basal ganglia, producing their extrapyramidal effects. A drug may block reuptake of neurotransmitter molecules from the synaptic cleft. In doing so, it increases neurotransmitter availability at the postsynaptic receptors. Cocaine, for example, interferes with the reuptake of dopamine, norepinephrine, and serotonin. Finally, a drug may facilitate release of neurotransmitter from the presynaptic vesicles. Amantadine (Symmetrel) may stimulate the release of dopamine from presynaptic vesicles.[11]

Upregulation and Downregulation

Upregulation and downregulation involve the development of increased or decreased numbers of postsynaptic receptors, respectively. As an example of upregulation, consider the following: Some psychotic patients require antipsychotic medications, such as chlorpromazine, for years, producing a prolonged dopamine receptor blockade. This may cause the development of additional postsynaptic receptors in an attempt to return synaptic transmission toward normal. If removal of the neuroleptic blockade occurs, a patient may develop tardive dyskinesia, a movement disorder, because normal amounts of dopamine activate the excess receptors.[12]

When excessive activation of postsynaptic receptors occurs over time, such as with heroin dependence, a decrease in the number of receptors occurs in an attempt to return synaptic transmission toward normal. This phenomenon is known as *downregulation*.[12]

Kindling

If a drug is capable of producing a symptom, regular use of the drug at the original dose level may evoke the symptom not after the first dose but after multiple doses, a phenomenon known as *kindling*. The paranoid schizophreniform reaction to cocaine is an example of kindling. It may not occur with the first dose, the second dose, or even the third dose, but it develops after many doses over a period of time.[12]

Neurotransmitters Affected by Psychoactive Substances

Six neurotransmitters (gamma-aminobutyric acid [GABA], acetylcholine, norepinephrine, dopamine, serotonin, beta-endorphin) account for most of the symptoms seen with the most commonly abused drugs in the United States (Table 7.1).[13]

TABLE 7.1. Neurotransmitters affected by commonly abused drugs.

Neurotransmitter	Central action	Drugs that affect neurotransmitter actions
GABA	central inhibition of other neurotransmitters	alcohol barbiturates benzodiazepines chloral hydrate ethchlorvynol meprobamate methaqualone (?) phencyclidine
Acetylcholine	counterbalances dopamine maintains memory initiates short-term memory	phencyclidine
Norepinephrine	modulates mood maintains sleeping state	amphetamines cocaine opioids phencyclidine
Dopamine	counterbalances acetylcholine stimulates pleasure center modulates mood affects intellectual processes inhibits prolactin release	amphetamines cocaine phencyclidine
Serotonin	modulates mood initiates sleep involved in REM sleep	hallucinogens phencyclidine
Beta-endorphin	modulates mood modulates pain perception inhibits norepinephrine release	opioids phencyclidine

Based on A.J. Giannini and N.S. Miller, Drug abuse: A biopsychiatric model, *American Family Physician*, 40:173–182, 1989, published by the American Academy of Family Physicians.

Primitive Survival-Brain Concept of Chemical Dependence

The primitive survival-brain concept of chemical dependence is based on the premise that millions of years ago on the evolutionary tree, man did not possess a reasoning, thinking brain—the cerebral cortex—but instead depended entirely on a rudimentary brain whose single-minded purpose was survival. This primitive brain served to find food and water, flee or fight when the occasion arose, and to have sex for survival of the species. The limbic system, discussed in Chapter 1, is a part of this primitive brain. As time passed, the cerebral cortex evolved around it. Because scientists believe that chemical dependence to many drugs takes place by alteration of neurotransmitters in the hypothalmus, chemical dependence is thought of as being a reversion to survival of the individual. During the use and abuse phases, the cerebral cortex is in charge. One may say, having processed the thought in his cerebral cortex, "I think I'll use some cocaine." Once chemical dependence occurs, the cerebral cortex is no longer in

Wall

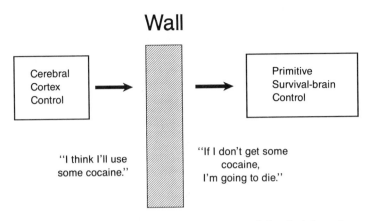

FIGURE 7.6. Primitive survival-brain concept of chemical dependence.

charge, and the primitive brain sends the message, "If I don't get some cocaine, I'm going to die." Getting cocaine becomes a matter of survival. The movement of control from the cerebral cortex to the primitive brain is the point at which researchers believe neurotransmitters in the hypothalmus are sufficiently deranged to signal dependence. Movement of control from the cerebral cortex to the primitive survival brain (Figure 7.6) is analogous to the crossing the wall concept discussed in Chapter 1.[14]

Tolerance

Tolerance

Most, if not all, psychoactive drugs lose some effect with repeated use. Individuals who wish to achieve a specific effect, such as becoming high, must use larger and larger doses, a phenomenon known as *tolerance*. Tolerance is traditionally divided into dispositional and pharmacodynamic tolerance. *Dispositional tolerance* involves an increased rate of metabolism, almost always because of hepatic microenzyme induction. This probably plays a small role in the development of tolerance to drugs. The major cause of tolerance, *pharmacodynamic tolerance*, takes place at the cellular level in the brain, perhaps resulting in part from neurotransmitter downregulation. Dependent individuals simply function better at a given serum level of a drug than nontolerant individuals do. An alcoholic with a blood alcohol level greater than 0.4 gm/100 ml may still be walking and talking while most nontolerant individuals would be approaching a comatose state at this level.[2-3,12]

Tolerance is not an all-or-none phenomenon. Drug users develop it to some aspects of drug actions but not to others. Amphetamine abusers, for example, may develop tolerance to the cardiovascular and euphoric effects of the drug but remain at high risk for the psychotic effects.[2-3]

TABLE 7.2. Abstinence syndrome.

Drug group	Abstinence syndrome
CNS depressants	$++++$
Opioids	$+++$
CNS stimulants	$++$
Phencyclidines	$++$
Cannabinoids	$+$
Hallucinogens	$-$
Inhalants	$-$

Cross-Tolerance

The development of tolerance to drugs in the same class as an abused drug, *cross-tolerance* occurs without actual use of other drugs. Heroin addicts, for example, automatically develop tolerance to other opioid drugs, such as morphine, hydromorphone, or codeine, as they become tolerant to the effects of heroin. Heroin addicts on methadone who are injured, for example, will not respond to the usual dose of narcotic pain medication. Alcoholics develop cross-tolerance to other central nervous system depressant drugs, such as barbiturates, benzodiazepines, meprobamate, and gaseous anesthetics. Cross-tolerance can occur among drugs of other classes as well.[2-3]

Physical Dependence and Abstinence Syndrome

The term *physical dependence* is used to distinguish drugs that, when patients stop using them, cause an *abstinence syndrome*—that is, they cause patients to develop withdrawal symptoms (Table 7.2). The most dramatic abstinence syndrome is produced by drugs that depress the central nervous system (alcohol, barbiturates, benzodiazepines). It results from central nervous system hyperactivity, which produces tachycardia, hypertension, anxiety, insomnia, and sometimes seizures. Death occasionally occurs, particularly when the syndrome develops in addicts who are not under medical supervision. When addicts stop using other drugs (cocaine, amphetamines, phencyclidine), they have much less dramatic withdrawal symptoms. In fact, for many years cocaine was thought not to produce physical dependence because doctors did not recognize its rather mild abstinence syndrome. Opioid drugs (heroin, morphine) produce an intermediate abstinence syndrome, with some central nervous system hyperactivity, but not as marked as CNS depressant drugs produce. It is not life-threatening to users. Some drugs are not associated with an abstinence syndrome.[2-3]

As we saw in Chapter 1, physical dependence is not a necessary requirement for chemical dependence. Similarly, physical dependence by itself does not mean that a person has the disease of chemical dependence.

References

1. Benet, L. Z., and L. B. Sheiner. Pharmacokinetics: The dynamics of drug absorption, distribution, and elimination. In *The Pharmacological Basis of Therapeutics*. Ed. by A. G. Gilman, L. S. Goodman, T. W. Rall, and F. Murad. Macmillan, New York, 1985, pp. 3–34.
2. Wilford, B. B. (Ed.). Pharmacology. In *AMSAODD Review Course Syllabus*. American Medical Society on Alcoholism and Other Drug Dependencies, New York, 1987, pp. 13–47.
3. Morgan, J. P. *Alcohol and Drug Abuse Curriculum Guide for Pharmacology Faculty*. National Institute of Drug Abuse, Rockville, Maryland, 1985.
4. Shlafer, M., and E. N. Marieb (Eds.) Absorption, distribution, metabolism, and excretion. In *The Nurse, Pharmacology, and Drug Therapy*. Addison-Wesley, Redwood City, California, 1989, pp. 46–65.
5. Benet, L. Z. Pharmacokinetics I: Absorption, distribution, and excretion. In *Basic and Clinical Pharmacology*. Ed. by B. J. Katzung. Appleton and Lange, Norwalk, Connecticut, 1987, pp. 23–35.
6. Correlia, M. A., and N. Castognolia, Jr. Pharmocokinetics II: Drug biotransformation. In *Basic and Clinical Pharmacology*. Ed. by B. J. Katzung. Appleton and Lange, Norwalk, Connecticut, 1987, pp. 36–43.
7. Shlafer, M., and E. N. Marieb (Eds.). Time-response aspects of drug actions. In *The Nurse, Pharmacology, and Drug Therapy*. Addison-Wesley, Redwood City, California, 1989, pp. 66–75.
8. Bourne, A. R., and J. M. Roberts. Drug receptors and pharmacodynamics. In *Basic and Clinical Pharmacology*. Ed. by B. J. Katsung. Appleton and Lange, Norwalk, Connecticut, 1987, pp. 9–22.
9. Ross, E. M., and Alfred G. Gilman. Pharmacodynamics: Mechanisms of drug action and the relationship between drug concentration and effect. In *The Pharmacological Basis of Therapeutics*. Ed. by A. G. Gilman, L. S. Goodman, T. W. Rall, and F. Murad. Macmillan, New York, 1985, pp. 35–48.
10. Shlafer, M., and E. N. Marieb (Eds.). Mechanisms of drug action. In *The Nurse, Pharmacology, and Drug Therapy*, Addison-Wesley, Redwood City, California, 1989, pp. 76–89.
11. Cohen, S. Neurotransmitters, neuropeptides, and neurohormones. In *The Chemical Brain: The Neurochemistry of Addictive Disorders*. Care Institute, Irvine, California, 1988, pp. 11–56.
12. Cohen, S. The chemistry of addiction. In *The Chemical Brain: Neurochemistry of Addictive Disorders*. Care Institute, Irvine, California, 1988, pp. 57–74.
13. Giannini, A. J., and N. S. Miller. Drug abuse: A biopsychiatric model. *America Family Physician*, 40:173–182, 1989.
14. Talbott, G. D. Alcoholism and other drug addictions: A primary disease entity. *Journal of the Medical Association of Georgia*, August 1986, pp. 490–494.

CHAPTER 8

CNS Depressants: Alcohol

History

Alcoholic beverages have been used by man since the dawn of history. Breweries can be traced back about 6,000 years to ancient Egypt and Babylonia. The oldest alcoholic drinks were fermented beers and wines of relatively low alcohol content. The Arabs introduced distillation into Europe in the Middle Ages to increase alcohol content in beverages. Alcohol was believed to be a remedy for practically all diseases, as indicated by the Gaelic term *whiskey*, which means "water of life."[1-2]

Early American colonists commonly drank beer and wine with meals. At that time, people consumed 95 percent of beverage alcohol in the form of beer (90 percent) or wine (5 percent). They did not tolerate drunkenness. However, a dramatic shift occurred after 1725. People increasingly drank distilled beverages, to the point where such beverages were the major form of alcohol consumed. Along with this came a major increase in intemperate drinking. Excessive drinking became not only tolerated but admired: It was immoral, but it was manly. As early as 1789, a movement began to oppose widespread intemperance. It did not oppose wine and beer, only distilled spirits. The movement at first promoted intemperance, but later promoted abstinence, culminating in the passage in 1920 of the Eighteenth Amendment to the U.S. Constitution, which prohibited the manufacture, sale, or transportation of intoxicating beverages except for medical or sacramental purposes. A massive struggle began between the people and law enforcement authorities. Prohibition simply did not work. Pressures for repeal resulted in 1933 in a redefinition of "intoxicating beverage" to allow the sale and consumption of beer with 3.2 percent alcohol content; in 1934 the Twenty-first Amendment repealed the Eighteenth Amendment, and Prohibition came to an end.[3]

In 1935, Dr. Bob Smith and Bill Wilson, two hopeless alcoholics, discovered that they could stay sober by helping each other and founded Alcoholics Anonymous. In 1945, Mrs. Marty Mann founded the National Council on Alcoholism (NCA), a volunteer group dedicated to eradicating the stigma of alcoholism and educating the general public about treatment and prevention. The World Health Organization acknowledged alcoholism to be a medical problem in 1951. In 1956, the American Medical Association declared alcoholism to be an illness, and the next year the American Hospital Association accepted it as an illness treatable in general hospitals. Jellinek published his landmark book *The Disease Concept of Alcoholism* in 1960, and the American Psychiatric Association recognized alcoholism as a disease in 1965.[3]

In 1970 the Hughes Act established the National Institute of Alcohol Abuse and Alcoholism (NIAAA); authorized financial assistance to states, communities, organizations, institutions, and individuals; funded research, education and training, and a variety of treatment and rehabilitation programs; withdrew federal funds from hospitals that refused to treat alcoholics; and required a comprehensive program for military and civilian federal employees with alcoholism. In 1974, the Internal Revenue Service ruled that not only is treatment for alcoholism a deductible medical expense but even transportation to and from Alcoholics Anonymous meetings or clubhouses could qualify.[3]

Pharmacology

Ethyl alcohol (ethanol) is a sedative-hypnotic drug commonly referred to as beverage alcohol. Toxicity from two other alcohols, methyl alcohol (methanol) and ethylene glycol, occurs with sufficient frequency to warrant discussion in this chapter as well. We will use the terms *ethanol* and *alcohol* interchangeably in this chapter.

Production of Alcoholic Beverages

Fermentation

Certain microorganisms—the yeasts—act on natural vegetable sugars. Enzymes the yeasts produce to provide them energy break down the sugars and produce a waste product, ethanol. This process is called *fermentation*. A variety of alcoholic beverages are produced in this way, depending on the original sugar base— wine from fruit juices, beer from malted grains, and mead from honey. The yeast action is inhibited by the increasing concentration of alcohol, and fermentation ceases when the concentration reaches about 14 percent.[4]

Distillation

Alcoholic beverages with a concentration higher than 14 percent are the result of *distillation*. The fermented liquid is heated and, because alcohol boils at a lower temperature than water, is evaporated off. It is then condensed in a coil and collected. Different distillates result from the fermented product used. Brandy is distilled wine, and whiskey is distilled from malted grains.[4]

Alcohol Content

The concentration of alcohol in beverages varies greatly. Beer has the lowest alcohol content, around 5 percent; wines range from 9 to 12.5 percent, and liquors and whiskeys are highest at 40 percent or more. Twelve ounces of beer contain about the same amount of alcohol as 5 ounces of wine, 3 ounces of port or sherry, or 1.5 ounces of whiskey or liquor. *Proof* equals twice the alcohol concentration; for example, 80 proof whiskey contains 40 percent alcohol by volume.[4]

Pharmacokinetics

Ethanol (CH_3CH_2OH) consists of small, water-soluble molecules that are absorbed rapidly and completely from the stomach (20 percent) and small intestine (80 percent). After a person ingests alcohol on an empty stomach, it reaches its peak blood level within 40 minutes. Food in the gut delays alcohol's absorption. Distribution is rapid, with tissue levels rapidly approximating the blood concentration. The volume of distribution is about 50 liters in a 70-kilogram person.[5]

Over 90 percent of alcohol a person consumes is metabolized in the liver; the rest is excreted unchanged by the lungs and in the urine. The rate of metabolism follows zero-order kinetics — that is, it is independent of the drug's concentration. The typical adult can metabolize between 7 and 10 grams of alcohol an hour (30 milliliters of 80 proof whiskey). However, the alcohol disappears from the body much more slowly in someone with liver damage. Two major pathways for metabolizing alcohol exist: the alcohol dehydrogenase pathway and the microsomal ethanol oxidizing system (MEOS).[5]

Alcohol Dehydrogenase Pathway

The main pathway for ethanol metabolism involves alcohol dehydrogenase (AD), an enzyme that catalyzes the conversion of ethanol to acetaldehyde (CH_3CHO) according to the following reaction:

$$CH_3CH_2OH + NAD^+ \xrightarrow{AD} CH_3CHO + NADH + H^+$$

In this reaction, hydrogen ion is transferred from alcohol to the cofactor nicotinamide adenine dinucleotide (NAD) to form NADH. The increased rate of blood alcohol clearance in alcoholics is thought to be due to increased alcohol dehydrogenase activity.[5]

Microsomal Ethanol Oxidizing System

This enzyme system uses NADPH instead of NAD as a cofactor according to the following reaction:

$$CH_3CH_2OH + NADPH + H^+ + O_2 \xrightarrow{MEOS} CH_3CHO + NADP^+ + H_2O$$

It is thought that at low concentrations of ethanol, alcohol dehydrogenase is the main oxidizing system and that at higher concentrations MEOS plays the more significant role. During chronic alcohol consumption, MEOS activity increases significantly due to enzyme induction. Other inducing drugs, such as barbiturates, may enhance the rate of blood alcohol clearance.[5]

Acetaldehyde Metabolism

Over 90 percent of the acetaldehyde formed by the above reactions is also metabolized in the liver. Aldehyde dehydrogenase is the main pathway for aldehyde oxidation. The product of this reaction is acetate, which is further metabolized and excreted as carbon dioxide and water.[5]

Pharmacological Actions

Central Nervous System

The central nervous system is more acutely affected by alcohol than any other organ system. Alcohol can cause sedation, relief of anxiety, slurred speech, ataxia, impaired judgement, and uninhibited behavior—that is, it causes intoxication. Many people think alcohol is stimulating; however, like other general anesthetics, alcohol is a central nervous system depressant. The apparent stimulation, which occurs at low doses, results from the activity of various parts of the brain that have been freed from inhibition as a result of depression of inhibitory control mechanisms.[1,5]

One of the most significant sites of action of alcohol is the cell membrane. Alcohol readily dissolves in the lipid layer, thereby reducing the viscosity of the cell membrane. This membrane-fluidizing effect has been related to changes in specific membrane functions, including neurotransmitter receptors, various enzymes, the mitochondrial transport chain, and ion channels, such as those for calcium. Ethanol exposure has been reported to increase the number of GABA receptors, which is consistent with the ability of drugs known to affect the GABA system (such as benzodiazepines) to mimic or intensify many of the acute effects of alcohol.[5]

The psychological and behavioral effects of various blood alcohol levels are given in Table 8.1. They range from feeling warm and relaxed after one or two drinks (a blood alcohol level of 0.02) to death from respiratory depression (a blood alcohol level of 0.50). Individual reactions to given blood alcohol levels vary considerably. Tolerance due to persistent and excessive alcohol consumption increases the levels at which the reactions occur. The effects are more marked when the concentration is rising than when it is falling.[4]

Circulatory System

The immediate effects of alcohol on the circulation are relatively minor. Blood pressure, cardiac output, and myocardial contraction do not change greatly in

TABLE 8.1. Effects of alcohol consumption in the nontolerant individual.

Blood alcohol level (gm/100 ml)	Effects
0:02	Reached after approximately one drink; light or moderate drinkers feel some effect—warmth and relaxation.
0.04	Most people feel relaxed, talkative, and happy; skin may become flushed.
0.05	First sizable changes begin to occur; lightheartedness, giddiness, lowered inhibitions, and less control of thoughts may be experienced; both restraint and judgment are lowered; coordination may be slightly altered.
0.06	Judgment is somewhat impaired; ability to make rational decisions about personal capabilities is affected (such as in being able to drive).
0.08	Definite impairment of muscle coordination and a slower reaction time occurs; driving ability becomes suspect; sensory feelings of numbness of the cheeks and lips occur; hands, arms, and legs may tingle and then feel numb (this level constitutes legal impairment in Canada and in some U.S. states).
0.10	Clumsiness, speech may become fuzzy; clear deterioration of reaction time and muscle control (this level constitutes drunkenness in most U.S. states).
0.15	Definite impairment of balance and movement.
0.20	Motor and emotional control centers are measurably affected; slurred speech, staggering, loss of balance, and double vision can all be present.
0.30	Lack of understanding of what is seen or heard occurs; individuals are confused or stuporous and may lose consciousness.
0.40	Usually unconscious; the skin becomes clammy.
0.45	Respiration slows and may stop altogether.
0.50	Death occurs

Based on W. Poley, G. Lee, and G. Vibe, Alcohol and its effects on the individual, in *Alcoholism Treatment Manual*, Gardner Press, New York, 1979, pp. 17–31.

most people after they consume a moderate amount of alcohol. However, significant decrease in myocardial contractility has been observed in some.[1,5]

Alcohol in moderate doses causes vasodilation, especially of the cutaneous vessels. This produces a warm and flushed skin. The vasodilation occurs partly from central nervous system vasomotor depression and partly from a direct vasodilating action of alcohol on blood vessels.[1]

In individuals with classical stable angina and proven coronary artery disease, alcohol decreases the duration of exercise required to produce angina and produces changes in electrocardiograms that are characteristic of myocardial ischemia.[1]

Several studies have shown a negative correlation between chronic ingestion of small amounts of alcohol and the incidence of coronary artery disease. The protective effect was originally thought to occur because ethanol increased the concentration of high-density lipoproteins and decreased the concentration of low-density lipoproteins in plasma. However, the particular HDL subfraction elevated is HDL-3, whereas decreased risk is associated with HDL-2.[1,6]

Gastrointestinal Tract

Alcohol in a concentration of about 10 percent physically stimulates the salivary and gastric secretions, especially if an individual likes its taste. The gastric juice is rich in acid and normal in pepsin. Alcohol may also stimulate the release of salivary and gastric secretions by directly stimulating sensory endings in the buccal and gastric mucosa. Finally, alcohol may stimulate gastric secretion by causing the release of gastrin. Ingested beverages with alcohol concentrations of about 20 percent tend to depress gastric secretions. Drinks of 40 percent alcohol and over are very irritating to the gastric mucosa and cause congestive hyperemia and inflammation and may produce an errosive gastritis.[1]

Alcohol consumed in moderate amounts does not significantly influence the colon's motor activity, but consumed to the point of intoxication, it stops gastrointestinal motor function. Absorption is delayed, and pylorospasm and vomiting may occur independent of the local irritant effect.[1]

The Kidneys

Alcohol exerts a diuretic effect on the kidneys. Although the large amount of fluid ordinarily ingested with alcoholic beverages undoubtedly contributes to the increased urine flow, alcohol itself produces a marked diuretic response because of decreased renal tubular reabsorption of water. Most likely, this effect is due to a direct action of alcohol on the neurohyphophyseal system to decrease the secretion of antidiuretic hormone (ADH). The diuretic effect is roughly proportional to the blood alcohol concentration.[1]

Temperature Regulation

After ingestion of ethanol, a feeling of warmth occurs because of enhanced cutaneous blood flow. Increased sweating may also occur. The body, therefore, loses heat more rapidly, and its internal temperature tends to fall. With large amounts of alcohol consumed, the central temperature regulating system becomes depressed and the fall in body temperature may be pronounced. Heavy alcohol consumption during exposure to cold is clearly dangerous.[1]

Interaction With Other Drugs

The impairment of muscular coordination and judgment that is associated with the ingestion of a moderate amount of alcohol is enhanced if people take other sedative-hypnotics, anticonvulsants, antidepressants, antianxiety agents, or narcotics. In addition, unusual side effects may occur when people take alcohol with other drugs. Patients treated with oral hypoglycemics may after drinking alcohol experience unpleasant symptoms similar to those patients who take disulfiram experience. Similar interactions may occur with some antibiotics and some anti-inflammatory drugs (see Chapter 4).[1,7]

The combination of alcohol and an oral hypoglycemic may cause unpredictable fluctuations of plasma glucose concentrations, apparently because of an additive hypoglycemic effect of alcohol and because chronic consumption of ethanol can decrease the half-life of some of these drugs. The hypoglycemic effect of insulin can also be markedly increased. Alcohol can interfere with the therapeutic actions of a wide variety of drugs by altering their metabolism. For example, acute ingestion of ethanol reduces the clearance of phenytoin because both drugs compete for the same MEOS enzymes. However, in the chronic drinker, enzyme induction by alcohol occurs, with the result that a period of abstinence leads to an enhanced rate of clearance of phenytoin.[1,7]

Toxicity

Acute alcohol overdose may cause depression of the respiratory system and can lead to death from respiratory failure, aspiration pneumonia, or cardiac arrhythmias. The lethal dose of alcohol varies widely because of the development of tolerance. Individuals who have not developed tolerance may lose consciousness at a blood alcohol level of 0.30. Respiratory depression usually occurs at a blood alcohol level of 0.45, and death at a blood alcohol level of 0.50 in individuals who have not developed tolerance. Metabolic alterations, such as alcoholic ketoacidosis, may occur as well as dehydration, hypoglycemia, and electrolyte alterations.

Tolerance

The repeated use of alcohol leads to the development of tolerance so that larger doses must be taken to produce the desired effects. Although chronic use results in an increased capacity to metabolize alcohol, it also results in increased pharmacodynamic tolerance so that a higher blood alcohol level is required to produce intoxication in the tolerant individual.[1]

Dependence

Both psychological and physical dependence can be produced by persistent and excessive consumption of alcohol.[1]

Abstinence Syndrome

Persistent and excessive consumption of alcohol can produce physical dependence and its associated abstinence syndrome. The acute phase of the alcohol abstinence syndrome has traditionally been divided into four stages (Table 8.2). However, the signs, symptoms, and temporal sequence of these stages may vary.

Stage 1: Most commonly occurring after an overnight abstinence from alcohol (approximately eight hours), Stage 1 is characterized by mild tremulousness, nervousness, mild tachycardia, and nausea. Usually these symptoms last less than 24 hours, or they become more pronounced and patients progress to the second stage.[8-9]

Stage 2: All the signs and symptoms of Stage 1 are magnified in intensity in Stage 2. Tremors are marked, insomnia occurs, patients are hyperalert and easily startled. Tachycardia becomes more pronounced, and tachypnea appears. Patients crave alcohol, and some have nightmares, illusions, or hallucinations. The hallucinations are usually visual, but they can be auditory or tactile.

TABLE 8.2. The alcohol abstinence syndrome.

Stage	Onset	Signs and symptoms
1	Approximately 8 hours after cessation or reduction in drinking (overnight abstinence)	Mild tremulousness, nervousness, mild tachycardia, nausea
2	Approximately 24 hours; occasionally up to 8 days	Marked tremors, hyperactivity, hyperalertness, increased startle response, pronounced tachycardia, insomnia, nightmares, illusions, hallucinations, alcohol craving
3	From 12 to 48 hours	Same as stage 2, only more marked; the distinguishing feature is grand mal seizures
4	Usually 3 to 5 days, sometimes up to 12 days	Delirium tremens—confusion, agitation, gross tremor, insomnia, tachycardia (120–140 beats/min), profuse sweating, hyperpyrexia (104°F or higher)

Based on H. Behnke, Recognition and management of alcohol withdrawal syndrome, *Hospital Practice,* vol. 11, issue 77, November, 1976, pp. 79–84.

Despite being oriented to time, place, and person, patients may admit to seeing bugs on the wall or a snake in the corner, although they may not seem particularly frightened by the experience. These visual hallucinations in the presence of a relatively clear mind are called *alcoholic hallucinosis.* Auditory hallucinations, however, may produce anxiety or outright panic. Although Stage 2 may take up to six to eight days to manifest itself, it usually appears within 24 hours of significant reduction of alcohol consumption.[8-9]

Stage 3: Characterized by increased severity of the signs and symptoms in Stage 2, Stage 3 is distinguished by seizures, which occur in 3 to 4 percent of patients. More than 90 percent of the seizures occur from 7 to 48 hours after the last drink. The attacks, which may be simple or multiple, resemble classic grand mal seizures but usually do not involve loss of bowel or bladder control. If abstinence syndromes in patients with seizures are not treated, 30 to 40 percent will develop delirium tremens (DTs).[8-9]

Stage 4: Stage 4 is marked by the appearance of delirium tremens, which usually begins on the third to fifth day of withdrawal, but may begin as late as the twelfth day. Although the risk of DTs is less than 8 percent, it is high in patients who have had seizures during withdrawal. DTs consist of confusion, agitation, gross tremor, insomnia, and increased psychomotor and autonomic activity. Patients often have pulse rates in the range of 120 to 140 beats a minute, suffer hypertension and profuse sweating, and may have high body temperatures (104°F or higher). In 80 percent of patients, the delirium resolves in less than three days. DTs is associated with significant mortality rate (between 5 and 20 percent). Deaths occur from electrolyte disturbances, seizures with respiratory insufficiency, aspiration pneumonia, cardiac dysrhythmias, dehydration, and cardiac failure.[8-9]

The alcohol postacute withdrawal syndrome consists of depression that may last a few days to weeks and Korsakoff's syndrome, which may take months to years to clear.

Alcoholism

Definition

Alcohol dependence (alcoholism) is a chronic, progressive disease characterized by significant impairment that is directly associated with persistent and excessive alcohol consumption. Impairment may involve physiological, psychological, or social dysfunction.[10]

Genetic Disposition

It has been known for years that alcoholism, like diabetes, runs in families. Several studies suggest that a disposition for developing alcoholism is transmitted genetically.[11,13] Males with alcoholic fathers have been found at highest risk.[14]

A search is under way to identify predisposing factors for alcoholism. Schuckit found that men with family histories of alcoholism had a greater tolerance to alcohol.[15] He also found that men with alcoholic relatives had a more pronounced dopaminergic response to alcohol than did controls.[16] Begleiter found that the electroencephalographic patterns of sons of alcoholics are measurably different from men with no family history of alcoholism.[17] Tabakoff found that, in general, alcohol tends to produce a more severe inhibition of monomine oxidase activity in platelets of alcoholics than in those of nonalcoholic controls.[18]

Types of Alcoholism

Jellinek in 1960 identified five categories of alcoholism, which he referred to as Alpha, Beta, Delta, Gamma, and Epsilon.[19]

1. *Alpha alcoholism.* This type represents a psychological dependence on alcohol to relieve emotional or bodily pain. It is sometimes known as problem drinking. It can progress but often continues in the same way for years. Loss of control and withdrawal symptoms do not occur.
2. *Beta alcoholism.* The person who suffers from this type of alcoholism, for some unknown reason, eventually develops medical complications such as cirrhosis or peripheral neuropathy. Beta alcoholism is not associated with dependence; it can progress.
3. *Gamma alcoholism.* This is the dominant type of alcoholism seen in the United States and is the type recognized by Alcoholics Anonymous. It is characterized by loss of control and physical dependence.
4. *Delta alcoholism.* This is the predominant type of alcoholism in France and other countries where significant wine consumption occurs. People gradually develop tolerance and can control the level of their drinking but cannot stop.

5. *Epsilon alcoholism.* This term refers to periodic alcoholism. Less is known about it than about other types.[19]

Later studies showed that Gamma alcoholism could be divided into two types. Type I individuals develop alcoholism after age 25. They infrequently seek alcohol and are able to abstain. They do not fight or get arrested when drinking. They frequently lose control and suffer from guilt and fear about alcohol dependence. They seldom seek novelty, tend to avoid situations that could result in harm, and respond positively to rewards. In contrast, Type 2 alcoholism usually begins before age 25. These alcoholics commonly seek alcohol spontaneously and are unable to abstain from it. They frequently fight and get arrested when drinking but lose control infrequently. They seldom feel guilt or fear about their alcohol dependence, often seek novelty, do not avoid harm, and respond poorly to rewards. Women tend to develop Type 1 alcoholism; men, on the other hand, develop both types.[14]

Health Consequences

The health consequences of persistent and excessive use of alcohol are numerous and involve virtually every organ system (Table 8.3).

Neurological

Neurological consequences of alcoholism include Wernicke-Korsakoff syndrome, alcoholic dementia, hepatic encephalopathy, cerebellar degeneration, and peripheral neuropathy. Rarer disorders are Marchiafava-Bignami disease and central pontine myelinolysis.

Wernicke-Korsakoff syndrome. Wernicke's encephalopathy most often has an acute onset and is characterized by nystagmus, sixth-nerve palsy, and paralysis of conjugate gaze. Ataxia may be manifested by a wide-based gait, falling, or inability to walk or stand. Patients appear confused. Korsakoff's psychosis is marked by a memory disorder and confabulation in an attempt to cover it up. Patient's are unable to learn new material, such as their physician's name.[20]

Wernicke-Korsakoff's syndrome usually follows years of drinking. Treatment consists of thiamine replacement and supportive care. The oculomotor dysfunction may resolve within minutes to hours, and Wernicke's syndrome may be reversed. Most improvement in Korsakoff's psychosis occurs in the first three months of abstinence but may continue up to five years.[20]

Alcoholic dementia. Characterized by a gradual decline in intellectual function, probably due to neuronal death secondary to long-term alcohol abuse, alcoholic dementia is irreversible. However, its progression ceases with abstinence.[21]

Hepatic encephalopathy. Occurring with severe liver disease, the exact cause of hepatic encephalopathy is unknown but is thought to be failure of the liver to detoxify a group of toxins, including ammonia, that increase cerebral sensitivity. Early signs of hepatic encephalopathy include inappropriate behavior,

TABLE 8.3. Disorders/conditions associated with alcohol dependence.

Neurological	*Metabolic and renal*
Wernicke-Korsakoff syndrome	alcoholic ketoacidosis
alcoholic dementia	hypomagnesemia
cerebellar degeneration	hypocalcemia
hepatic encephalopathy	hypophosphatemia
Marchiafava-Bignami disease	hepatorenal syndrome
central pontine myelinolysis	
peripheral neuropathy	*Dermatological*
	red face and nose
Gastrointestinal	edematous eyelids and injected conjunctiva
fatty liver	intensification of rosacea and rhinophyma
alcoholic hepatitis	scaly skin
cirrhosis	seborrheic dermatitis
gastritis/gastric ulcers	palmar erythema
malabsorption	spider angiomata and ecchymoses
pancreatitis	bruises and cigarette burns
Cardiovascular	*Nutritional*
hypertension	beriberi
cardiomyopathy	riboflavin deficiency
	pyridoxine deficiency
Muscoloskeletal	pellegra
myopathy	scurvy
aseptic necrosis of the hip	
gout	*Cancer*
	oral cavity
Hematological/immunological	esophagus
elevated MCV	liver
anemia	possibly pancreas, colon, rectum, prostate,
leukopenia	stomach, and thyroid gland
coagulation disorders	
increased infection rate	
Endocrine/reproductive	
depressed ADH level	
pseudo–Cushing syndrome	
hypoglycemia	
feminization of males	
loss of libido	
impotency	
altered sperm function	

change in sleep habits, and mood swings, including agitation, depression, and apathy. If early hepatic encephalopathy is left untreated, confusion, disorientation, depressed mental status, asterixis, and coma occur. Neurological signs include tremor, rigidity, and hyperreflexia. Signs of chronic liver disease (caput medusa, spider angiomata, palmar erythema) are present. Laboratory data that may be helpful include abnormal liver enzyme values, hypoalbuminemia, and prolonged prothrombin time. The arterial ammonia level may not correspond to the degree of encephalopathy.[21]

Hepatic encephalopathy is reversible in most patients, although the mortality rate is high once coma develops. Treatment includes avoidance of sedative-hypnotic medications, dietary protein restriction to 30 to 40 grams a day, neomycin to reduce the number of colonic bacteria that produce ammonia, and lactulose, which acidifies bowel contents and reduces back diffusion of ammonia. Lactulose is given in sufficient dose to achieve three to four loose bowel movements per day.[21]

Cerebellar degeneration. Alcoholic cerebellar degeneration is characterized by truncal ataxia and a wide-based stance and gait. The upper extremities are less affected than the lower ones. The exact cause is unknown. Nutritional deficiencies may play a role. Abstinence from alcohol and treatment of the nutritional deficiencies may result in some improvement over several months.[21]

Marchiafavi-Bignami disease. This is a rare disease involving primary degeneration of the corpus callosum. It occurs almost exclusively in middle-aged or elderly alcoholic Italian men who drink wine. It is characterized by severe, nonspecific mental symptoms. The diagnosis is usually made at autopsy.[20]

Central pontine myelinolysis. Patients who have central pontine myelinolysis have pseudobulbar palsy and quadriplegia. Death usually occurs within a few days or weeks. The disease is not limited to alcoholics.[20]

Peripheral neuropathy. The peripheral neuropathy of alcohol dependence commonly occurs as a polyneuropathy. Symmetric impairment or loss of tendon reflexes, sensation, and motor function occurs. The proximal portions of the limbs are usually less affected than the distal segments, especially the legs. The cause may be the toxic effect of ingested alcohol, nutritional deficiency, or both. The neuropathy usually appears after many years of excessive drinking. The first symptom is often a dull or burning pain in the feet, which may be accompanied by muscle tenderness and superficial hyperesthesia. Stroking the soles may produce exquisite pain, and even the touch of bedcovers may be painful. The initial phase of pain and hyperalgesia is followed by a decrease in tactile and deep sensibility, sometimes progressing to a complete sensory loss in a stocking-glove distribution. Weakness of the legs, foot drop, and ataxic walking usually follow the original sensory manifestations. Deep tendon reflexes disappear, especially at the ankles.[20]

Despite treatment (abstinence, balanced diet, thiamine) improvement of alcoholic peripheral neuropathy is slow.[20]

Alcoholics may also suffer from a local pressure neuropathy when they pass out with their limbs in an unusual position. The radial and peroneal nerves are particularly susceptible. Wristdrop is a common manifestation of pressure neuropathy.[20]

Gastrointestinal

Gastrointestinal manifestations of alcohol dependence may involve the liver, stomach, esophagus, small bowel, and pancreas.

Fatty liver. Fat accumulation in the liver is an early effect of alcohol and can occur with modest consumption. It is thought to result from alteration of the NADH/NAD ratio that occurs when alcohol is metabolized by the alcohol dehydrogenase pathway. Patients with fatty liver may have no complaints or may complain of right upper quadrant tenderness, nausea, vomiting, or anorexia. Most patients have hepatomegally. It is reversible with abstinence; however, in alcoholics who continue to drink, it may progress to alcoholic hepatitis.[22]

Alcoholic hepatitis. Alcoholic hepatitis occurs after chronic, excessive consumption of alcohol. It frequently coexists with fatty liver or cirrhosis. Patients may be asymptomatic or ill with anorexia, weight loss, abdominal pain, fever, and chills. Most have hepatomegally. Less often, they exhibit jaundice, ascites, and spider angiomata. Laboratory data may reveal a mildly to moderately elevated bilirubin, elevated transaminases with AST in the range of 100 to 500, and an elevated alkaline phosphatase. Serum proteins are frequently depressed and serum globulins elevated. Prothrombin time may be prolonged.[22]

Therapy for alcoholic hepatitis is primarily supportive. Most patients have a mild course and recover in six weeks to six months with abstinence. As many as 50 percent of patients who continue to drink develop cirrhosis.[22]

Cirrhosis. Alcoholic (Laennec's) cirrhosis develops in a moderate percentage of alcoholics. It is distinguished histologically by fibrosis and regeneration of liver tissue. Signs and symptoms include anorexia, weight loss, weakness, fatigability, jaundice, low-grade fever, and abdominal discomfort. Hepatic encephalopathy, ascites, splenomegaly, esophageal varices, and hemorrhoids may occur.[7]

Laboratory studies are nonspecific. Transaminases are moderately elevated, serum albumin is low, and prothrombin time is prolonged.[10]

Complications of alcoholic cirrhosis are numerable. They include esophageal varices and variceal bleeding, ascites, portal hypertension, hepatorenal syndrome, spontaneous bacterial peritonitis, and hepatic encephalopathy.[22]

Treatment of the ascites includes bed rest, dietary restriction to 2 grams of sodium a day, fluid restriction to 2 liters a day, and treatment with spironolactone (Aldactone), 25 to 50 mg orally four times a day, to achieve a daily weight loss of 1 kilogram. The mortality from cirrhosis is significant. The most important treatment is for the patient to stop drinking.[23]

Esophagitis. Alcohol exposure causes lower esophageal sphincter pressure to decrease and esophageal peristalsis to be depressed. Alcohol also damages the esophageal mucosa. The impaired lower esophageal sphincter function increases the likelihood of gastroesophageal reflux that, coupled with defective esophageal clearance, predisposes alcoholics to chronic esophagitis and esophageal stricture. Treatment for esophagitis is abstinence and conventional antacid and antireflux regimens.[23]

Gastritis and gastric ulcers. High concentrations of alcohol suppress motor function of the stomach, resulting in delayed gastric emptying. This contributes to disruption of gastric mucosa by alcohol. As a result, gastritis is a frequent consequence of excessive alcohol ingestion. Patients may exhibit anorexia, vomiting, epigastric pain, and even hemorrhage. With treatment (abstinence, antacids, H_2 blocking agents), the symptoms of gastritis usually resolve in a few hours to two days.[23]

The relationship between alcohol consumption and gastric ulcers is less clear. A variety of other factors, including smoking, may be predisposing factors.[23]

The alcoholic with upper gastrointestinal bleeding presents a challenge. The differential diagnosis includes esophageal varices, esophagitis, Mallory-Weiss tears, gastritis, or peptic ulcer disease.[23]

Small intestine effects. Alcohol affects the small intestine in a number of ways. It increases small bowel motility and decreases transit time. It causes reversible disruption of the intestinal brush border enzyme system, with depression of disaccharidase activity. As a result, significant lactose intolerance may occur. Disruption of active transport occurs, with impaired absorption of water, sodium, glucose, and amino acids. Malabsorption of folate, vitamin B_{12}, thiamine and calcium are also common. Shortened intestinal transit time, lactose intolerance, and impaired water and electrolyte absorption account for the frequent occurrence of diarrhea in the alcoholic.[23]

Pancreatitis. Acute pancreatitis due to alcohol consumption is characterized by severe, poorly localized upper abdominal pain associated with nausea and vomiting. The pain may radiate to the back and may be relieved somewhat by leaning forward. It is usually precipitated by a drinking binge. Physical examination may reveal low-grade or moderate fever, tachycardia, and relatively mild abdominal tenderness to palpation, given the severity of the pain. Serum amylase may be elevated; however, it is not diagnostic. Serum lipase remains elevated longer and may be helpful when serum amylase is within normal limits.[23]

Chronic pancreatitis may be associated with severe episodes of abdominal pain or insidiously increasing abdominal discomfort. Malabsorption, abnormal glucose tolerance test, or diabetes may occur. Pancreatic calcification on plain abdominal X ray strongly suggests a diagnosis of chronic pancreatitis but is not diagnostic. The presentation of the patient must be considered.[23]

Management of mild cases of acute pancreatitis involves limiting the inflammatory process and controlling pain. Oral feedings are withheld to reduce pancreatic secretions. Nasogastric suction offers no added benefit in the absence of vomiting or abdominal distention. Narcotic analgesics are usually required to control pain. Conservative management leads to resolution of the acute attack in two to four days. More severe cases may be complicated by hypotension and shock, pancreatic abscesses, or pseudocysts; these last two complications may require surgery.[23]

Management of chronic pancreatitis centers around abstinence, pain control, and treatment of complications. Steatorrhea is improved with pancreatic enzyme replacement and dietary fat restriction.[23]

Cardiovascular

Cardiovascular complications of alcohol dependence include hypertension and cardiomyopathy.

Hypertension. Excessive alcohol consumption often is a factor in drinkers with mild to moderate hypertension. It may also interfere with the efficacy of medical therapy. It is not unusual for hypertensive alcoholic patients to become normotensive with abstinence. Alcohol should always be kept in mind as a correctable factor that may be contributing to a patient's hypertension or interfering with treatment.[6,10]

Cardiomyopathy. Development of alcoholic cardiac disease does not always depend on nutritional deficiencies. The well-nourished alcoholic may develop cardiac disease related directly to the biochemical and ultrastructural effects of alcohol. The clinical picture of alcoholic cardiomyopathy is nonspecific. Diagnosis is based on the alcohol history and the findings of biventricular enlargement, enlarged cardiac silhouette on chest X ray, and abnormal electrocardiogram.[6,10]

Alcoholic cardiomyopathy should be considered in all patients under 50 years of age who experience heart failure. Arrhythmias are common, particularly after heavy binges. The so-called holiday heart syndrome, typically occurring after weekend or holiday binges, refers to atrial fibrillation, atrial flutter, premature ventricular beats, or other evidence of cardiac irritability. Once the clinical picture of congestive cardiomyopathy appears, the damage is likely to be permanent.[6]

Musculoskeletal

Musculoskeletal effects of alcoholism include myopathy, aseptic necrosis of the hip, and gout.

Myopathy. Myopathy occurs in an acute and in a chronic form. Acute alcoholic myopathy is rare but may develop after a sustained episode of heavy drinking. It is characterized by swollen, extremely painful, and exquisitely tender muscles, as well as severe proximal muscle weakness. Myoglobinuria resulting from acute alcoholic myopathy is an uncommon but important cause of renal failure. The pain of acute alcoholic myopathy usually resolves after a few days, but the accompanying weakness may last longer. The damage to muscle cells results in leakage of cellular enzymes, reflected by elevation of serum aldolase, serum lactate dehydrogenase (LDH), and the MM izoenzyme of creatine kinase.[24]

Chronic alcoholic myopathy is a reversible atrophy of skeletal muscle fibers. It occurs after several years of heavy drinking. The condition is characterized by progressive, usually painless wasting and weakness of the proximal muscle groups, particularly in the lower extremities. Symptoms include difficulty in climbing stairs and in rising from a squatting position.[24]

In general, abstinence produces overall improvement in both acute and chronic alcohol-induced myopathies. An exercise program to improve strength and endurance, particularly in proximal muscles, can be helpful.[24]

Aseptic necrosis of the hip.   Although uncommon, this condition should be considered in alcoholics who have hip or knee pain unrelated to trauma, particularly if they are nonresponsive to anti-inflammatory drugs. The mechanism is uncertain. An X ray or bone scan will confirm the diagnosis.[24]

Gout.   Persistent and excessive consumption of alcohol raises the serum uric acid level and may precipitate gouty attacks or make preexisting gout difficult to control. Alcohol dependence should be considered in patients with gout.[10]

Hematological/Immunological

Hematological abnormalities encountered in alcoholics include elevated mean cell volume (MCV), anemia, leukopenia, and coagulation problems. The hematological consequences come from nutritional deficiencies, liver disease, and the toxic effect of alcohol on bone marrow. In addition, the increased infection rate among alcoholics may be, in part, due to suppression of the immune system.[25]

Elevated MCV.   An elevated MCV, in the absence of anemia, should alert the physician to the possibility of alcoholism. Typically an alcoholic's MCV may be in the range of 100 to 115 cu microns (normal 80 to 94). After heavy drinking ceases, the MCV may remain elevated for up to two months. The mechanism of the macrocytosis of alcoholism is unknown.[6,10]

Anemia.   Anemia in the alcoholic can be hemorrhagic, hemolytic, hypoplastic, or a combination of these. Bleeding can result from gastrointestinal complications or coagulation defects. Hemolytic anemia is the result of liver disease and portal hypertension. Anemia is compounded in alcoholics by the hypoplastic effect of alcohol on bone marrow suppression and folic acid deficiency. Unlike the macrocytosis discussed above, the macrocytosis of folic acid deficiency is accompanied by hypersegmented neutrophils. The anemia of folic acid deficiency rapidly responds to dietary therapy. Siderblastic anemia, with elevated serum iron levels, may also occur in the alcoholic. It may be associated with pyridoxine deficiency.[6,10]

Leukopenia.   Leukopenia secondary to alcoholism may occur as the result of folate deficiency, hypersplenism, or a direct effect of alcohol on the bone marrow. When the condition is due to suppression of the bone marrow, a patient's white count usually reaches a normal level in one to two weeks after he or she stops drinking alcohol.[6,10]

Coagulation disorders.   Coagulation disorders are common with cirrhosis because of the body's diminished production of the vitamin K–dependent factors (VII, IX, X, prothrombin). Disseminated intravascular coagulation (DIC) may also be a problem. Platelet counts may be suppressed secondary to hypersplenism, folic acid deficiency, and a direct effect of alcohol to decreased platelet production and shorten platelet survival time. When the thrombocytopenia is due to the direct effect of alcohol, the platelet count usually returns to normal within a week or two of cessation of alcohol consumption.[6,10]

Increased infection rate.   Alcohol impairs the immune system and lowers resistance to infection. It adversely affects the bactericidal activity of polymorphonuclear leukocytes and the ability of alveolar macrophages to cleanse the tracheobronchial tree. As a result, alcoholics are at an increased risk for pulmonary infections, in particular gram-negative and anaerobic aspiration pneumonias and lung abscesses. Tuberculosis is also associated with alcoholism.[6,10]

Endocrine/Reproductive

A variety of endocrine and reproductive disorders occur as a result of excessive alcohol consumption.

Endocrine.   Alcohol adversely affects the endocrine system; it inhibits the posterior-hypophyseal system. Following alcohol ingestion, antidiuretic hormone (ADH) level falls, accounting for the diuretic effect of alcohol. Alcohol ingestion can cause hypoglycemia by interfering with gluconeogenesis. Depleted glycogen stores from malnutrition may contribute to alcoholic hypoglycemia. Alcohol also causes a pseudo-Cushing's syndrome. These patients develop moon faces, truncal obesity, buffalo humps, proximal muscle weakness, and osteoporosis. The biochemical evidence of Cushing's syndrome disappears within days to weeks after drinking stops.[6,10]

Reproductive.   Alcohol is toxic to the testes, the pituitary, and the hypothalamus. This results in reduced beard growth, loss of libido, impotency, and abnormal sperm function. Menstrual disturbances and infertility may occur. Testicular atrophy occurs in severe cases. With the development of cirrhosis, feminization occurs, including gynecomastia and redistribution of body hair and fat.[6,10]

Metabolic and Renal

Metabolic disturbances from excessive alcohol consumption include alcoholic ketoacidosis, hypomagnesemia, hypocalcemia, and hypophosphotemia. The major renal effect is the hepatorenal syndrome.

Alcoholic ketoacidosis.   Alcoholic ketoacidosis is seen in heavy drinkers who have been vomiting and have eaten little or no food for several days. The acetaldehyde produced from alcohol by the liver stimulates the hepatic production of ketoacids (beta-hydroxybutyrate, acetoacetic acid). Since ketoacids are not readily determined, the diagnosis of ketoacidosis should be suspected in any alcoholic who has metabolic acidosis with an increased anion gap.[26]

Hypomagnesemia.   Hypomagnesemia often accompanies alcoholism. It may result in neuromuscular irritability, fatigue, and muscle weakness. Maintenance of a normal serum magnesium level depends on renal tubular absorption of a considerable amount of magnesium daily. Alcohol apparently interferes with this mechanism, allowing the loss of increased amounts of magnesium in the urine and a corresponding decline in serum magnesium concentration. Alcoholism also can cause phosphate depletion, which results in renal tubular magnesium wasting, further complicating the hypomagnesemia. Hypomagnesemia, in turn, causes renal potassium wasting.[26]

Hypocalcemia. The hypocalcemia of alcoholism results from at least three factors. First, magnesium depletion suppresses parathyroid hormone secretion, and the resulting hypoparathyroidism produces a fall in serum calcium concentration. Second, chronic liver disease can impair conversion of vitamin D to its active form, dihydroxycholecalciferol. Third, poor dietary intake can reduce the amount of vitamin D available for absorption in the small intestine.[26]

Hypophosphatemia. Phosphate depletion in alcoholics occurs for several reasons: gastrointestinal malabsorption of phosphate due to ketoacidosis, an increased parathyroid hormone secretion secondary to hypomagnesemia, and, most importantly, a shift of phosphate into cells when glucose is administered to correct hypoglycemia. Hypophosphatemia due to an isolated dietary deficiency does not occur. Severe hypophosphatemia (less than 1 mg/dL) results in severe neuromuscular symptoms. Ptosis, dysarthria, difficulty in swallowing, paresthesias, seizures, proximal muscle myopathy with rhabdomyolysis, depressed left ventricular function, hemolysis, and respiratory failure may occur. The phosphate depletion syndrome can mimic delirium tremens, but patients do not have hallucinations.[26]

Hepatorenal syndrome. Patients with advanced cirrhosis and hepatic insufficiency may develop renal failure — that is, the hepatorenal syndrome. When the kidneys of patients dying of hepatorenal syndrome are transplanted into hosts with normal hepatic function, they work normally. Conversely, when patients with hepatorenal syndrome undergo liver transplantation, the kidneys regain their normal function. The cause of hepatorenal syndrome is unknown but is thought to result from intense renal vasoconstriction. A small gastrointestinal bleed, sepsis, or injudicious use of a loop diuretic may precipitate the renal failure. Prognosis is extremely poor.[26]

Dermatological

A variety of dermatological problems are caused by alcoholism. A common manifestation is the reddened face and nose, the edematous eyelids, and injected conjunctiva so often seen in alcoholics. Rosacea and rhinophyma, characterized by rose-red papules and nodules distributed across the face and nose, are intensified by alcoholism. In addition, scaly skin and seborrheic dermatitis are common. Cigarette burns and bruises are common. Spider angiomata, palmar erethema, and ecchymoses occur with advanced liver disease.[6,10]

Nutritional

Alcohol impairs nutrition in a variety of ways. It suppresses the appetite, both directly and as a result of gastritis, and it damages the organs of digestion — the liver, the pancreas, and the small intestine.

Alcohol is highly caloric. For example, a shot of liquor ($1\frac{1}{2}$ ounces) has 105 calories. These are empty calories—that is, they contain none of the nutritive vitamins, minerals, or amino acids required by the body. It is not unusual for half of an alcoholic's calories to be obtained from alcohol. This contributes to malnutrition.[2]

In advanced stages of alcoholism many specific syndromes resulting from vitamin deficiencies can be identified.

Beriberi.   Thiamine deficiency can cause neurological disease (dry beriberi) and cardiac disease (wet beriberi). The neurological findings of thiamine deficiency include peripheral neuropathy and Wernicke-Korsakoff syndrome. The cardiac manifestations are the result of peripheral vasodilation, leading to vascular congestion, edema, and effusions.[6]

Riboflavin deficiency.   Riboflavin deficiency results in cheilosis, stomatitis, seborrheic dermatitis, and conjunctivitis. Photophobia, lacrimation, and corneal neovascularization may occur.[6]

Pyridoxine deficiency.   Alcohol interferes with the metabolism of pyridoxine, resulting in sideroblastic anemia and neuritis.[6]

Pellagra.   Pellagra is due to niacin deficiency and is characterized by dermatitis, diarrhea, and dementia. The dermatitis is due to a photosensitivity reaction, and the diarrhea results from a generalized inflammation of the gastrointestinal tract. In women, it may also involve the vagina. The intellectual changes of pellegra are nonspecific. A patient may be disoriented or psychotic.[6]

Scurvy.   Scurvy results from vitamin C deficiency. Symptoms include lassitude, irritability, and generalized aches and pains. Characteristic changes in the skin occur. These consist of perifollicular hyperkeratotic papules, especially on the posterior thighs. The hairs within these follicles coil inward and become buried, and the perifolicular zones become hemorrhagic. Generalized bleeding into the skin and soft tissue is present in advanced scurvy. Gums become swollen, spongy, friable, and bleed easily.[6]

Cancer

Many mechanisms have been proposed to explain the role of alcohol in producing cancer in specific sites in the body. These include the suggestion that alcohol itself is a carcinogen or that it is a cocarcinogen that enhances the effects of carcinogens. Alternately, the cirrhotic liver may not be able to detoxify circulating carcinogens. Finally, there is the possibility that alcohol itself does not promote the development of cancer but that, instead, some contaminant in alcoholic beverages acts as the carcinogen.[6]

The fact that 85 percent of alcoholics smoke complicates the question of etiology of many cancers. Oral and esophageal cancers seem to be related more to drinking than smoking. However, smoking acts synergistically in producing these tumors. The risk of developing laryngeal cancer, on the other hand, is more strongly associated with smoking. Alcohol may act as a cocarcinogen with hepatitis B virus in producing hepatocellular carcinoma (hepatoma), and alcohol may increase the risk of breast cancer in women. The role of alcohol in the development of pancreatic, colon, rectum, prostate, stomach, and thyroid cancers is unclear.[6]

Diagnosis and Management

Intoxication

Diagnosis

Almost everyone recognizes the signs and symptoms of alcohol intoxication. They consist of slurred speech, confusion, disorientation, sedation, difficulty thinking, slowness of speech and comprehension, and the smell of alcohol on the breath. A breathalyzer test or blood alcohol level may be helpful. In most states individuals with a blood alcohol level of 0.10 gm/100 ml or higher are considered legally drunk.

Management

Treatment of alcohol intoxication usually consists of allowing the individual to sleep it off.

Overdose

Diagnosis

Patients suffering from alcohol overdose may be stuporous or comatose. In sufficiently high levels, alcohol depresses the respiratory center, and respiratory and cardiovascular collapse may occur. The smell of alcohol is virtually always present, and a blood alcohol level is significantly elevated.

Management

Management of alcohol overdose consists of respiratory and cardiovascular support. Metabolic acidosis and hypoglycemia, when present, should be corrected. Hemodialysis effectively removes alcohol from the body. To date, no agent has been found to reverse the acute effects of alcohol.

Alcohol Dependence

Diagnosis

Patients who meet the definition of alcohol dependence given earlier are considered to be alcoholic. Screening tests, medical history, drinking history, family history, physical examination, and laboratory studies may be helpful (see Chapter 2).[10]

Management

Treatment of alcohol dependence involves detoxification, treatment of medical consequences, rehabilitation, and aftercare (see Chapter 3).

Abstinence Syndrome

The major goals in the management of alcohol abstinence syndrome are to prevent progression to more serious stages of withdrawal, thereby preventing delirium, seizures, or cardiac arrhythmias; to make patients more comfortable; and to correct nutritional deficiencies.

Detoxification

Vital signs (pulse, blood pressure, temperature) should be monitored closely. Patients should be given a multivitamin tablet containing zinc once or twice a day. The zinc may ensure continued function of alcohol dehydrogenase. Patients are given thiamine immediately in a dose of 100 mg intramuscularly and then orally once or twice a day for the duration of detoxification. They should be given thiamine initially prior to a glucose load to prevent precipitation of Wernicke-Korsakoff syndrome. Folic acid, 1 mg orally, may be given daily to correct folate deficiency. Magnesium deficiency, in the presence of good renal function, can be corrected by administration of a 50 percent solution of magnesium sulfate, 2 ml intramuscularly every 6 hours for 48 hours. If a patient requires an intravenous line, magnesium sulfate can be given by this route. Magnesium can also be given orally as the glucoheptonate salt, 15 ml three times a day. Magnesium replacement may help to prevent seizures. Hypocalcemia can be corrected by administration of 10 ml of 10 percent calcium gluconate solution or until symptoms clear or the serum calcium level rises above 7.5 mg/dL. Hypophosphatemia can be corrected by adding 20 to 40 mmol of potassium phosphate to each liter of intravenous fluid. Most alcoholics are initially overhydrated and, thus, do not require parenteral hydration. Patients usually experience diuresis during the first two days of detoxification and may lose 1 to 2 kg of body weight. Those with excessive vomiting, however, may be dehydrated and require fluid replacement.[5,8,26-28]

Drug treatment for detoxification involves two basic principles: substituting another sedative-hynotic agent for alcohol (benzodiazepine, barbiturate, paraldehyde) and gradually tapering the dose. Substituting another sedative-hynotic for alcohol is based on the principle of cross-tolerance—that is, benzodiazepines, barbiturates, and paraldehyde are pharmacological substitutes for alcohol. Therapy should be initiated early in the course of withdrawal. Chlordiazepoxide (Librium), a long-acting benzodiazepine, is the most commonly used drug for detoxification. It should be given initially in doses of 75 to 100 mg orally every four to six hours as needed, and then tapered over the next three to five days. Diazepam (Valium), another benzodiazepine with a long half-life, is also very effective. The dose should be reduced and the dosing interval increased for elderly patients and patients with severe liver dysfunction. Alternatively, shorter-acting benzodiazepines, such as oxazepam (Serax) or lorazepam (Ativan), can be used. Most benzodiazepines, with the exception of lorazepam, are irradically absorbed from intramuscular sites. Therefore, intramuscular injection of most benzodiazepines should be limited to the first one or two doses. When patients cannot take medications orally, they can be given intravenously.[8-9,27]

Barbiturates, especially the longer acting ones such as phenobarbital, are good alternatives to benzodiazepines. When used, phenobarbital should be started in a dose of 30 to 60 mg every six hours and then tapered over three to five days. Paraldehyde, for the most part, has been replaced by benzodiazepines for treatment of the alcohol abstinence syndrome. When used, the dose is 10 ml orally in orange juice or 10 ml intramuscularly every four hours as needed. In addition to a benzodiazepine, elderly patients undergoing hard withdrawal or patients with a history of angina or myocardial infarction can be treated with propranalol (Inderal), 20 mg every 6 hours for 48 hours, to reduce the severity of the withdrawal syndrome. Propranalol is contraindicated in patients with congestive heart failure, asthma, and diabetes mellitus. Nausea and vomiting can be controlled with promethazine (Phenergan), 25 to 50 mg by mouth, by intramuscular injection, or by suppository every six hours as needed. Haloperidol (Haldol) can be used in small doses (1 to 2 mg orally every four hours) as needed to control alcoholic hallucinosis.[8-9,27]

Seizures

Patients may suffer withdrawal seizures in the first 48 hours after they cut down or take the last drink; patients rarely start having them after 96 hours from last taking a drink. In patients with no history of seizures, either withdrawal or idiopathic, the probability of having withdrawal seizures is so low that prophylaxis with anticonvulsant medication is unwarranted. Similarly, seizures can usually be prevented, even in patients with a history of withdrawal seizures, by liberal use of the benzodiazepine detoxifying agent and correction of magnesium deficiency if one is present. Prophylaxis with an anticonvulsant in addition to the benzodiazepine, however, may be somewhat more effective in preventing withdrawal seizures than the benzodiazepine alone. If desired, phenytoin (Dilantin), 100 mg orally every eight hours, can be administered. Patients with no prior history of withdrawal seizures who develop them need full neurological workups. Diazepam should be administered by slow intravenous push, 5 to 20 mg, in the rare patient who develops status epilepticus during withdrawal.[8]

Delirium Tremens

Delirium tremens (DTs) is a medical emergency. Patients with DTs should be admitted to intensive care units where they can be given respiratory and circulatory support if they need them. An intravenous access should be established.

Fluid and electrolyte disturbances, when present, should be corrected. Patients should not be restrained but should be sedated sufficiently to prevent them from harming themselves.[8]

Methyl Alcohol and Ethylene Glycol Toxicity

Other alcohols have wide applications, and alcoholics sometimes consume them when ethanol is not available. Two of the more common ones are methyl alcohol (methanol), which is found in canned heat and windshield washing materials, and ethylene glycol, which is most commonly found in antifreeze. Methanol is primarily oxidized to formaldehyde, formic acid, and carbon dioxide by the alcohol dehydrogenase pathway. Toxicity is due to products of metabolism rather than the methanol itself. Ethylene glycol is primarily oxidized to aldehydes, acids, and oxylate by the same pathway as methanol. The oxylate may deposit in the renal tubules, causing acute renal failure.[29]

Diagnosis

The diagnosis of methanol toxicity is usually based on a history of alcoholism and typical signs and symptoms. Patients commonly complain of visual disturbances, which they describe as like being in a snowstorm or as having blurred vision. The odor of formaldehyde may be present on patients' breath or in their urine. Metabolic acidosis, with elevated anion and osmolar gaps, may be present. The development of bradycardia, prolonged coma, seizures, and resistant acidosis all indicate a poor prognosis. A serum methanol level should be obtained.[5]

Ethylene glycol toxicity usually results in initial central nervous system excitation followed by depression. This may be followed by severe acidosis and then renal insufficiency. Increased muscle enzymes and hypocalcemia may occur. Anion and osmolar gaps may also be present, as well as oxylate crystals in the urine. Visual symptoms do not occur.[5,29]

Management

Treatment of methanol and ethylene glycol toxicity includes suppression of their metabolism by ethanol infusion, dialysis, and alkalinization to counteract the metabolic acidosis. Ethanol competes with methanol and ethylene glycol in the alcohol dehydrogenase pathway to reduce production of the toxic breakdown products. It may be infused intravenously to maintain the serum ethanol level at 0.10 gm/100 ml. Blood sugar should be monitored and glucose infused when necessary.[5,29]

References

1. Ritchie, J. M. The aliphatic alcohols. In *Goodman and Gilman's The Pharmacological Basis of Therapeutics*. Ed. by A. G. Gilman, L. S. Goodman, T. W. Rall, F. Murad. Macmillan, New York, 1985, pp. 372–384.

2. Poley, W., G. Lea, and G. Vibe. Alcohol in society. In *Alcoholism Treatment Manual.* Gardner Press, New York, 1979, pp. 1–15.

3. Royce, J. E. Sociocultural aspects. In *Alcohol Problems and Alcoholism.* Free Press, New York, 1981, pp. 33–47.

4. Poley, W., G. Lea, and G. Vibe. Alcohol and its effects on the individual. In *Alcoholism Treatment Manual.* Gardner Press, New York, 1979, pp. 17–31.

5. Lee, N. M., and C. E. Becker. The alcohols. In *Basic and Clinical Pharmacology.* Ed. by B. G. Katzung. Appleton and Lange, Norwalk, Connecticut, 1987, pp. 254–261.

6. Ende, J. Nutritional status, cardiovascular, hematologic, reproductive, and musculoskeletal systems. In *Alcoholism: A Guide for the Primary Care Physician.* Springer-Verlag, New York, 1987, pp. 134–144.

7. Saxe, T. G. Drug-alcohol interactions. *American Family Physician,* 33:159–162, 1986.

8. Landers, D. F. Alcohol withdrawal syndrome. *American Family Physician,* 27:114–118, 1983.

9. Behnke, H. Recognition and management of alcohol withdrawal syndrome. *Hospital Practice,* November, 1976, pp. 79–84.

10. Milhorn, H. T., Jr. The diagnosis of alcoholism. *American Family Physician,* 37:175–193, 1988.

11. Schuckit, M. A. Genetics and the risk of alcoholism. *Journal of the American Medical Association,* 254:2614–2617, 1988.

12. Schuckit, M. A. The importance of genetic factors in alcoholism. *Drug Abuse and Alcoholism Newsletter,* Vista Hill Foundation, vol. 18, no. 1, 1989.

13. Blum, K., E. P. Noble, P. J. Sheridan, et al. Allelic association of human dopamine D_2 receptor gene in alcoholism. *JAMA,* 263:2055–2060, 1990.

14. Cloninger, C. R. Neurogenetic adaptive mechanisms in alcoholism. *Science,* 236:410–416, 1987.

15. Schuckit, M. A., and E. O. Gold. A simultaneous evaluation of multiple markers of ethanol/placebo challenges in sons of alcoholics and controls. *General Psychiatry,* 45:211–216, 1988.

16. Schuckit, M. A., D. C. Parker, and L. R. Rossman. Ethanol-related prolactin responses and risk for alcoholism. *Biological Psychiatry,* 18:1153–1159, 1983.

17. Begleider, H., B. Porjesz, B. Bihari, and B. Kissin. Event-related brain potentials in boys at risk for alcoholism. *Science,* 225:1493–1495, 1984.

18. Tabokoff, B., P. L. Hoffman, J. M. Lee, T. Saito, B. Willard, and F. DeLeon-Jones. Differences in platelet enzyme activity between alcoholics and nonalcoholics. *New England Journal of Medicine,* 318:134–139, 1988.

19. Jellinek, E. M. *The Disease Concept of Alcoholism.* Hillhouse, New Haven, Connecticut, 1960.

20. Packard, R. C. The neurological consequences of alcoholism. *American Family Physician,* 14:111–115, 1976.

21. Hesse, K., and J. Savitsky. The elderly. In *Alcoholism: A Guide for the Primary Care Physician.* Ed. by H. N. Barnes, M. D. Aronson, and T. L. Delbanco. Springer-Verlag, New York, 1987, pp. 167–175.

22. Moulton, A. W., and M. G. Cyr. The liver. In *Alcoholism: A Guide for the Primary Care Physician.* Ed. by H. N. Barnes, M. D. Aronson, and T. L. Delbanco. Springer-Verlag, 1987, pp. 119–126.

23. Cyr, M. G., and A. W. Moulton. The gastrointestinal tract and pancreas. In *Alcoholism: A Practical Treatment Guide.* Ed. by H. N. Barnes, M. D. Aronson, and T. L. Delbanco. Springer-Verlag, 1987, pp. 119–126.

24. Hodges, D. L., V. N. Kumar, and J. B. Redford. Effects of Alcohol on Bone, Muscle and Nerve. *American Family Physician,* 34:149–156, 1986.
25. Cohen, S. Alcohol and the immune system. *Drug Abuse and Alcoholism Newsletter,* Vista Hill Foundation, vol. 16, no. 5, 1987.
26. Daley, J., and J. T. Harrington. Metabolic and renal effects of alcohol. In *Alcoholism: A Guide for the Primary Care Physician.* Ed. by H. N. Barnes, M. D. Aronson, and T. L. Delbanco. Springer-Verlag, New York, 1987, pp. 145–150.
27. Miller, G. W. Principles of alcohol detoxification. *American Family Physician,* 30:145–148, 1984.
28. Embry, C. K., and S. Lippmann. Use of magnesium sulfate in alcohol withdrawal. *American Family Physician,* 35:167–170, 1987.
29. Brown, C. G., T. Trumbull, W. Klein-Schwartz, and J. D. Walker. Ethylene glycol poisoning. *Annals of Emergency Medicine,* 12:501–506, 1983.

CHAPTER 9

CNS Depressants: Barbiturates, Barbiturate-like Drugs, Meprobamate, Chloral Hydrate, Paraldehyde

In addition to alcohol, drugs that depress the central nervous system include the barbiturates, barbiturate-like drugs, meprobamate, chloral hydrate, paraldehyde, and benzodiazepines. These drugs are mainly used to calm and relax patients (sedatives) or to induce sleep in them (hynotics). They are collectively known as sedative-hynotics. The benzodiazepines are discussed in Chapter 10.

Barbiturates

History

The first barbiturate, barbital, was sensitized from barbituric acid in 1864. It was first manufactured and used in medicine in 1882 and was released under the trade name Veronal in 1903. It was used to induce sleep. Phenobarbital, a second derivative of barbituric acid, was introduced under the trade name Luminal in 1912. In the 1930s, barbiturates were widely prescribed in the United States. In the 1940s studies began to show that they were addicting and could cause withdrawal symptoms when patients stopped taking them. In 1942, states began passing laws against nonprescription barbiturate use, and the black market became profitable. In the 1950s, barbiturates became one of the major abused drugs in the United States, and in the 1960s their use spread to young people. Despite a decline in their use, they were still widely prescribed and abused in the 1970s and 1980s. The benzodiazepines, for the most part, have replaced barbiturates for most medicinal uses.[1-2]

Pharmacology

Classifications

A large number of barbiturates are in use today (Table 9.1). They are classified as ultrashort-acting (thiopental, methohexital), short- to intermediate-acting (amobarbital, aprobarbital, butabarbital, butalbital, pentobarbital, secobarbital), and long-acting (phenobarbital, mephobarbital). Tuinal is a combination of

TABLE 9.1. The barbiturates.

Generic name	Trade name	Half-life (hours)
Ultrashort-acting		
thiopental	Pentothal	3–4
methohexital	Brevital	3–4
Short- to intermediate-acting		
amobarbital	Amytal	8–42
aprobarbital	Alurate	14–34
butabarbital	Butisol	34–42
butalbital	Fiorinal, Esgic, Axotal	35 (avg.)
pentobarbital	Nembutal	15–48
secobarbital	Seconal	15–40
amobarbital + secobarbital	Tuinal	8–42
Long-acting		
mephobarbital	Mebaral	11–67
phenobarbital	Luminal	80–120

amobarbital and secobarbital. The ultrashort-acting barbiturates produce anesthesia within one minute of administration. Their rapid onset and brief duration of action make them undesirable as drugs of abuse. The intermediate-acting barbiturates are the most abused. With oral administration, their onset of action is 20 to 40 minutes and their effects last four to six hours. They are medically useful as sedatives and hypnotics. The long-acting barbiturates have onset times of up to one to two hours and are effective for up to 16 hours. They are medically useful as sedatives, hypnotics, and anticonvulsants. They are not usually abused because of their slow onset of action. Barbiturates are known in the drug culture by a variety of names (Table 9.2).

Pharmacokinetics

The barbiturates are usually administered orally, except when they are given intravenously to control seizures and as general anesthetics. When taken orally, the drugs are absorbed in the intestines; food in the stomach decreases absorp-

TABLE 9.2. Street/slang names for barbiturates.

Drug	Street/slang names
Amytal	bluebirds, blue devils, blue heavens, blues, blue tips, blue dolls, blue bullets
Luminal	purple hearts
Nembutal	nebbies, nimbies, yellow jackets, yellows, yellow dolls, yellow bullets
Seconal	reds, redbirds, red devils, Mexican reds, R.D., seccies
Tuinal	Christmas trees, rainbows, tooies, trees, double trouble

Other street names: barbs, beans, blockbusters, downers, foolpills, goofballs, green dragons, pajao rojo, pink ladies, pinks, reds and blues, sleeping pills, stumblers.

tion. Intramuscular injection is painful and causes necrosis at injection sites. Binding to plasma albumin varies from 80 percent for thiopental to 5 percent for barbital. The highly lipid-soluble barbiturates, such as thiopental, rapidly cross the blood-brain barrier to induce sleep. The ultra-short duration of these drugs is due to rapid distribution in the body rather than elimination from it. The less lipid-soluble barbiturates equilibrate more slowly. Those with high partition coefficients are readily absorbed from the lumen of the renal tubules and therefore must be metabolized to metabolites with lower partition coefficients to be excreted. Renal excretion of barbiturates can be enhanced by osmotic diuresis or alkalinization of the urine. The barbiturates are metabolized in the liver by a variety of mechanisms, including oxidation to alcohols, phenols, ketones, and carboxylic acid.[4]

Pharmacological Actions

The reticular activating system is exquisitely sensitive to sedative-hynotic drugs. As a result, barbiturates can produce all degrees of central nervous system depression, ranging from mild sedation to anesthesia. The effect appears to be mediated, at least in part, by the ability of barbiturates to potentiate gamma amino butyric acid (GABA) inhibition. The antianxiety properties of barbiturates are not equivalent to those of the benzodiazepines, and they produce a greater degree of sedation. A paradoxical excitement occurs in some people. Barbiturates suppress rapid eye movement (REM) sleep and depress both the respiratory drive and the mechanism responsible for the rhythmic character of respiration. The degree of respiratory depression is dose-related. In the liver, chronic use causes enzyme induction in the MEOS system. In therapeutic doses, the drugs have little effect on cardiac, skeletal, and smooth muscle.[4]

Interactions With Other Drugs

Barbiturates act synergistically with other CNS depressant drugs, including alcohol, to cause cerebral and respiratory depression. Most drug interactions result from induction of hepatic microenzymes, causing significant increase in clearance of corticosteroids, oral anticoagulants, digitoxin, beta-adrenergic antagonists (propranalol, metoprolol), doxycycline, oral contraceptives, griseofulvin, quinidine, phenytoin, and tricyclic antidepressants. Elderly patients may have low plasma calcium concentrations because of a probable result of acceleration of vitamin D elimination. Hepatic enzyme induction lowers endogenous steroid hormone concentrations, which may cause endocrine disturbances. Barbiturates also competitively inhibit the metabolism of certain other drugs, most importantly tricyclic antidepressants.[4]

Toxicity

Barbiturate overdose can result in stupor or coma. The Babinski sign may be present, and an EEG may show periods of brief silence. Patients' pupils may initially be constricted and react to light, but later hypoxic dilation may occur. Breathing may be either slow, or rapid and shallow. Respiratory insufficiency, as well as Cheyne-Stokes breathing, may occur. Eventually, blood pressure fails due to hypoxia and to the direct effect of the drug on the medullary vasomotor center. Depression of cardiac contractibility, sympathetic ganglia, and vascular smooth muscle also contributes to the hypotension, which may progress to shock and hypothermia. Death sometimes occurs.[4]

Tolerance

Both dispositional and pharmacodynamic tolerance to barbiturates can develop; the latter is the more important. With chronic administration of gradually increasing doses, pharmacodynamic tolerance continues to develop over a period of weeks to months. Dispositional tolerance, on the other hand, reaches a peak in a few days. Despite the development of tolerance, the lethal dose of barbiturates essentially remains the same. Therefore, the dose necessary for an addict to get high may approach a lethal dose. Tolerance to barbiturates confers tolerance to other CNS depressant drugs. They share cross-tolerance with other drugs in this class, including alcohol.[4]

Dependence

Like other CNS depressant drugs, barbiturates tend to be abused, and patients can develop physical dependence.[4]

Abstinence Syndrome

The barbiturate abstinence syndrome may be life-threatening. Withdrawal symptoms include restlessness, tremors, anxiety, weakness, orthostatic hypotension, insomnia, hyperactive reflexes, psychosis, and generalized seizures. The severity depends on the particular drug and the dose used. Symptoms are less pronounced with longer-acting drugs, which may be in part due to self-detoxification because of their slow elimination. Symptoms from intermediate-acting barbiturate withdrawal peak at 48 to 72 hours; they peak later for long-acting barbiturates, and seizures may occur a week after the last dose.[5-6]

Health Consequences of Barbiturate Abuse

The medical consequences of barbiturate dependence include depression, injuries from falls and other accidents, altered metabolism of certain prescribed medications, and depressed respiration and death in overdose. Addicts who inject drugs may get local necrosis, cellulitis, abscesses, bacterial endocarditis, hepatitis B, and AIDS. Overdose has been associated with necrosis of sweat glands and bullous cutaneous lesions that heal slowly.[4,6]

Diagnosis and Management
Intoxication

Physicians can usually diagnose barbiturate intoxication when patients have slurred speech, short attention spans, emotional lability, ataxia, and nystagmus; when they are unable to think clearly, have no alcohol on their breath, and when physicians know that they have a history of barbiturate abuse. A toxicology screen can be helpful.

Management of barbiturate intoxication, like alcohol intoxication, consists of letting the person sleep it off.[4,6]

Overdose

Physicians can diagnose barbiturate overdose in patients with central nervous system and cardiovascular depression. With severe overdose, patients are stuporous or comatose, and their EEG may show periods of silence. Their pupils may be constricted, and their pupillary and corneal reflexes may be diminished or absent. Delayed gastric emptying may occur. Later, hypoxic pupillary dilatation may occur. Breathing may be either slow, or rapid and shallow. Cheyne-Stokes breathing may be present. Eventually, shock and hypothermia may develop.[4,6]

The treatment of barbiturate overdose consists mainly of respiratory and cardiac support. Dialysis is effective but seldom needed. Gastric lavage should be considered if the overdose has occurred within 24 hours. Activated charcoal and a cathartic, such as magnesium citrate, may be helpful. Alkalinization of the urine will increase the excretion of most barbiturates.[4,6]

Dependence

The diagnosis of barbiturate dependence is based on the definition of chemical dependence given in Chapter 2. The treatment of barbiturate dependence is the same as for dependence on any other drug (see Chapter 3).

Abstinence Syndrome

Physicians can diagnose barbiturate abstinence syndrome in patients having typical withdrawal symptoms or positive drug screens, or when they know of patients' barbiturate abuse.

Treatment of barbiturate abstinence syndrome involves estimating the usual daily barbiturate dose a patient has been taking, substituting phenobarbital for the abused drug, stabilizing the patient at the equivalent phenobarbital dose, and tapering the dose over four to five days. Amobarbital, butabarbital, butalbital, pentobarbital, and secobarbital in 100 mg doses are equivalent to 30 mg of phenobarbital. As an example of this approach, suppose a patient has been taking 1200 mg/day of secobarbital. The initial daily detoxification dose of phenobarbital would be $12 \times 30 = 360$ mg. This would be given as 90 mg every six hours. The maximum daily dose of phenobarbital should not exceed 500 mg.[7-8]

TABLE 9.3. The pentobarbital challenge test.

Patient's condition	Degree of tolerance	Estimated dose (mg)
asleep but arousable	none or minimal	none
drowsy, slurred speech, coarse nystagmus, ataxia, marked intoxication	definite	400–600
comfortable, fine lateral nystagmus only sign of intoxication	marked	800
no sign of drug effect	extreme	1000–1200

From B.B. Wilford (Ed.), Sub-acute care, in *Review Course Syllabus,* American Medical Society on Alcoholism and Other Drug Dependencies, New York, 1987, p. 195.

Classically, when physicians cannot estimate a daily dose, they have used the pentobarbital challenge test. They give a patient 200 milligrams of pentobarbital orally and assess his or her mental state in one hour. The patient's condition at the end of the hour determines his or her estimated initial daily dose of pentobarbital (Table 9.3). If a patient is asleep but arousable, he or she needs no detoxification medication. Conversely, if at the end of the hour a patient shows no sign of drug effect at all, the equivalent daily dose of pentobarbital is estimated to be between 1,000 and 1,200 mg. This dose is then converted to an equivalent phenobarbital dose and given in four daily divided doses.[7-8]

Barbiturate-like Drugs

The barbiturate-like drugs were developed in an attempt to avoid some of the common side effects of barbiturates, including their potential for lethal overdose. Most of them, however, share the dangers and the abuse potential of the barbiturates. The barbiturate-like drugs (Table 9.4) are methaqualone (Quaalude), ethchlorvynol (Placidyl), glutethimide (Doriden), methyprylon (Noludar), and ethinamate (Valmid). They are used clinically to induce sleep and have essentially been replaced by the benzodiazepines. The barbiturate-like drugs can produce tolerance, dependence, and an abstinence syndrome similar to that produced by the barbiturates.[3]

Methaqualone

Methaqualone (Quaalude) was first synthesized in India in 1951 as an antimalarial drug. It was introduced in the United States in 1965 as a treatment for anxiety and insomnia and was believed to possess none of the abuse potential of the barbiturates. It did, however, become a very popular abused drug, partly because it gained a reputation for enhancing sexual performance (there is little evidence that it actually does this). Intoxication with methaqualone is similar to barbiturate intoxication. In addition, a prickling of the fingers, lips, and tongue may occur. The risks are the same—death by overdose and accidents due to confusion

TABLE 9.4. Other CNS depressants.

Generic name	Trade name	Half-life (hours)
Barbiturate-like drugs		
methaqualone	Quaalude	10–40
ethchlorvynol	Placidyl	10–20
glutethimide	Doriden	8–12
methyprylon	Noludar	9.2
ethinamate	Valmid	———
Others		
meprobamate	Equinil, Miltown	6–17
chloral hydrate	Noctec	4–8
paraldehyde	–	4–12

and impaired motor coordination. Like barbiturates, methaqualone has a synergistic effect when used with alcohol or other CNS depressants. It was removed from the market in the early 1980s because of its widespread abuse. Withdrawal symptoms are similar to those of the barbiturate abstinence syndrome. Tolerance to the drug's euphoric effects develops at a more rapid rate than its respiratory depressant effect, increasing the danger of overdose. Street/slang names for methaqualone include ludes, quads, quas, soapers, and sopes.[1,3-4,9]

Ethchlorvynol

Ethchlorvynol (Placidyl) has a rapid onset and short duration of action. In addition to its hypnotic effect, it has anticonvulsant and muscle relaxant properties. Overdose is characterized by a prolonged coma, severe respiratory depression, hypotension, bradycardia, hypothermia, and cutaneous bullae. Intravenous injection is sometimes associated with pulmonary edema. It is especially dangerous in overdose because it is highly fat-soluble and resistant to excretion. In addition, it tends to remain in the stomach longer than the barbiturates. Withdrawal symptoms in the severest form may resemble delirium tremens.[4,6,10]

Glutethimide

Glutethimide (Doriden) was introduced in 1954 as a nonbarbiturate that did not produce dependence. However, it was soon found to have no advantages over the barbiturates and to have some disadvantages, particularly its long duration of action. It is difficult to dialyze out of the body, making it exceptionally difficult to reverse overdoses. Because it produces pronounced anticholinergic activity, ileus, atony of the urinary bladder, mydriasis and hyperpyrexia may occur. Respiratory depression is usually less severe than that caused by barbiturates, but its depressive effects on the circulatory system are equivalent. Bouts of tonic muscular contraction, twitching, and even convulsions can occur with overdose.

Patients tend to show a cyclic level of consciousness because of rise and fall of plasma concentration as the drug is absorbed from the intestinal tract. Glutethimide does not have anticonvulsant or muscle relaxant properties.[4,6]

Methyprylon

Methyprylon (Noludar) has been in clinical use since 1956. Overdose resembles that caused by barbiturates, and the general principles of management are the same. Hypotension, shock, and pulmonary edema may occur. Because the drug is quite water-soluble, hemodialysis is an effective component of treatment. The abstinence syndrome is similar to that of the barbiturates and can include insomnia, confusion, psychosis, and convulsions.[4,6,11]

Ethinamate

Ethinamate (Valmid) has a rapid onset and a short duration of action. Overdose and withdrawal symptoms resemble those of the barbiturates. Deaths from overdose have been reported.[4,6,11]

Detoxification from Barbiturate-like Drug Dependence

Detoxification from barbiturate-like drugs is probably best accomplished by switching patients to phenobarbital and tapering the dose over four to five days. Doses equivalent to 30 mg of phenobarbital are methaqualone (300 mg), methyprylon (100 mg), and glutethimide (250 mg). Equivalent doses for other barbiturate-like drugs are not well established. The pentobarbital challenge test can be used when the abused dose is unknown.[7-8]

Meprobamate

Meprobamate (Equinil, Miltown) was first synthesized in 1951 as a potential muscle relaxant. It was subsequently found to have anticonvulsant and sedative-hynotic activity. It became available in the United States in 1955 and at one time was widely prescribed as a tranquilizer and hynotic. However, it has essentially been replaced by the benzodiazepines. The liver is the primary site of degradation, and the drug is capable of stimulating the hepatic microenzyme system. The predominant manifestations of meprobamate overdose include stupor, vomiting, paresthesias, seizures, and coma. Profound and persistent hypotension may occur following large ingestions. Forced diuresis, dialysis, and hemoprofusion are effective in removing the drug from the body. Repeated oral charcoal administration may be effective.[12]

Withdrawal symptoms include tremors, insomnia, anxiety, gastrointestinal distress, psychosis, and seizures.[4,12-13] Detoxification from meprobamate dependence can be accomplished with phenobarbital. A 400 mg dose of meprobamate is equivalent to 30 mg of phenobarbital.[7-8]

Chloral Hydrate

First synthesized in 1869, chloral hydrate (Noctec) was the first synthetic sedative-hynotic. Today it has been largely replaced by the benzodiazepines. In therapeutic doses, chloral hydrate has little effect on respiration and blood pressure; however, toxic doses can produce severe respiratory depression and hypotension. It is reduced to trichlorethanol largely by the alcohol dehydrogenase pathway in the liver. Ethanol accelerates the reduction because its own oxidation provides NADH to drive the reduction of chloral hydrate.[1,4-5]

The irritant effects of chloral hydrate give rise to an unpleasant taste, epigastric distress, nausea, occasional vomiting, and flatulence. The tendency of hypnotics to cause persistent effects in the elderly is less pronounced with chloral hydrate than with agents that are metabolized by the hepatic microenzyme system. In addition, chloral hydrate interferes very little with REM sleep.[1,4-5]

Chloral hydrate causes displacement of oral anticoagulants from binding sites, thereby increasing their activity. The combination of chloral hydrate and furosemide (Lasix) in some individuals causes vasodilation and flushing, tachycardia, hypotension or hypertension, and sweating. The combination of chloral hydrate and alcohol acts synergistically to produce sedation. The combination is known as knock-out drops or a Mickey Finn. The mechanism, in addition to the combined sedative effects, is probably the inhibition of ethanol metabolism by chloral hydrate and the enhancement of the generation of trichlorethylene by ethanol.[1,4-5]

Chloral hydrate overdose resembles acute barbiturate toxicity, and the same supportive management is indicated for it. Patients may have gastric irritation that may result in vomiting and gastric necrosis and may have pinpoint pupils. Hemodialysis and hemoperfusion may be effective. If patients survive, icterus due to hepatic damage and albuminuria from renal irritation may occur.[1,4-5]

Sudden withdrawal from chloral hydrate results in symptoms similar to those of alcohol abstinence syndrome. Delirium and seizures may occur.[1,4-5] Detoxification from chloral hydrate dependence can be accomplished with a long-acting barbiturate or a long-acting benzodiazepine. The equivalent dose to 30 mg of phenobarbital is 250 mg and to 25 mg of chlordiazepoxide is 200 mg.[8]

Paraldehyde

Introduced into medicine in 1884, paraldehyde has been used in a variety of clinical situations, including the emergency treatment of seizures associated with tetanus, eclampsia, status epilepticus, and obstetric anesthesia. Currently, it has only limited use in managing delirium tremens. It is a rapidly acting hypnotic that has little effect on respiration and blood pressure in therapeutic doses. However, in large doses it produces respiratory depression and hypotension. When exposed to air, it oxidizes to acetic acid. Because its decomposition products are very dangerous, sometimes causing death, strict guidelines must be followed when administering it. It should be stored in amounts no greater than 30 ml and at temperatures no higher than 25°C. It must be discarded if not used within 24 hours of opening.[1,4,14]

Paraldehyde is metabolized to acetaldehyde and then oxidized by aldehyde dehydrogenase to acetic acid, which is ultimately metabolized to carbon dioxide and water. It has a strong odor and disagreeable taste. Orally, it is irritating to the throat and stomach; intramuscularly, it may cause necrosis and nerve injury. Intravenously, it is associated with cyanosis, cough, pulmonary edema, venous thrombosis, and hypotension. It can be given in a retention enema. To do so, the drug is usually mixed with two parts of olive oil. Overdose produces very rapid, labored respiratory movements. Acidosis, bleeding gastritis, muscular irritability, azotemia, oliguria, albuminuria, leukocytosis, fatty changes in the liver and kidney with toxic hepatitis and nephrosis, pulmonary hemorrhages and edema, and dilation of the right ventricle have all been observed in severe toxicity.[4,14]

Paraldehyde addiction resembles alcoholism, and delirium tremens may occur with sudden withdrawal.[4,14] Paraldehyde dependence is extremely rare. Detoxification can be accomplished with a long-acting barbiturate or a long-acting benzodiazepine.

References

1. O'Brien, R., and S. Cohen. Barbiturates. In *The Encyclopedia of Drug Abuse*. Facts on File, New York, 1984, pp. 35–38.
2. Cohen, S. The barbiturates: Has their time gone? In *The Substance Abuse Problems: Volume One*. Haworth Press, New York, 1981, pp. 119–124.
3. Wilford, B. B. (Ed.). Major drugs of abuse. In *Drug Abuse: A Guide for the Primary Care Physician*. American Medical Association, Chicago 1981, pp. 21–84.
4. Harvey, S. Hypnotics and sedatives. In *Goodman and Gilman's The Pharmacological Basis of Therapeutics*. Ed. by A. G. Gilman, L. S. Goodman, T. W. Rall, and F. Murad, Macmillan, New York, 1985, pp. 339–369.
5. Trevor, A. J., and W. L. Way. Sedative-hypnotics. In *Basic and Clinical Pharmacology*. Ed. by B. G. Katzung. Appleton and Lange, Norwalk, Connecticut, 1987, pp. 241–253.
6. Schonberg, S. K. (Ed.). Specific drugs. In *Substance Abuse: A Guide for Health Professionals*. American Academy of Pediatrics, Elk Grove Village, Illinois, 1988, pp. 115–182.
7. Smith, D. E., and D. R. Wesson. A new method for treatment of barbiturate dependence. *Journal of the American Medical Association*, 213:294–295, 1970.
8. Wilford, B. B. (Ed.). Sub-acute care. In *Review Course Syllabus*. American Medical Society on Alcohol and Other Drug Dependencies, New York, 1987, pp. 189–218.
9. Kulberg, A. Substance abuse: Clinical identification and management. *Pediatric Toxicology*, 33:325–361, 1986.
10. Conces, D. J., D. L. Kreipke, and R. D. Tarver. Pulmonary edema associated with intravenous ethchlorvynol. *American Journal of Emergency Medicine*, 4:549–551, 1986.
11. Gwilt, P. R., M. D. Pankaskie, R. Zustiak, and D. R. Shoenthal. Pharmacokinetics of methyprylon following a single oral dose. *Journal of Pharmaceutical Science*, 74:1001–1003, 1985.

12. Hasson, E. Treatment of meprobamate overdose with repeated oral doses of activated charcoal. *Annals of Emergency Medicine,* 15:73–76, 1986.
13. Bertino, J. S., Jr., and M. D. Reed. Barbiturate and nonbarbiturate sedative hypnotic intoxication in children. *Pediatric Clinics of North America,* 33:703–722, 1986.
14. Ananthakopan, S. Severe lactic acidosis following paraldehyde administration. *British Journal of Psychiatry,* 149:650–651, 1986.

CHAPTER 10

CNS Depressants: Benzodiazepines

History

The first benzodiazepine, chlordiazepoxide (Librium), was synthesized in 1955 and marketed in 1960. Since that time, benzodiazepines have become some of the most widely prescribed drugs in the United States and throughout the world. In 1971 alone, physicians wrote 50 million prescriptions for diazepam (Valium) and 24 million for chlordiazepoxide, representing approximately 3.6 billion pills and $200 million in sales. The use of benzodiazepines in the United States steadily increased through 1975 to a peak level of approximately 100 million prescriptions annually. In the mid-1970s, diazepam was the most commonly prescribed drug of any kind. Subsequently, benzodiazepine prescriptions decreased to approximately 65 million. In the last few years they have again been on the increase, and in 1985, 81 million prescriptions were filled. In a household survey in 1985, 7.1 percent of the adult population reported using benzodiazepines. Of the various medical specialties, family physicians and internists are the major prescribers of benzodiazepines. Individuals using benzodiazepines for nonmedical purposes usually abuse more than one drug.[1-4]

Pharmacology

Classification

A number of benzodiazepines are marketed in the United States. They are usually divided into short-acting, intermediate-acting, and long-acting (Table 10.1).

Pharmacokinetics

The benzodiazepines are completely absorbed after ingestion, except for chlorazepate (Tranxene), which is converted to its active metabolite (nordazepam) by gastric juices in the stomach prior to absorption. With the exception of lorazepam (Ativan), the absorption of benzodiazepines tends to be erratic after intramuscular injection. They and their active metabolites bind to plasma proteins to an

TABLE 10.1. The benzodiazepines.

Generic name	Trade name	Half-life (hours)
Short-acting		
temazepam	Restoril	5–12
triazolam	Halcion	3–8
Intermediate-acting		
aprazolam	Xanax	12–15
lorazepam	Ativan	12–18
oxazepam	Serax	12–20
Long-acting		
chlordiazepoxide	Librium	18–80
chlorazepate	Tranzene	30–100
diazepam	Valium	32–100
flurazepam	Dalmane	47–100
halazepam	Paxipam	14–100
prazepam	Centrax	30–100
clonazepam	Clonopen	40 (avg)

extent that correlates strongly with lipid solubility and ranges from about 70 percent for aprazolam (Xanax) to nearly 99 percent for diazepam. Rapid uptake of benzodiazepines by the brain occurs after ingestion because of their high lipid solubilities (high partition coefficient) and the high perfusion rate.[5]

The benzodiazepines are metabolized by several different microenzyme systems in the liver. All undergo glucuronidation by the liver prior to urinary excretion. Most have active metabolites, which, because they may have half-lives longer than the parent benzodiazepine, may have durations of action that bear little resemblance to the half-life of the original drug. Benzodiazepines do not produce enzyme induction.[5]

Pharmacological Actions

The benzodiazepines act on the central nervous system to produce sedation, hypnosis, decreased anxiety, muscle relaxation, and anticonvulsant activity. They depress REM sleep. Aprazolam, lorazepam, oxazepam, chlordiazepoxide, chlorazepate, diazepam, halazepam, and prazepam are mainly used as sedatives; temazepam, triazolam, and flurazepam are used as hypnotics. In addition, diazepam has muscle relaxant and anticonvulsant activity, and clonazepam is sometimes used to treat petit mal seizures.[5]

The actions of benzodiazepines appear to be due to potentiation of neural inhibition, which is mediated by GABA. In therapeutic doses the drugs have little effect on the respiratory, cardiovascular, and gastrointestinal systems. They do not cause a true general anesthesia as do the barbiturates. Paradoxical reactions, although uncommon, do occur. When used for sedation, they are often referred to as minor tranquilizers.[5-7]

Patients often use benzodiazepines as substitutes for learning to cope with normal life situations. But they need to learn that anxiety is not a disease; in most cases it is a normal response to an acute situation. Physicians should not routinely prescribe benzodiazepines for anxiety. Instead, the drugs should be used for recognized anxiety disorders when indicated.[1]

Interactions with Other Drugs

The benzodiazepines act synergistically with other drugs — including alcohol — that depress the central nervous system.

Toxicity

Oral benzodiazepines do not produce the degree of respiratory and cardiovascular depression that barbiturates do. They are, therefore, considered to be much safer drugs. Oral overdose causes varying degrees of light-headedness, lassitude, paresthesias, motor incoordination, ataxia, mental impairment, dysarthria, and antegrade amnesia. In greater dose, they cause stupor to mild coma, but they rarely cause death when taken by themselves. Overdose with intravenous diazepam, as used to treat status epilepticus, can cause respiratory depression and death.[5]

Tolerance

With protracted use, patients develop tolerance to the sedative effect of benzodiazepines. However, it is doubtful that anyone develops tolerance to the drugs' antianxiety effect.[2,9]

Dependence

Development of dependence to high doses of benzodiazepines (two to five times the therapeutic dose) is well-known. Many people can take these drugs in therapeutic doses for months to years without developing dependence. However, other individuals develop dependence on therapeutic (low-doses.) The likelihood of developing dependence on therapeutic doses increases for up to twelve months of continuous use, but dependence does not tend to develop after this. However, low-dose dependence may develop in less than three months of use. Benzodiazepines with shorter half-lives (aprazolam, lorazepam, oxazepam) appear to have the highest potential for abuse.[2,9-12]

Abstinence Syndrome

Based on how they are used, three abstinence syndromes for benzodiazepines have been identified: high-dose, short-duration; low-dose, long-duration; and high-dose, long-duration (Figure 10.1).[12]

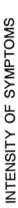
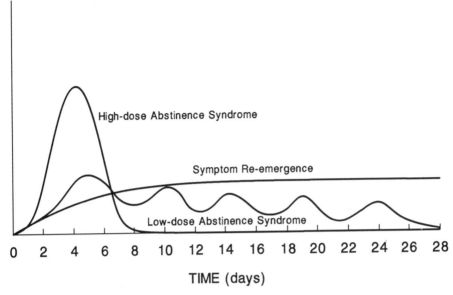

FIGURE 10.1. Benzodiazepine abstinence syndromes. Based on D.E. Smith and D.R. Wesson, Benzodiazepine withdrawal syndromes, *Journal of Psychoactive Drugs*, 15:85–95, 1983.

High-dose, short-duration abstinence syndrome. The high-dose, short-duration abstinence syndrome is very similar to the barbiturate abstinence syndrome. Symptoms include intense anxiety, insomnia, sensitivity to light and sound, and irritability. These may progress to tremulousness, diaphoresis, muscle twitching, tachycardia, elevated blood pressure, confusion, psychosis, hyperpyrexia, and seizures. Onset varies from a few hours to several days, depending on the half-life of the drug. Similarly, symptoms peak in two to four days for shorter-acting benzodiazepines and in five to six days for longer-acting ones. Seizures, for the long-acting ones, can occur up to a week after the last dose.[1-2,7,12]

Low-dose, long-duration abstinence syndrome. The low-dose, long-duration abstinence syndrome consists of many of the minor symptoms of the high-dose, short-duration abstinence syndrome—anxiety, insomnia, sensitivity to light and sound, muscle spasm, and irritability. Psychosis occasionally occurs. Panic attacks are extremely troublesome symptoms. Disturbing nightmares may also occur. These symptoms may wax and wane, gradually decreasing in intensity for up to six months, making it very difficult for many patients to discontinue benzodiazepine use.[12-13]

High-dose, long-duration abstinence syndrome. The high-dose, long-duration abstinence syndrome consists of an initial barbiturate-like syndrome, which lasts a few days, followed by a low-dose, long duration syndrome lasting several months.[12]

Other syndromes. Two other syndromes that follow the discontinuation of benzodiazepines should be mentioned. The first is a rebound phenomenon that occurs after discontinuation of short-term, low-dose benzodiazepine use. This consists of an exacerbation of the original symptoms (anxiety, insomnia) and lasts only a day or two. The second phenomenon is symptom reemergence, in which the original symptoms occur again after cessation of benzodiazepine use. Unlike the rebound phenomenon, these symptoms persist and do not fluctuate, as do the low-dose, long-duration symptoms (Figure 10.1).[13]

Health Consequences of Benzodiazepine Abuse

In addition to decreasing motivation, the benzodiazepines can, when used regularly, cause depression that is sometimes severe and may result in suicide attempts. Intravenous use can cause the same complications as use of barbiturates or other drugs by that route.[1]

Diagnosis and Management

Intoxication

Diagnosis

Individuals intoxicated on benzodiazepines may appear sedated and have slurred speech, an unsteady gait, and altered perception and sensations. Although such people appear to be inebriated, their breath does not smell of alcohol. A history of benzodiazepine abuse or a toxicology screen is helpful.[2]

Management

Treatment for benzodiazepine intoxication is the same as for alcohol and barbiturate intoxication. Patients are allowed to sleep it off.

Overdose

Diagnosis

The diagnosis of benzodiazepine overdose depends on the typical picture of depressed sensorium in the absence of hypotension or alcohol on the breath. Quite often physicians find that patients have been taking prescribed benzodiazepines or find empty prescription bottles. However, this will not be the case when patients have obtained a drug illicitly. A toxicology screen may help.

Management

Treatment of benzodiazepine overdose involves hospital admission and careful monitoring of vital signs. In the unusual instance when a dose has been massive, general respiratory and cardiovascular support may be needed. Gastric lavage, activated charcoal, and magnesium citrate may be helpful.[7]

Dependence

Diagnosis

The diagnosis of benzodiazepine dependence is made by the criteria for chemical dependence discussed in Chapter 2.

Management

Treatment of benzodiazepine dependence is basically the same as described for chemical dependence in Chapter 3. Many patients, because of the duration of their abstinence syndrome, require a great deal of education and emotional support.

Abstinence Syndrome

Diagnosis

Diagnosis of benzodiazepine abstinence syndrome depends on the appearance of typical withdrawal symptoms and knowledge that patients have been using or abusing benzodiazepines. Positive toxicology screens are helpful.

Management

Treatment of the benzodiazepine abstinence syndrome is simply not adequate for many patients. The intensity of the symptoms coupled with the protracted course makes it a difficult problem to treat. Because withdrawal symptoms tend to be worse with the shorter-acting benzodiazepines (aprazolam, lorazepam, oxazepam), patients should be switched to and stabilized on one of the longer-acting ones (chlordiazepoxide, diazepam). The longer-acting benzodiazepines are then tapered over a period of time. Patients addicted to therapeutic doses can try outpatient detoxification. Typically, the tapering is done over six to twelve weeks. Despite this, many patients cannot tolerate the withdrawal symptoms and must be admitted for inpatient treatment. Inpatient detoxification from the short-acting to intermediate-acting benzodiazepines may take up to seven days; detoxification from the longer-acting ones may take up to fourteen days. The main goals of detoxification are to make patients more comfortable and to prevent psychosis and seizures.[1,7-8,10]

In switching to a longer-acting benzodiazepine, equivalent doses are used: 25 mg of chlordiazepoxide is equivalent to 15 mg of chlorazepate, flurazepam, and temazepam; to 10 mg of diazepam, oxazepam, and prazepam; to 4 mg of clonazepam; to 2 mg of lorazepam; and to 1 mg of aprazolam. Alternatively, phenobarbital can be used for detoxification: A dose of 30 mg is equivalent to the doses of benzodiazepines just mentioned.[12]

In addition, on the third to the fifth day, propranolol (Inderal), 20 mg every six hours, can be added to moderate the tachycardia, increased blood pressure, and anxiety. Propranolol is discontinued after two weeks, except for PRN doses.[1,12]

References

1. Laux, G., and D.A. Puryear. Benzodiazepines: Misuse, abuse, and dependency. *American Family Physician*, 30:139–147, 1984.
2. Preskorn, S.H., and L.J. Denner. Benzodiazepines and withdrawal psychosis. *Journal of the American Medical Association*, 237:36–38, 1977.
3. Miller, N.S., and M.S. Gold. Identification and treatment of benzodiazepine abuse. *American Family Physician*, 40:175–183, 1989.
4. National household survey on drug abuse: Main findings. Department of Health and Human Services, Publication No. (ADM)88-1586, Rockville, Maryland, 1985.
5. Harvey, S. Hypnotics and sedatives. In *Goodman and Gilman's The Pharmacological Basis of Therapeutics*. Ed. by A.G. Gilman, L.S. Goodman, T.W. Rall, and F. Murad. Macmillan, New York, 1985, pp. 339–369.
6. Trevor, A.J., and W.L. Way. Sedative-hypnotics. In *Basic and Clinical Pharmacology*. Ed. by B.G. Katzung, Appleton and Lange, Norwalk, Connecticut, 1987, pp. 241–253.
7. Schonberg, S.K. (Ed.). Specific drugs. In *Substance Abuse: A Guide for Health Professionals*, American Academy of Pediatrics, Elk Grove Village, Illinois, 1988, pp. 115–182.
8. Cohen, S. Benzodiazepine withdrawal. *Vista Hill Foundation Drug Abuse and Alcoholism Newsletter*, vol. 16 January, 1987.
9. Rickels, K., W.G. Case, R.W. Downing, and A. Winokur. Long-term diazepam therapy and clinical outcome. *Journal of the American Medical Association*, 250:767–771, 1983.
10. Lemane, K.J. Treatment of benzodiazepine dependence. *Medical Journal of Australia*, 144:594–597, 1986.
11. Lader, M. Dependence on benzodiazepines. *Journal of Clinical Psychiatry*, 44:121–127, 1983.
12. Smith, D.E., and D.R. Wesson. Benzodiazepine withdrawal syndromes. *Journal of Psychoactive Drugs*, 15:85–95, 1983.
13. Winokur, A., K. Rickels, D.J. Greenblatt, P.J. Snyder, and N.J. Schatz. Withdrawal reaction from long-term, low-dosage administration of diazepam. *Archive General Psychiatry*, 37:101–105, 1980.

CHAPTER 11

Opioids

Introduction

The term *opioid* is used to designate a group of drugs that are, to varying degrees, morphine-like in their properties. Opioids include naturally occurring, semisynthetic, synthetic, agonist-antagonist, and pure antagonist drugs. The term *opiate* is often used to refer only to the naturally occurring opioids and their semisynthetic derivatives. Because of the ability of opioid analgesics to produce somnolence, they are often referred to as *narcotics*, a word that comes from *narcosis*—meaning "sleep."[7,10]

Pharmacology

Endogenous Opioids and Receptors

Three distinct families of endogenous opioid peptides have been identified: the enkephalins, the endorphins, and the dynorphins. By interacting with specific receptors, they appear to function as neurotransmitters, modulators of neurotransmission, or neurohormones. Firm evidence exists for four major categories of endogenous opioid receptors, designated as μ (mu), κ (kappa), δ (delta), and σ (sigma). The μ receptor is thought to mediate supraspinal analgesia, respiratory depression, euphoria, and physical dependence. The κ receptor is thought to mediate spinal anesthesia, miosis, and sedation. Dysphoria and hallucinations are thought to be related to the σ receptors, and affective behavior to the δ receptor.[1]

The various opioid drugs react with opioid receptors. At a specific receptor, a given agent may act as an agonist, a partial agonist, or an antagonist. The receptors with which individual opioids interact determine the actions of the drug.[1,3]

Classification of Opioid Drugs

Opioids are classified as naturally occurring, semisynthetic, synthetic, agonist-antagonist, and pure antagonist drugs (Table 11.1). The naturally occurring opioids are opium, morphine, codeine, and thebaine. They are extracted from the poppy plant (*Papaver somniferum*). The semisynthetic opioids are drugs that are made by relatively simple modifications of morphine and thebaine molecules. They include heroin, hydromorphone, oxymorphone, hydrocodone, and oxycodone. The synthetic opioids are drugs that, although structurally unrelated to it, apparently act by the same mechanism as morphine does. They have analgesic properties, are cross-tolerant with morphine, and relieve the symptoms of morphine withdrawal. They include meperidine, levorphanol, fentanyl, methadone, propoxyphene, alphaprodine, loperamide, and diphenoxylate.[1,3-4]

The agonist-antagonist opioids are pentazocine, nalbuphine, butorphanol, and buprenorphine. The pure antagonist opioids are naloxone and naltrexone.[3-4]

Opioids are known by a variety of names in the drug culture (Table 11.2).

Pharmacokinetics

Most opioid analgesics are well absorbed from subcutaneous and intramuscular sites, as well as from the nose and gastrointestinal tract. Despite rapid absorption from the gastrointestinal tract, some opioid drugs (morphine, hydromorphone, oxymorphone) are far less potent when absorbed that way than they are when administered parenterally because of a significant first-pass effect by the liver. Therefore, the oral dose of these compounds is considerably greater than the parenteral dose. On the other hand, some opioids (methadone, levorphanol, codeine) do not undergo significant first-pass effect so that their oral dose is close to their parenteral dose. Yet others are intermediary in oral to parenteral potency.[1,3]

Opioids bind to plasma proteins with varying degrees of affinity. However, they rapidly leave the blood and localize in highest concentration in parenchymatous tissues such as lungs, liver, kidneys, and spleen. Although these drugs maintain low concentrations in skeletal muscle, this tissue serves as the main reservoir for the drugs because of its bulk. Brain concentrations are usually relatively low when compared to concentrations in other tissues.[1,3]

The opioids are converted in large part by the liver to metabolites that are readily excreted by the kidneys. Compounds that have a free hydroxyl group (for example, morphine and levorphanol) are conjugated with glucuronic acid. Esters, such as meperidine and heroin, are hydrolyzed by esterases.[1,3]

Pharmacological Actions

The opioid analgesics cause central nervous system, cardiovascular, respiratory, gastrointestinal, genitourinary, endocrine, and skin effects (Table 11.3).

Central nervous system.   The opioid analgesics reduce both a patient's perception of pain and reaction to it. They also produce euphoria, which leads to their abuse. In addition, they reduce anxiety and stress and produce sleep. Respiratory depression can occur because the drugs inhibit the respiratory brain stem

TABLE 11.1. The opioid drugs.

Generic name	Trade name
Naturally occurring	
opium	Paregoric, Paripectolin, Pantopon, B & O Supprettes, Donnagel-PG
morpine	Morphine sulfate, Duramorph, Roxanol
codeine (methylmorphine)	Empirin with codeine, Tylenol with codeine, Phenergan with codeine, Robitussin AC and other cough compounds
Semisynthetic	
heroin (diacetylmorphine)	—
hydromorphone	Dilaudid
oxymorphone	Numorphone
hydrocodone	Hycodan, Hycomine, Lorcet-HD, Vicodin
oxycodone	Percodan, Percocet, Tylox
Synthetic	
meperidine	Demerol
levorphanol	Levo-dromoran
fentanyl	Sublimaze
methadone	Dolophine
propoxyphene	Darvon, Darvon-N, Lorcet, SK-65, Wygesic
alphaprodine	Nisentil
loperamide	Imodium
diphenoxylate	Lomotil (diphenoxylate + atropine)
Agonist-Antagonist	
pentazocine	Talwin
nalbuphine	Nubain
butorphanol	Stadol
buprenorphine	Buprenex
Antagonist	
naloxone	Narcan
altrexone	Trexan

mechanism, in particular the body's responsiveness to carbon dioxide, which is dose-related. Suppression of the cough reflex is a well-recognized effect of the opioids. All opioid agonists constrict the pupils except meperidine, which in large doses may dilate the pupils. Opioids also activate the brain stem chemoreceptor trigger zone to produce nausea and vomiting.[1,3]

Cardiovascular. Most opioid analgesics do not have significant effects on the heart, cardiac rate and rhythm, or blood pressure in the supine position. However, they do produce peripheral vasodilation, reduced peripheral resistance, and inhibition of the baroreceptor reflex. Therefore, when supine patients raise their heads up they may suffer orthostatic hypotension and may faint.[1,3]

Repiratory. The opioid analgesics decrease both the rate and depth of respiration.[2]

TABLE 11.2. Street/slang names for opioids.

Drug	Street/slang names
opium	O, Op, black pills, black stuff, gum, hop, tar, blue velvet (paregoric)
morphine	M, morph, M.S., dreamer, Miss Emma
codeine	schoolboys, pops
heroin	H, big H, horse, hairy, Harry, junk, joy powder, Mexican brown, mud, smack, white stuff, thing, duster (heroin + tobacco), A-bomb (heroin + marijuana), speedball (heroin + cocaine)
hydromorphone	fours, D, dillies, lords
methadone	dollies, dolls, wafers, 10-8-20
propoxyphene	pinks and grays
pentazocine	Ts and blues (Talwin + pyribenzamine)
fentanyl	China white

Gastrointestinal. The opioids constrict biliary smooth muscle, which may cause biliary colic. Constriction of the sphincter of Oddi may result in reflux of biliary secretions and elevated plasma amylase and lipase levels. In addition, the drugs decrease intestinal motility, leading to constipation.[1,3]

Genitourinary tract. The opioids depress renal function, probably because they decrease renal plasma flow. Ureteral and bladder tone are increased, and increased urethral sphincter tone may lead to urinary retention. The opioids also reduce uterine tone and may prolong labor.[1,3]

TABLE 11.3. Major pharmacological effects of opioid analgesics.

System	Effects
central nervous system	analgesia, sedation, drowsiness, ataxia, euphoria or dysphoria, impaired reflexes and coordination, dizziness, syncope, nausea, vomiting, and miosis (meperidine may cause mydriasis)
cardiovascular	only slight reduction in blood pressure and heart rate in supine position, orthostatic hypotension in head-up position
respiratory	decreased respiratory rate and depth
gastrointestinal	increased tone of the antrum of the stomach, increased tone and decreased propulsive movements of the intestines, and increased tone of the anal sphincter
genitourinary	increased tone of detruser, bladder sphincter, and ureter, slight decrease of uterine muscle tone
endocrine	increased release of ACTH, antidiuretic hormone, and prolactin; decreased release of luteinizing hormone and thyrotropin
skin	flushing and warm feeling, especially on the face, neck, and upper thorax (the effect is thought to be due to histamine release)

Endocrine.   The opioid analgesics stimulate the release of antidiuretic hormone, prolactin, and somatatropin but may inhibit the release of luteinizing hormone.[1,3]

Skin.   Opioids produce flushing and warming of the skin, sometimes accompanied by sweating and itching. The effect may be mediated by the release of histamine.[1,3]

Interactions With Other Drugs

Opioids act synergistically with CNS depressants to depress the sensorium and respiration. Hyperpyrexia, hypertension, and coma have been reported when opioids are used with monoamine oxidase (MAO) inhibitors.[3]

Toxicity

By the time people who have overdosed on opioids see physicians, they are usually stuporous or comatose. If they have taken large overdoses, they cannot be aroused from deep comas. Their respiratory rate is often very low (two to four breaths a minute), and they may suffer cyanosis. As respiratory function declines, blood pressure begins to fall. The pupils are symmetrical and pinpoint until hypoxia occurs; then they may be dilated. (The pupils may be dilated with large doses of meperidine.) Urine formation is depressed. Body temperature falls, and the skin becomes cold and clammy. Seizures may occur, particularly with meperidine and propoxyphene. Pulmonary edema is sometimes a complicating factor. Death usually results from respiratory failure or complications such as aspiration pneumonia and shock.[1]

Tolerance

Patients develop a high tolerance to the opioids' analgesic, euphoric, mental clouding, sedation, respiratory depression, antidiuresis, nausea and vomiting, and cough suppression effects. They develop moderate tolerance to bradycardia but minimal or no tolerance to miosis, constipation, and seizures. Tolerance to the euphoriant and respiratory effects dissipates within a few days after patients stop taking the drugs. However, tolerance to the emetic effects may persist for several months.[1,3]

Patients develop tolerance to the agonist-antagonist opioids to a much lesser extent. They do not develop tolerance to the antagonist actions of agonist-antagonist drugs or to the pure antagonists.[1,3]

Dependence

Some opioids (heroin, morphine, hydromorphone, oxymorphone, methadone, meperidine, alphaprodine, fentanyl, levorphanol) have high abuse/dependence potential, whereas others (propoxyphene, pentazocine, nalbuphine, buprenorphine, butorphanol) are said to have low abuse/dependence potential. However, some individuals do abuse and become dependent on these latter drugs. Patients with histories of chemical dependence cannot safely take them without precautions.[1,3]

Abstinence Syndrome

Opioid withdrawal signs and symptoms include rhinorrhea, lacrimation, yawning, chills, goose pimples, hyperventilation, hypothermia, mydriasis, muscle aches and spasm, bone pain, vomiting, diarrhea, anxiety, and hostility. Goose pimples give the skin the appearance of gooseflesh, from which we get the expression "quitting cold turkey." The expression "kicking the habit" probably comes from the movements that result from patients' muscle spasms. About twelve to fourteen hours after their last dose, opioid addicts may fall into a tossing, restless sleep known as the "yen," from which they awaken several hours later even more miserable than they were before.[1,5]

The abstinence syndrome's time of onset, intensity, and duration are related to the half-life of the abused drug. With morphine or heroin, withdrawal signs and symptoms start within six to ten hours after the last dose, peak in 36 to 48 hours, and then gradually subside. By five days most of the effects have disappeared. A secondary phase of protracted symptoms lasts several months and is characterized by hypotension, bradycardia, hypothermia, mydriasis, and decreased responsiveness to carbon dioxide. With longer-acting drugs, such as methadone, patients may take several days to reach the peak of the abstinence syndrome, and it may last as long as two weeks. Because of its longer course, it tends to be less severe.[1,5]

A transient, explosive abstinence syndrome can be precipitated by the administration of naloxone or other antagonist. Within five minutes of injection of the antagonist, withdrawal signs and symptoms appear, peak in ten to twenty minutes, and subside in about an hour.[1,3,6]

The neonatal abstinence syndrome is discussed in Chapter 19.

Medical Uses and Contraindications

Opioid drugs have a variety of medical uses. In addition, they are contraindicated in several situations.

Uses

In addition to pain relief, intravenous morphine is used to treat pulmonary edema. It appears to reduce anxiety and decreases cardiac preload (venous return) and afterload (peripheral resistance). Codeine is used in many preparations for its antitussive properties. The antitussive dose is less than the analgesic dose. Opium preparations, such as paregoric, have long been used to treat diarrhea. In recent years, opioids (loperamide, diphenoxylate) have been developed with more specific gastrointestinal effects. Some (morphine, fentanyl) are used as preanesthetic agents, intraoperative adjuncts to anesthetic agents, and in high doses as anesthetics themselves.[1,3]

Contraindications

Pregnant women should not use opioids chronically because they can adversely affect the fetus. Opioid administration may lead to acute respiratory failure in patients with impaired pulmonary function. Patients with liver failure, adrenal insufficiency, and hypothyroidism may have prolonged and exaggerated responses to opioids. Patients taking opioid agonists should not take agonist-antagonist agents because, in the presence of dependence, they may precipitate an abstinence syndrome.[3]

Specific Opioid Drugs

Naturally Occurring Opioids

The naturally occurring opioids include opium, morphine, codeine, and thebaine.

Opium

Opium is made by air drying the juice of the unripe seed pods of the Oriental poppy. It has been used since ancient times. Recorded use dates back to 5000 B.C. in Mesopotamia. It was used in 1500 B.C. as an anesthetic by Egyptian physicians. In 1200 A.D. it was used in the Middle East as a medicine and an intoxicant. A tincture of opium (laudanum) was used as early as 1541 to relieve pain, to control dysentery, to suppress cough, and to sedate. By 1650 opium smoking had become rampant in China. As a result, the Chinese government tried to control its importation, sale, and use. The British opposed this because it interfered with their profitable trade of opium grown in India. This led to the Opium War (1835–1842), which the British won. As a result, Chinese immigrants carried the habit of opium smoking to the United States and elsewhere.[7]

During the 1870s patent medicines containing opium proliferated in Europe and America. The most important of these was paregoric, a tincture of opium combined with camphor still used today to control diarrhea. It is a Schedule III drug, and heroin addicts sometime use it when they cannot get heroin (they call it "blue velvet"). Other drugs that contain opium are Pantopon, which is given parenterally as a morphine substitute, and B&O Supprettes, which are rectal suppositories for relief of moderate to severe ureteral pain.[7]

The Harrison Narcotic Act in 1914 placed opium under strict federal control, and the Controlled Substance Act of 1970 placed it in Schedule II.[7]

Morphine was extracted from opium in 1803, and opium's medical use began to decline. Heroin, a derivative or morphine, was developed in 1898. By the early 1900s heroin had replaced opium and morphine on the streets. Opium is still smoked in China, Hong Kong, and Southeast Asia. Physical dependence, pharmacological effects, and an abstinence syndrome like that of morphine occur with its use.[4]

Street/slang names for opium include O, Op, black pills, black stuff, gum, hop, tar, and blue velvet (paregoric).[7]

Morphine

Morphine, the principal alkaloid of opium, was extracted in 1803 and named for Morpheus, the god of sleep and dreams. It constitutes about 10 percent of opium. Morphine sulfate is used for moderate to severe pain. When taken orally, it is only about one-tenth as effective as when given intramuscularly. It can also be used intravenously, subcutaneously, and as a rectal suppository.[7]

When morphine was introduced to the medical profession in 1825, it was hailed as a powerful analgesic and, falsely, as a cure for opium addiction. The advent of the hypodermic needle in 1853 made possible almost immediate relief from pain and anxiety. Physicians prescribed morphine liberally. It could be purchased from the local drugstore or ordered through the mail without a prescription. Hypodermic needles were also readily available.[7]

During the American Civil War (1861–1865) morphine was used as a surgical anesthetic and analgesic. Physicians distributed the drug, along with hypodermic needles, to soldiers for use at home to ease the continued pain of battle injuries. It is estimated that as many as 400,000 morphine addicts were created in this manner—many of them physicians. Morphine was synthesized independent of opium in 1925, making its supply almost endless. Today, opioid addicts prefer the shorter-acting heroin to morphine.[7]

Currently morphine is used medically to relieve severe pain, to treat pulmonary edema, and as a preanesthetic to reduce the fear and anxiety associated with surgery and to reduce the amount of anesthetic needed.[1,4]

Morphine is a Schedule II drug. Street/slang names include M, morph, M.S., dreamer, and Miss Emma.[7]

Codeine

A naturally occurring opium alkaloid, codeine, was discovered in 1832. It gets its name from the Greek word *kodeia*, meaning "poppyhead." The natural yield from opium is only about 0.5 percent, so it is also synthesized by the methylization of morphine. It is sometimes called methylmorphine.[7]

Codeine appears in two forms. Codeine phosphate is an odorless, white crystalline powder soluble in water. Codeine sulfate consists of white crystals that are soluble in alcohol. Therefore, codeine phosphate is used in elixirs and in injectable form, and codeine sulfate is used in tablet form.[7]

Taken orally, codeine's peak effect occurs in about 30 to 60 minutes and lasts three to four hours. About 10 percent of codeine is converted to morphine by the liver. Codeine can be taken orally, intramuscularly, or subcutaneously. It has about one-sixth to one-tenth of morphine's analgesic potency, so it is used for minor pain. It is considered to be only moderately addictive, and withdrawal symptoms are relatively mild.[7]

Codeine's most common medical use is as an antitussive in cough syrups (10 to 15 mg dose), often in combination with nonnarcotic analgesics such as aspirin or acetaminophen, which is also commonly used to relieve minor pain. Because of its limited potency and because of its use with nonnarcotic drugs, codeine has not been greatly abused. By itself, it is a Schedule II drug. Street/slang names include schoolboys and pops.[7]

Thebaine

Thebaine, a principal alkaloid of opium, was isolated in 1835. Because of its toxicity, it has no medical use. Its conversion products include the opioid antagonists naloxone and naltrexone and some codeine. Other conversion products are used in veterinary medicine.[7]

Semisynthetic Opioids

The semisynthetic opioids include heroin, hydromorphone, oxymorphone, hydrocodone, and oxycodone.

Heroin

Heroin (diacetylmorphine) was derived from morphine in 1874 and produced commercially in 1898. It is rapidly converted to morphine by the liver. Its actions greatly resemble those of morphine and last three to five hours. Heroin's name comes from the German word *heroisch*, meaning "powerful." It was originally thought to be a cure for morphine and opium addiction. It rapidly replaced opium and morphine as drugs of abuse in the United States. In 1924 its manufacture was prohibited. Soon after, it became available on the black market.[4,7]

Pure heroin is a white, crystalline, water-soluble powder with a bitter taste. Originally, most of the heroin that was smuggled into the United States came from Southeast Asia. Later, Mexico became a major source (Mexican heroin is brownish). Most of the heroin on the U.S. market today comes from Southwest Asia.[7]

Depending on the method of administration, heroin produces varying degrees of euphoria. After a "fix," a sudden high occurs (the rush), followed by a period of sleep (the nod). Addicts usually inject heroin into veins (this is called "shooting up" or "mainlining"). It can also be injected subcutaneously ("skin popping"), swallowed, snorted, placed under the tongue, or smoked. Addicts need a number of fixes a day to keep from having withdrawal symptoms.[7]

A heroin dose can be difficult to estimate because the heroin on the street is adulterated (cut) many times as it passes down the line from the large distributor to the street pusher. Adulterants include quinine, sugar, starch, and powdered milk. Talcum powder is sometimes used to cut heroin and can be extremely dangerous because it does not dissolve in the bloodstream.[4,7]

To prepare heroin for injection, addicts dilute the powder in a little water, put it in a spoon, and boil it over a flame from a match or cigarette lighter for a few seconds. They then filter the liquid through a piece of cloth and draw it up in a syringe for injection.

Heroin is a Schedule I drug. Its potential for abuse and dependence is extremely high, and it has no medical value.[7]

Street/slang names for heroin include H, big H, horse, Harry, hairy, junk, joy powder, Mexican brown, mud, smack, white stuff, and thing.[7]

Hydromorphone

A morphine derivative, hydromorphone (Dilaudid) is used for moderate to severe pain and is about eight times as potent as morphine. Its potential for abuse and dependence is high, and it has become a common street drug. Although it is more potent and has the same activity as morphine, many of its side effects, such as nausea and vomiting, are not as severe. It is available for injection, in oral form, and in rectal suppositories. Street/slang names include fours, D, dillies, and lords.[7]

Oxymorphone

A morphine derivative whose potency is much greater than morphine's, oxymorphone (Numorphan) causes little suppression of the cough reflex, which makes it particularly useful in postoperative patients.[4]

Hydrocodone

Hydrocodone's usefulness as an antitussive is similar to that of codeine, although it is three times as potent. The dependency potential is greater than codeine's. When used alone it is classified as a Schedule II drug; when used in combination with nonscheduled drugs (Hycodan, Tussend, Tussionex) it is classified as a Schedule III drug.[4]

Oxycodone

A morphine derivative whose potency is similar to that of morphine, oxycodone is an ingredient in Percocet (which also contains acetaminophen) and in Percodan (which contains both oxycodone hydrochloride and oxycodone terephthalate along with aspirin).[7]

Synthetic Opioids

Synthetic opioids include meperidine, levorphanol, alphaprodine, fentanyl, methadone, propoxyphene, loperamide, and diphenoxylate.

Meperidine

Similar pharmacologically but not in structure to morphine, meperidine (Demerol) is about one-tenth as potent as morphine. It was introduced to the medical profession in 1939 for reducing spasms of the smooth muscle of the stomach and small intestine. With the discovery of its analgesic property came the belief that a drug had been found with morphine's effects but without its addictive potential. This, of course, proved to be false.[7]

Meperidine is a fine white crystalline powder that is odorless and soluble in water and alcohol. It can be administered orally or parenterally. Its effects last two to four hours, which is briefer than morphine's effects. It is used medically for the relief of moderate to severe pain and in combination with other drugs as a preoperative analgesic. After morphine, meperidine is the second most widely used drug for severe pain. Meperidine (25 mg) in combination with promethazine (25 mg) is called Mepergan. Medical professionals—particularly nurses—may abuse meperidine and become addicted to it.[2,7]

Levorphanol

The pharmacological actions of levorphanol (Levo-dromoran) closely parallel those of morphine, although it may produce less nausea and vomiting. It has a half-life of about eleven hours. Its nonanalgesic isomer dextromethorphan possesses considerable antitussive action and is used clinically for this property.[1,3]

Alphaprodine

Alphaprodine (Nisentil) is a Schedule II drug that produces morphine-like effects but is neither as potent or as long-acting as morphine. It is mainly used in obstetrics and dentistry.[3,7]

Fentanyl

Between 50 and 100 times as potent as morphine, fentanyl (Sublimaze) is used intravenously as a preoperative anesthetic, for brief anesthesia, and for postoperative pain. It has a rapid onset and brief duration of action (45 minutes). Anesthesiologists and nurse anesthetists sometimes abuse and become addicted to fentanyl.[4]

Related drugs are alfentanyl (Alfenta) and sufentanyl (Sufenta). Alfentanyl is an ultra-short-acting opioid, having a duration of action about one-third to one-half that of fentanyl (5 to 15 minutes). It has only about one-fourth the potency of fentanyl. It is frequently administered by intravenous infusion to maintain a persistent action. Sufentanyl is five to ten times as potent as fentanyl and has the same duration of action.[5,7]

Methadone

Developed by the Germans during World War II, methadone (Dolophine) is structurally unlike morphine but shares its effects. It is best known for its use in methadone maintenance programs (see Chapter 4). It is as likely as morphine to produce dependence, but its abstinence syndrome is more prolonged and less severe. Methadone is an odorless, white crystalline powder that is soluble in water and alcohol. It can be used as an antitussive and to relieve moderate to severe pain. It is used orally in methadone maintenance programs and for controlling coughing but can be given parenterally. It has a half-life of 1 to 1.5 days. Methadone is a Schedule II drug. Street/slang names include dollies, dolls, wafers, and 10-8-20.[1,7-8]

Levo-alpha-acetylmethadol (LAAM) is an opioid that has been tried as an alternative to methadone. Unlike methadone, which must be taken daily, LAAM is taken only three times a week.[7]

Propoxyphene

Synthesized in 1953 and marketed in 1957, propoxyphene (Darvon) was claimed to be as effective as codeine but to lack its potential for abuse and dependence. In reality, it is only about half as effective as codeine as an analgesic and is addicting. It is similar to methadone in structure and action except that it lacks an antitussive effect. It is one of the most prescribed opioid analgesics in the United States. It is used for mild pain and occasionally for withdrawal from morphine or heroin addiction. It is not prescribed for parenteral use because it is very irritating and damages veins and soft tissue. In addition to the hydrochloride form, it also is supplied as propoxyphene napsylate (Darvon-N), which is longer-acting. Propoxyphene is a Schedule IV drug.[1,7]

Loperamide

Loperamide (Imodium) is used to treat diarrhea. Its potential for abuse and dependence is low because it has limited ability to gain access to the brain.[3,7]

Diphenoxylate

Chemically related to meperidine, diphenoxylate combined with atropine (called Lomotil) is used to treat diarrhea. It shares the same abuse and dependence potential as meperidine. Lomotil is a Schedule V preparation.[1,7]

Agonist-Antagonists

The agonist-antagonist group of drugs include pentazocine, nalbuphine, butorphanol, and buprenorphine.

Pentazocine

A potent analgesic that was synthesized in 1961, pentazocine (Talwin) resembles morphine in most of its properties and is used for moderate pain. It can be given orally or parenterally. Like propoxyphene, it can cause confusion, disorientation, and hallucinations. It is abused on the street; addicts usually dissolve tablets and inject them intravenously in combination with pyribenzamine (Ts and Blues). The tablets have been reformulated to include naloxone (Talwin NX) to make intravenous use undesirable because it precipitates withdrawal symptoms in those addicted to opioid analgesics. Pentazocine is a Schedule IV drug.[7]

Nalbuphine

Chemically related to oxymorphone and naloxone, nalbuphine (Nubain) is used for relief of moderate to severe pain, as a preoperative analgesic, and as a supplement to surgical anesthesia. It is administered intravenously and has a duration of action from three to six hours. When respiratory depression occurs, it may be relatively resistant to naloxone reversal.[7]

Butorphanol

Butorphanol (Stadol) produces analgesia equivalent to nalbuphine and buprenorphine but appears to produce more sedation. The duration of action is three to four hours.[3,7]

Buprenorphine

Buprenorphine (Buprenex) is a potent opioid. Its clinical applications are much like those of nalbuphine.[1] After intramuscular injection, its action lasts up to six hours.[3]

Antagonists

The opioid antagonists (naloxone, naltrexone) have no analgesic effects. They reverse the effect of the opioid analgesic drugs and can precipitate withdrawal symptoms in those addicted to opioids.

Naloxone

Naloxone (Narcan) is a pure narcotic antagonist that is used to reverse the depressive effects of opioid analgesics. It does not depress respiration. In the absence of an opioid analgesic, it has very little pharmacological activity. It is given intravenously and has a duration of action of one to four hours. It will reverse the effects of opioid analgesics in one to two minutes.[3,7]

Naltrexone

A pure antagonist that was developed in 1963, naltrexone (Trexan) is well absorbed when taken orally. It is used as a preventive agent for opioid addicts. A single oral dose will block the effects of injected heroin for up to 48 hours. It, thus, is given every other day (see Chapter 4).[3,9]

Designer Opioids

Designer drugs are substances that have psychoactive properties and which had the molecular structures of their parent drugs changed by their makers specifically to avoid prosecution for manufacturing scheduled drugs. There are two types of designer opioid drugs: fentanyl analogs and meperidine analogs.[10]

Fentanyl Analogs

In street drug mythology, "China White" is an extremely pure and potent form of heroin that comes from Southeast Asia and produces the perfect high. Designer fentanyl drugs became associated with this myth and are known on the street as China White.[10]

By the end of 1980, ten people had died mysteriously of drug overdoses in the United States. In each case, the victim showed all the classic signs of opioid toxicity, and yet no trace of an opioid drug could be found. The new drug was eventually identified as alpha-metylfentanyl (AMF). It was 200 times as potent as morphine. Since the Controlled Substances Act of 1970 based scheduling and control on specific drugs, AMF was legal. It was eventually classified as a Schedule I drug. Then, a second analog of fentanyl appeared on the streets. This was para-fleurofentanyl, with only half the potency of AMF. It, too, was temporarily legal. In 1983, 3-methylfentanyl showed up on the streets. It was one of the most potent opioid analgesics known, being 700 to 1,000 times as potent as morphine. This was followed in the spring of 1984 by the discovery of alpha-methyl acetyl fentanyl, which was only 10 times as potent as morphine but had a duration of action as long as morphine itself.[10]

Meperidine Analogs

In 1982, Parkinson-like symptoms and paralysis began showing up in California addicts who had injected a drug referred to as synthetic heroin. The drug was supposed to be 1-methyl-4-phenyl-4-proprionoxypiperidine (MPPP). Instead, due to sloppy basement chemistry, a toxic contaminant of MPPP production, 1-methyl-4-phenyl-1,2,5,6-tetrahydropyridine (MPTP), caused the problem. Too much heat or acid can turn an entire batch of MPPP into MPTP. In the brain, MPTP converts to a substance that destroys brain cells in the substantia nigra, thus leading to decreased dopamine synthesis in the area. Subsequently, batches of MPTP were identified in Texas and Florida.[10]

In 1984 another meperidine analog appeared on the street with a contaminant similar to MPTP. The drug was PEPAOP. Its contaminant, PEPTP, caused spastic movements of the limbs and facial muscles similar to those seen in people with Huntington's chorea. Both MPPP and PEPAOP were placed on emergency Schedule I status in 1985.[10]

Health Consequences of Opioid Abuse

The adverse health effects of opioid abuse are related not only to the pharmacological actions of the drugs themselves but also to the methods used to administer them and to the life-styles of the abusers. Addicts get serious infections because they lack aseptic techniques and share needles and syringes. Cellulitis, skin abscesses, thrombophlebitis, endocarditis, intracranial and pulmonary abscesses, bacterial endocarditis, hepatitis B, and AIDS are common among them.[4,11-12]

Overdose can result in respiratory depression, pulmonary edema, hypotension, circulatory collapse, and death. Peripheral neural complications include transverse myelitis and brachial and lumbar plexitis, which sometimes occur when heroin addicts are reexposed to the drug after a period of abstinence. Ankle or wrist drop may occur secondary to injection into or adjacent to a peripheral nerve.[4,12]

Although the opioid drugs decrease libido, young drug abusers have high rates of sexually transmitted diseases because of promiscuity and prostitution. Female addicts may frequently experience amenorrhea and anovulatory cycles, so that they have low pregnancy rates despite promiscuity. The VDRL may be falsely positive with opioid abuse. Chronic constipation is commonly a problem.[4,12]

Diagnosis and Management

Intoxication

Diagnosis

The diagnosis of opioid intoxication is made on the basis of the CNS depressant effects of the drug (slurred speech, ataxia), pinpoint pupils, and knowledge of a patient's history of opioid abuse. In the absence of such a history, a toxicology screen can be helpful.

Management

Management of opioid intoxication consists of merely allowing the effects to wear off.

Overdose

Diagnosis

The classic triad of coma, pinpoint pupils, and depressed respiration strongly suggests opioid toxicity. With meperidine overdose, however, the pupils may be dilated. Body temperature tends to fall, and the skin becomes cold and clammy. Skeletal muscles are flaccid, and the tongue may fall back and block the airway. Needle tracts may be present. A toxicology screen is helpful.[4-5,12]

Management

The first step in managing an opioid overdose is establishing an adequate airway to ventilate the patient. Pulmonary edema, when present, must be treated vigorously. Administration of naloxone (0.4 to 0.8 mg) can produce a dramatic reversal of respiratory depression. The dose is repeated every two to three minutes until a patient responds or until 10 mg has been given. The dose has to be repeated periodically because its duration of action is much shorter than those of the opioid analgesics. The antagonist sometimes precipitates a severe abstinence syndrome that in some cases may be more life-threatening than the overdose itself. It is usually possible to titrate the naloxone dose to restore respiration without producing severe withdrawal symptoms. Grand mal seizures, produced primarily by meperidine and propoxyphene, are relieved by administration of naloxone.[1,4,12]

Dependence

Diagnosis

The diagnosis of opioid dependence is made based on the principles outlined in Chapter 2.

Management

The treatment of opioid dependence obeys the same principles as outlined in Chapter 3. The special cases of methadone maintenance and naltrexone treatment are discussed in Chapter 4.

Abstinence Syndrome

Diagnosis

The diagnosis of opioid abstinence syndrome is made on the basis of typical withdrawal symptoms and knowledge of opioid abuse, or on a positive drug screen.

Management

Several approaches are available for opioid detoxification. Classically, methadone has been the agent of choice. The abused drug is converted to a daily methadone equivalent that is given orally in a divided dose twice a day and tapered over four to five days. Doses of opioid drugs equivalent to 1 mg of methadone include heroin (1 to 2 mg), morphine (3 to 4 mg), hydromorphone (0.5 mg), and meperidine (20 mg). Alternatively, the daily dose of the abused drug itself can be tapered. Detoxification from methadone, because of its large half-life, is probably best done by tapering the methadone itself over two weeks.

A current popular opioid detoxification agent is clonidine (Catapres), which decreases sympathetic nervous system overactivity during withdrawal.[8] I have found clonidine to be effective when combined with a benzodiazepine such as chlordiazepoxide. The clonidine dose is 0.1 to 0.2 mg every four to six hours and is continued at this level for four to five days. The dose is held if a patient's systolic pressure is less than 90 mmHg. The chlordiazepoxide dose is initially 50 mg every four to six hours, is given on a PRN basis, and is tapered over four to five days. Promethazine (Phergan), 25 to 50 mg every four to six hours PRN, can be given for nausea or vomiting, loperamide (Imodium), two capsules initially, followed by one PRN (not to exceed eight in 24 hours) can be given for diarrhea, and ibuprofen (Motrin), 400 mg every four hours PRN, can be given for pain. Neonatal detoxification is discussed in Chapter 19.

Outpatient detoxification from opioid drugs is prohibited by federal statute. Prescriptions can be written daily, for up to three days, while making arrangements to get an addict into treatment.

References

1. Jaffe, J.H., and W.R. Martin. Opioid analgesics and antagonists. In *Goodman and Gilman's Pharmacological Basis of Therapeutics*. Ed. by A.G. Gilman, L.S. Goodman, T.W. Rall, and F. Murad. Macmillan, New York, 1985, pp. 491–531.

2. Shlafer, M., and E. Marieb. Narcotic analgesics and their antagonists. In *The Nurse, Pharmacology, and Drug Therapy*. Addison-Wesley, Redwood City, California, 1989, pp. 332–355.

3. Way, W.L., and E.L. Way. Opioid analgesics and antagonists. In *Basic and Clinical Pharmacology*. Ed. by B.G. Katzung. Appleton and Lange, Norwalk, Connecticut, 1987, pp. 336–349.

4. Wilford, B.B. (Ed.). Major drugs of abuse. In *Drug Abuse: A Guide for Primary Care Physicians*. American Medical Association, Chicago, 1981, pp. 21–84.

5. Jaffe, J.H. Drug addiction and drug abuse. In *Goodman and Gilman's Pharmacological Basis of Therapeutics*. Ed. by A.G. Goodman, L.S. Goodman, T.W. Rall, and F. Murad. Macmillan, New York, 1985, pp. 532–576.

6. Hollister, L. Drugs of abuse. In *Basic and Clinical Pharmacology*. Ed. by B.G. Katzung. Appleton and Lange, Norwalk, Connecticut, 1987, pp. 350–361.

7. O'Brien, R., and S. Cohen. *The Encyclopedia of Drug Abuse*. Facts on File, New York, 1984.

8. Digregorio, G.J., and M.A. Bukovinsky. Clonidine for narcotic withdrawal. *American Family Physician*, 14:203–204, 1981.

9. Gonzole, J.P., and R.N. Brogden. Naltrexone: A review of its pharmacodynamic and pharmacokinetic properties and therapeutic efficacy in the management of opioid dependence. *Drugs*, 35:192–213, 1988.

10. Seymour, R., D. Smith, D. Inaba, and M. Landsy. Analogs of sedative-hypnotics, and treatment issues. In *The New Drugs: Look-alike, Drugs of Deception, and Designer Drugs*. Hazelden, Center City, Minnesota, 1989, pp. 39–54.

11. Wilford, B.B. (Ed.). Sub-acute care. In *Review Course Syllabus*. American Medical Society on Alcoholism and Other Drug Dependencies, New York, 1987, pp. 189–218.

12. Schonberg, S.K. (Ed.). Specific drugs. In *Substance Abuse: A Guide for Health Professionals*. American Academy of Pediatrics. Elk Grove Village, Illinois, 1988, pp. 115–182.

CHAPTER 12

CNS Stimulants: Amphetamines, Amphetamine Cogeners, Caffeine, Others

The central nervous system stimulants include amphetamines, amphetamine cogeners, caffeine, methylphenidate, pemoline, phenylpropanolamine, cocaine, and nicotine (Table 12.1). Cocaine is discussed in Chapter 13, and nicotine in Chapter 14.

Amphetamines

History

Amphetamine was first synthesized in 1887 and was first used in medicine in 1927 as a stimulant and as a decongestant. Benzedrine was marketed as an inhaler in 1932. In 1937 amphetamine was first used to calm hyperactive children. It was issued to soldiers in World War II to counteract fatigue, elevate mood, and increase endurance. The amphetamine black market began, and students and truck drivers used them to stay awake. In 1949 benzedrine inhalers were associated with amphetamine overdoses. In the 1950s, U.S. soldiers in Korea mixed amphetamines with heroin to create the first speedballs. Amphetamines began to be prescribed for narcolepsy, chronic fatigue, and obesity. In the 1960s widespread abuse began. Intravenous methamphetamine became a popular drug of abuse, and speed freaks injected large amounts of the drug. The black market flourished. In the 1970s and 1980s cocaine abuse replaced much of the amphetamine abuse. Today, amphetamines have very limited medical indications.[1]

Pharmacology

Classifications

Current amphetamines on the market include dextroamphetamine, amphetamine sulfate, and methamphetamine (Table 12.1). These are used as secondary drugs to treat several disorders, including obesity, attention deficit disorder (ADD), and narcolepsy. They are classified as Schedule II drugs. Illicit amphetamines are manufactured in basements and garage laboratories. In the drug culture, amphetamines are known by many names (Table 12.2).[2,3]

TABLE 12.1. Central nervous system stimulants.

Generic name	Trade name	Medical use
Amphetamines		
dextroamphetamine	Dexedrine	obesity, ADD, narcolepsy
amphetamine sulfate	Benzedrine	obesity, ADD, narcolepsy
dextroamphetamine plus		
amphetamine sulfate	Biphetamine	
methamphetamine	Desoxyn	obesity, ADD
Amphetamine cogeners		
benzphetamine	Didrex	obesity
diethylproprion	Tenuate, Tepanil	obesity
fenfluramine	Pondimin	obesity
mazindol	Mozanor, Sanorex	obesity
phendimetrazine	Plegine, Prelu-2, Trimstat	obesity
phenmetrazine	Preluden	obesity
phentermine	Fastin, Adipex-P, Teramine	obesity
Other		
caffeine	Vivarin, No Doz, component in multiple analgesic medications	to stay awake, potentiation of analgesic drugs
methylphenidate	Ritalin	ADD, narcolepsy
pemoline	Cylert	ADD
phenylpropanolamine	multiple decongestants and diet pills	congestion, obesity
cocaine	—	local anesthetic and vasoconstrictor
nicotine	multiple brand names	no medical use

Pharmacokinetics

The amphetamines are absorbed well from the gastrointestinal tract, which is their only legal route of administration. They are distributed throughout the body and enter the CNS easily. Both central and peripheral effects occur in 30 to 60 minutes. Amphetamines are excreted in the urine unchanged. Excretion is significantly increased in acidic urine.[4]

TABLE 12.2. Street/slang names for amphetamines.

Drug	Street/slang names
amphetamine sulfate	bennies, peaches, splash, whites
dextroamphetamine	copilots, dexies, oranges, footballs
methamphetamine	crystal, crank, glass, ice, meth, quartz, speed
Biphetamine	black beauties, black birds, black mollies

Other names for amphetamines are crosses, double crosses, hearts, pep pills, wake-ups, and uppers.

Pharmacological Actions

Both the central and peripheral effects of amphetamines are due mainly to their release of norepinephrine from adrenergic nerve endings and, to a lesser extent, their inhibition of norepinephrine reuptake into the presynaptic vesicles. Alteration of dopamine concentration in synaptic clefts in neurons in the pleasure center of the brain may be responsible for their euphoric effects.[2,4]

Centrally, amphetamines stimulate the cerebral cortex, the brain stem, and the reticular activating system. Major responses include elevated mood, mydriasis, increased ability to concentrate, hyperalertness, increased motor activity, decreased fatigue, and suppressed appetite. For reasons not totally understood, these drugs often produce a calming effect in hyperactive children.[1,4]

The peripherial effects of amphetamines include increased respiratory rate, rise in blood pressure and pulse rate, brisk reflexes, and fine tremors of the limbs. Heart rate may be slowed reflexively with small doses.[1,4-5]

Injection of amphetamine, usually methamphetamine, produces an almost instant rush or flash. Users compare this to the sensation of orgasm. After shooting up, users feel energetic and self-confident. They become more social, and they have feelings of enhanced sexuality. Orgasm is delayed in both men and women, prolonging and intensifying sexual intercourse. Because users are eager to reexperience the initial sensation, they develop a pattern of use called a "run." Users inject the drug over and over again, each injection separated from the proceeding one only by a few hours. A run may last for several days. During this time users do not eat or sleep and may experience frightening visions or feel that bugs are crawling on their skin. They may develop paranoid symptoms, sometimes leading to violence. At the end of the run, users sink into an exhausted sleep (the crash), which may last for several days.[1,3]

Recently, a new form of methamphetamine, called ice, has been encountered on the U.S. mainland. Originating in Hawaii, it is a smokable form of methamphetamine, much like crack is a smokable form of cocaine. The pharmacokinetics of this drug are similar to intravenous methamphetamine.[6]

Abuse of amphetamine sulfate (Benzedrine) and propylhexedrine (Benzedrex) nasal inhalers has been reported. To use the drugs, abusers prepared a solution by dripping a weak solution of hydrochloric (muriatic) acid over a wick from one of the inhalers and then injected the mixture intravenously. More recently, abuse of Vicks nasal inhalers in the same manner has been reported. The principle ingredient in these inhalers is L-desoxyephedrine. I have seen some severe necrotic reactions in local tissues when addicts missed veins.[7]

Interactions with Other Drugs

By increasing urinary excretion, acidifying agents, such as ascorbic acid, decrease the effects of amphetamines. Similarly, by decreasing urinary excretion, alkalinizing agents (sodium bicarbonate, sodium lactate) increase the effects of amphetamines. Amphetamines increase tricyclic antidepressant blood levels and decrease the effects of antihypertensive agents. They alter blood sugar levels in patients on hypoglycemic agents (insulin, oral hypoglycemics) and make diabetes difficult to control. They decrease the effect of lithium, causing poor control of manic-depressive illness. When used with MAO inhibiters, they increase the risk of a severe hypertensive episode and stroke. Foods that contain tyramine (Chianti wines, aged cheeses, liver) in combination with amphetamines increase blood pressure, central nervous system stimulation, and cardiac activity. Finally, amphetamines, when used with other sympathomimetic preparations, including over-the-counter ones, increase potentially serious cardiovascular and central nervous system risks.[4]

Toxicity

Amphetamine overdose produces responses similar to but more intense than its pharmacological effects. Common signs and symptoms are restlessness, tremors, exaggerated reflexes, panic states, dizziness, confusion, and extreme irritability. Patients are hyperalert, talkative, and may have been sleepless for several days. They may have headache, excessive sweating, nausea, vomiting, diarrhea, and abdominal cramps and may develop paranoia, hallucinations, and violent behavior. Amphetamine psychosis may be indistinguishable from paranoid schizophrenia. In its full-blown state, it is characterized by vivid visual, auditory, and olfactory hallucinations, delusions of persecution, body-image changes, bruxism, and sometimes picking and excoriating of the skin. Tachyarrhythmias, profound hypertension, hyperpyrexia, cerebral hemorrhage, coma, seizures, and death may occur.[2-4]

Tolerance

Tolerance to amphetamine effects develops rapidly, often after only a few doses. Tolerance to the lethal effects also develops, so that individuals addicted to amphetamines may experience only moderate effects after taking doses that are hundreds of times greater than the therapeutic dose. Tolerance does not develop to the ability of amphetamines to produce psychosis. One cause of tolerance is depletion of norepinephrine from presynaptic vesicles. Because amphetamines cause anorexia, ketone bodies are excreted in the urine, acidifying it and increasing the rate of amphetamine excretion. This contributes to tolerance.[1,3-4]

Dependence

Amphetamines have a high potential for abuse and dependence.[3]

Abstinence Syndrome

For years, an abstinence syndrome following cessation of amphetamine abuse was not appreciated, primarily because of its mild nature compared to CNS depressant and opioid withdrawal. An amphetamine abstinence syndrome does exist and consists of sleepiness, hunger, irritability, depression, and amphetamine craving. The depression may last for months, often leading to relapse or suicide.[4]

Health Consequences of Amphetamine Abuse

A number of health problems arise from amphetamine abuse. Weight loss of 20 to 30 pounds is common; nonhealing ulcers and brittle fingernails may develop, possibly from malnutrition. Violent behavior and psychotic symptoms may occur (the psychosis usually resolves within a week after patients stop taking drugs). Fatalities from amphetamine overdose are relatively rare. When they do occur, they usually result from myocardial infarction or cerebral hemorrhage. Grand mal seizures can occur. Injecting amphetamines can lead to infections such as local abscesses, bacterial endocardititis, hepatitis B, and AIDS.[1]

Diagnosis and Management

Intoxication

The diagnosis of amphetamine intoxication consists of recognizing typical signs of CNS and peripheral overstimulation in patients with histories of amphetamine abuse. A drug screen can be helpful.

For mild intoxication, treatment consists of decreasing environmental stimuli and giving reassurance. For greater degrees of intoxication, a benzodiazepine, such as diazepam 10 to 20 mgs orally, may be required.

Overdose

The diagnosis of amphetamine overdose is made based on the greatly exaggerated CNS and peripheral signs. An empty prescription bottle or a toxiology screen can be very helpful.

Emesis should be induced if patients are not stuporous or comatose; if they are, gastric lavage is indicated. Other standard procedures to reduce drug absorption (activated charcoal, magnesium citrate) should be instituted. Forced diuresis and urinary acidification may hasten elimination of the amphetamines. Phentolamine (Regitine) or nitroprusside may be needed to control blood pressure. Psychosis may require the use of Haldol 2.5 to 5 mg intramuscularly. Seizures may require intravenous diazepam for control, and hyperpyrexia may require a cooling blanket.[4-5]

Dependence

The diagnosis of amphetamine dependence obeys the principles outlined in Chapter 2. Treatment is for chemical dependence in general, discussed in Chapter 3.

Abstinence Syndrome

Diagnosis of amphetamine abstinence syndrome is based on typical symptoms and knowledge that patients have been abusing amphetamines but have recently stopped.

Treatment consists of letting patients sleep and supplying them adequate nutrition. The protracted depression may respond to antidepressants such as desipramine (Norpramin, Pertofrane) prescribed for two to three months.

Amphetamine Cogeners

Drugs that qualitatively have the same CNS and peripheral effects as amphetamines (Table 12.1), amphetamine cogeners, are used as anorexics more frequently than amphetamines because they produce less euphoria and are less likely to be abused. Phenmetrazine is classified in Schedule II, benzphetamine and phendimetrazine in Schedule III, and diethylproprion, fenphetamine, mazindol, and phentermine in Schedule IV. The effects of benzphetamine, mazindol, phenmetrazine, and phentermine are not dramatically different from those of amphetamines. Diethylproprion produces less cardiovascular stimulation; however, it is more likely to cause seizures in seizure-prone patients. Fenfluramine tends to depress the CNS and may cause psychiatric symptoms, particularly in combination with alcohol. Its side effects tend to be more severe than those of other nonamphetamine anorexics.[4]

Caffeine

A natural alkaloid found in many plants throughout the world, caffeine is an ingredient in coffee, tea, and carbonated soft drinks. It is also an ingredient in some over-the-counter headache remedies, cold medications, appetite suppressants, and stimulants. It is related to the bronchodilator drugs aminophylline and theophylline. A related drug, theobromine, is found in cocoa and chocolate. Caffeine is used in some form by 80 to 90 percent of North American adults, who on average consume 220 mg a day.[1,4,8]

Caffeine is readily absorbed from the gastrointestinal tract and has a half-life of three to four hours. Its half-life is shorter in cigarette smokers and is prolonged in pregnant women, the elderly, patients with cirrhosis, and patients taking cimetidine (Tagamet). It is partially metabolized by the liver and excreted in the urine. It stimulates the central nervous system and heart and relaxes smooth muscle in the blood vessels and bronchi. Increased renal blood flow leads to diuresis; gastric acid secretion is increased.[1,4,9]

Caffeine is clearly addicting when consumed in sufficient quantities. It is associated with an abstinence syndrome consisting of sleepiness, anxiety, nervousness, irritability, lethargy, palpatations, nausea, headaches, inability to work effectively, and caffeine craving. The caffeine withdrawal headache is usually a generalized, throbbing headache that occurs 8 to 18 hours after the last caffeine ingestion. It is thought to relate to caffeine's cerebral vasoconstrictor property and the rebound vasodilation that occurs when the drug is abruptly discontinued.[1,4,9]

Caffeine has few medical uses. It is used in doses of 30 to 60 mg in over-the-counter headache remedies that contain aspirin or acetaminophen and in Cafergot, which contains 100 mg per tablet. Nonprescription stimulants (Vivarin, No Doz) contain 100 to 200 mg of caffeine per dose. Brewed coffee contains 60 to 180 mg per cup, and tea contains about half that much. Colas contain about 50 mg per 12 ounces. Contrary to popular belief, caffeine does not significantly alter the effects of alcohol on the central nervous system.[4,9]

Caffeine in excess may cause jitteriness, restlessness, nervousness, excitement, and insomnia. Flushed face, arrhythmias, and diuresis are common. Gastrointestinal distress can occur because caffeine irritates the gastric mucosa and stimulates gastric acid secretion. Overdose may produce periods of inexhaustibility, psychomotor agitation, rambling thoughts and speech, tinnitus, and hallucinations. Peripheral effects include muscle twitching, tachypnea or respiratory distress, severe nausea and vomiting, and cardiac arrhythmias.[4]

Caffeinism (consumption of 500 mg per day or more) afflicts about 10 percent of Americans and is recognized as a disorder in DSM-III-R. Characteristics include marked anxiety, affective symptoms, and psychological complaints. Patients may have signs and symptoms that resemble manic episodes, panic disorder, or generalized anxiety disorder. Doses of caffeine in excess of 10 grams may precipitate seizures that may require intravenous diazepam for control.[4,9]

Individuals taking MAO inhibitors should not ingest caffeine in significant amounts because of the risk of hypertensive episodes. Caffeine may increase renal excretion of lithium, leading to flare-up of manic episodes.[4]

Other CNS Stimulants

Other CNS stimulants (Table 12.1) include methylphenidate, pemoline, and phenylpropanolamine.

Methylphenidate

Structurally related to amphetamine, methylphenidate (Ritalin) is well absorbed from the gastrointestinal tract. Its actions appear about an hour after ingestion and last from three to six hours. The drug is completely metabolized in the liver to inactive products that are excreted in the urine. The main urinary metabolite is ritalinic acid. Methylphenidate produces milder effects than amphetamines. Because of its potential for abuse, it is classified as a Schedule II drug.[10]

Methylphenidate is the drug of choice for most children with attention deficit disorder. It is also used to treat narcolepsy. In sufficient dose, it can cause all the severe problems noted for amphetamines, including seizures and psychosis. Like the amphetamines, it can suppress growth during chronic therapy for ADD. Other side effects (insomnia, anorexia, irritability, abdominal pain, headache, tachycardia) often are only temporary.[3-4,10]

Pemoline

Used exclusively for the treatment of attention deficit disorder, pemoline (Cylert) is well absorbed after oral administration and has a duration of action of about 12 hours, which allows once-a-day dosing. About half is metabolized by the liver, and the other half is excreted unchanged. It apparently exerts its effects by increasing the storage or synthesis of dopamine. Pemoline causes less CNS stimulation than any other drug used for attention deficit disorder, and peripheral effects are minimal. However, it has occasionally been associated with hepatic damage. Side effects and toxicity are similar to those of amphetamines. Pemoline's potential for abuse and dependence is lower than amphetamines, most amphetamine cogeners, and methylphenidate. It is classified as a Schedule IV drug.[4]

Phenylpropanolamine

A common ingredient in many prescription and over-the-counter medications, phenylpropanolamine on the street may be sold as amphetamine. It has a half-life of three to four hours, and 80 to 90 percent of the drug is excreted unchanged in the urine in 24 hours.[11]

Phenylpropanolamine is the most common ingredient in nonprescription anorexics (Acutrim, Appedrine, Dexatrim, Ordinex), in which it may be the sole ingredient or combined with caffeine. The amount per capsule or tablet ranges from 25 to 75 mg. At lower doses, usually 12.5 mg, it is used as a decongestant in many over-the-counter cold, cough, and allergy medications (Allerest, Alkaselzer Plus, Contac, Coricidin-D, Naldecon, Sinarest).[11]

Phenylpropanolamine is not a benign drug. It may cause hypertension, throbbing bilateral headache, nausea and vomiting, anxiety, palpitations, seizures, tremor, tachycardia, and paranoid psychosis.[4,11]

References

1. O'Brien, R., and S. Cohen. *The Encyclopedia of Drug Abuse.* Facts on File, New York, 1984.
2. Jaffe, J.H. Drug addiction and drug abuse. In *Goodman and Gilman's The Pharmacological Basis of Therapeutics.* Ed. by A.G. Gilman, L.S. Goodman, T.W. Rall, and F. Murad. Macmillan, New York, 1985, pp. 537–581.
3. Wilford, B.B. (Ed.). Major drugs of abuse. In *Drug Abuse: A Guide for the Primary Care Physician.* American Medical Association, Chicago, 1981, pp. 21–84.
4. Shlafer, M., and E.N. Marieb. Substance use and misuse. In *The Nurse, Pharmacology, and Drug Therapy.* Addison-Wesley, Red Wood City, California, 1989, pp. 509–528.
5. Weiner, N. Norepinephrine, epinephrine, and the sympathomimetic amines. In *Goodman and Gilman's The Pharmacological Basis of Therapeutics.* Ed. by A.G. Gilman, L.S. Goodman, T.W. Rall, and F. Murad. Macmillan, New York, 1985, pp. 145–180.

6. Jackson, J.G. Hazards of smokable methamphetamine. *New England Journal of Medicine*, 321:907, 1989.
7. Halle, A.B., R. Kessler, and M. Alvarez. Drug abuse with Vicks Nasal Inhaler. *Southern Medical Journal*, 78:761–762, 1985.
8. Schuckit, M.A. Caffeine: The most widely used drug. *Vista Hill Foundation Drug Abuse and Alcoholism Newsletter*, vol. 18, May, 1989.
9. Clementz, G.L., and J.D. Dailey. Psychotropic effects of caffeine. *American Family Physician*, 37:167–172, 1988.
10. Franz, D.N. Central nervous system stimulants. In *Goodman and Gilman's The Pharmacological Basis of Therapeutics*. Ed. by A.G. Gilman, L.S. Goodman, T.W. Rall, and F. Murad. Macmillan, New York, 1985, pp. 587–588.
11. Dilsaner, S.C., N.A. Votolato, and N.E. Alessi. Complications of phenylpropanolamine. *American Family Physician*, 39:201–206, 1989.

CHAPTER 13

CNS Stimulants: Cocaine

History

Cocaine (benzoylmethylecgonine) is a CNS stimulant whose effects greatly resemble those of amphetamines. It is a naturally occurring alkaloid extracted from the leaves of the *Erythroxylon coca* plant and has been used for its stimulant effects for hundreds of years. The coca plant was originally found mainly along the Andes in Bolivia and Peru. Andes Indians chewed coca leaves, and during the rule of the Incas (11th to 15th century), myths of the time suggested cocaine was of divine origin.[1-2]

When the Spanish came to America in the 16th century, they considered cocaine use to be idolatrous and banned it. However, they soon found it difficult to get the Incas to work in the mines and fields without cocaine. As a result, the Catholic Church began to cultivate the coca plant and, for a period of time, became the largest producer of coca in South America. Cocaine did not become popular in Europe because much of its potency was lost during the long sea voyage from the Americas. In 1859, Alfred Niemann extracted the alkoloid from the coca leaf and named it cocaine.[2-3]

Sigmund Freud, in 1884, after experimenting with it, began prescribing the drug to his patients. He thought it could treat a variety of ailments, including nervous exhaustion, hysteria, hypochodriasis, digestive disorders, alcoholism, syphilis, asthma, and altitude sickness. He also believed that it suppressed the craving for morphine and used it to treat the morphine addiction of one of his colleagues, who became a cocaine addict. He abandoned this practice when one of his patients died of a cocaine overdose.[2-3]

In the 1880s and 1890s Coca-Cola and patent medicines containing cocaine were marketed. Coca wine, Vin Mariani, was said to aid digestion and stimulate a fatigued body. The cocaine in Coca-Cola was replaced with caffeine in 1906. Because of rampant abuse of cocaine, it was incorrectly classified by Congress as a narcotic and banned by the Harrison Narcotic Act of 1914. Its use, thereafter, greatly declined. In the late 1960s and early 1970s, cocaine reemerged. Its primary route of administration was intranasal. In the late 1970s and early 1980s, the use of freebase cocaine spread rapidly, and in the mid-1980s, crack smoking became the predominant means of cocaine abuse. Cocaine has now become the largest source of illicit drug income in the United States.[2-4]

Because cocaine blocks nerve transmission and constricts blood vessels, it is useful for topical application in otolaryngology surgery. This is its only medical use. It is classified as a Schedule II drug.[4]

Pharmacology

Varieties

Cocaine can be used in several forms: coca leaves, coca paste, cocaine HCl, freebase cocaine, and crack or rock cocaine (Figure 13.1). Coca leaves are toasted and chewed along with an alkaline substance or powdered leaves are mixed with alkaline ash from other burned leaves and chewed. The alkaline material improves buccal absorption. This practice is limited to the Indians of the Andes Mountains.[2,5]

Coca paste is made by mixing coca leaves with gasoline, kerosene, or sulfuric acid to extract a crude paste containing 40 to 80 percent cocaine. It is smoked in the form of a brown cigarette and can be dangerous because of the impurities it contains. It has not become a popular method of cocaine use in the United States.[4-5]

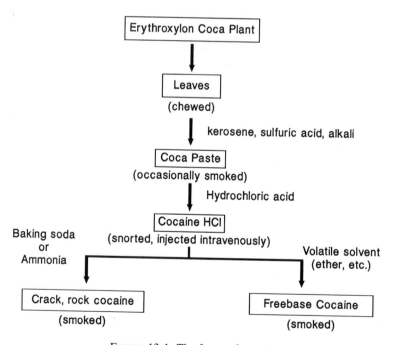

FIGURE 13.1. The forms of cocaine.

Cocaine HCl is the purified form of cocaine. Extracted from coca paste with hydrochloric acid, it is smuggled into the United States in a pure form, which is then cut with adulterants such as glucose, inositol, manitol, lactose, lidocaine, tetracaine, procaine, caffeine, or flour. It is snorted and injected intravenously. Cocaine HCl is not effective when smoked because it does not volatilize sufficiently. When snorted, cocaine HCl is placed on a hard, flat surface such as a mirror and chopped into lines with a razor blade to remove lumps. Lines are inhaled up the nose through a straw or a rolled-up bill. When used intravenously, it is sometimes combined with CNS depressant drugs to decrease its irritability. The combination of cocaine HCl and heroin is known as a speedball.[4-6]

With the aid of a volatile substance such as ether, the base form of cocaine can be freed and is called freebase cocaine. It is smoked. Another form of freebase cocaine is produced by combining cocaine HCl and baking soda or ammonia and heating the mixture. Because the end result is small pieces of material that resemble rocks, it is called rock cocaine. Because it makes a crackling sound when smoked, it is also referred to as crack cocaine. The most popular method of using crack is to smoke it in a pipe, but sometimes it is smoked by sprinkling it on tobacco or marijuana. Cocaine is known by a variety of names by users (Table 13.1).[4-5]

Pharmacokinetics

The rapidity of onset and duration of action depend on the form of cocaine used and its route of administration (Table 13.2).

Coca leaf chewing. Chewing coca leaves is a relatively safe practice because they contain only 0.5 to 1 percent cocaine. Although buccal absorption is initially effective, the local vasoconstrictive effect of cocaine greatly slows absorption. As a result, the peak blood level reached is relatively low. Time of

TABLE 13.1. Street/slang names for cocaine.

base	mujer
bernice	nose candy
C	nose powder
Charlie	paradise
coca	perico
coke	Peruvian flake
cola	polvo blanco
crack	rock
flake	snow
freebase	speedball (cocaine + heroin)
girl	toot
heaven	the champagne of drugs
heaven dust	
lady	
line	

TABLE 13.2. Cocaine effects by route of administration.

Form	Route	Onset	Peak effect	Duration of action
coca leaf	chewed	5–10 min	–	45–90 min
cocaine HCl	oral	10–30 min	60 min	–
	intranasal	2–3 min	15–20 min	30–45 min
	intravenous	15–25 sec	3–5 min	10–20 min
coca paste	smoked	8–10 sec	1–5 min	5–10 min
freebase	smoked	8–10 sec	1–5 min	5–10 min
crack, rock	smoked	8–10 sec	1–5 min	5–10 min

onset with chewing coca leaves is five to ten minutes, with a duration of effects of 45 to 90 minutes.[5,7]

Oral cocaine. Oral administration of cocaine HCl also results in relatively low peak blood levels. Between 70 and 80 percent of the dose is lost as a result of the first-pass effect of the liver. Onset of action occurs 10 to 30 minutes after ingestion, and the peak effect occurs in about an hour.[5,7]

Intranasal cocaine. Intranasal cocaine suffers from the drawback of vasoconstriction of nasal vessels, which limits absorption. After intranasal application, the onset of activity is two to three minutes, peaking in 15 to 20 minutes. The duration of action is 30 to 45 minutes. Because of its more rapid onset and greater peak blood level, intranasal cocaine has a higher potential for dependence than oral cocaine.[5,7]

Intravenous cocaine. The intravenous route is the most efficient of all the methods of cocaine administration, delivering 100 percent of the dose to the circulatory system. Following intravenous injection, onset of action is 15–25 seconds, and duration of action is 10 to 20 minutes. The peak effect occurs in three to five minutes. The quicker onset, shorter duration of action, and higher blood levels following intravenous administration make this mode of administration more addictive than intranasal use.[5,7]

Coca paste smoking. Coca paste smoking causes a rapid and intense high, which is short in duration. Effects begin in eight to ten seconds and last five to ten minutes. Its peak effect is in one to five minutes. The dependence potential for coca paste is high.[5,7]

Freebase cocaine smoking. Crack is not pharmacologically different from freebase cocaine. In fact, it is a form of freebase cocaine. The financial success of crack is due strictly to a marketing and packaging strategy that made a small quantity of high quality cocaine available to people of lower economic status and to high school students. The effects of smoking freebase cocaine occur rapidly and intensely because of four factors. First, the freebase form of cocaine has a lower temperature of volatilization than the HCl form. As a result, a large percentage of it enters the lungs. Second, the large surface area of the pulmonary membrane allows rapid access of freebase cocaine to the bloodstream. Third, the shorter distance to the brain that freebase cocaine has to traverse, when compared to the longer distance for intravenous injection, contributes to the rapidity of response. Fourth, freebase cocaine is much more lipid-soluble than the HCl form, allowing quick passage into the central nervous system. Onset of action occurs in eight to ten seconds after inhalation, compared to 15 to 25 seconds for intravenous injection.[2,7-8]

The duration of action of freebase cocaine is five to ten minutes, with the peak effect occurring in one to five minutes. Administration of the drug must be repeated about every 20 minutes to maintain the euphoria and avoid the crash. This often leads to a run that may last for days until the addict runs out of drug or collapses from exhaustion.[2,5,7]

Metabolism

Cocaine is metabolized by plasma and liver esterases to the metabolites benzoylecgonine and ecogonine methyl ester, which are excreted in the urine.[7]

Pharmacological Actions

Neurotransmitter Effects

Evidence indicates that cocaine euphoria results from the acute activation of dopamine systems in the brain. Normally, action potentials travel down the presynaptic neuron to the nerve terminal, where they cause release of dopamine from presynaptic vesicles (Figure 13.2a). The dopamine then crosses the synaptic cleft to stimulate receptors on the postsynaptic neuron, where it initiates a secondary action potential that proceeds down the postsynaptic neuron. Most of the dopamine is then taken back up by the presynaptic vesicles for reuse. Some of it is metabolized by catecho-O-methyltransferase in the synaptic cleft.

With acute use, synaptic transmission in the dopamine pathways is enhanced by blockage of dopamine reuptake by cocaine, thus increasing the dopamine concentration in the synapse (Figure 13.2b). Repeated use of cocaine tends to decrease synaptic transmission by depleting dopamine stores because the portion that is normally reused is metabolized by catechol-O-methyltransferase (Figure 13.2c). It is thought that the dopamine depletion gives rise to cocaine craving, withdrawal symptoms, and dysphoria (the dopamine depletion hypothesis). Cocaine also blocks synaptic reuptake of norephinephrine and serotinin. The role this plays in cocaine dependence is uncertain.[9-10]

Acute and Chronic Effects

Cocaine use causes a variety of acute and chronic effects (Table 13.3), which are virtually indistinguishable from those amphetamines produce. The effects of intravenous or smoked cocaine, however, last only a few minutes, whereas those of methamphetamine may last for hours. Acute CNS effects of cocaine include euphoria, grandiosity, feelings of enhanced sexuality, feelings of enhanced strength, feelings of enhanced mental capacity, increased sociability, insomnia, decreased fatigue, increased energy, anorexia, heightened sensory awareness,

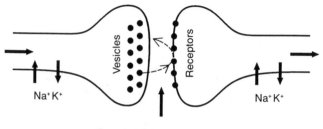

Catechol-O-Methyl transferase
A. Normal Dopamine Function

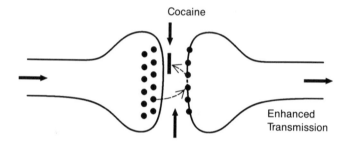

Catechol-O-Methyl transferase
B. Acute Cocaine Use
(Increased Synaptic Dopamine)

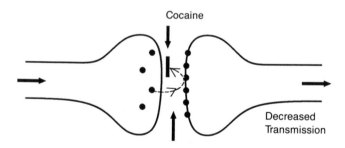

Catechol-O-Methyl transferase
C. Chronic Cocaine Use
(Decreased Synaptic Dopamine)

FIGURE 13.2. Effect of acute and chronic cocaine use on synaptic dopamine concentration.

indifference to pain, and increased pupil size. Peripherally, cocaine increases heart rate, blood pressure, and respiratory rate, and causes hyperactive reflexes. Small doses of cocaine may slow the heart rate as a result of central vagal stimula-

TABLE 13.3. Pharmacological effects of cocaine use.

	Acute use	Chronic use	Overdose
CNS	euphoria	dysphoria	acute anxiety
	grandiosity	depression	marked agitation
	feelings of enhanced sexuality	sexual disinterest	confusion
		impotence	delirium
	feelings of enhanced strength	irritability	nausea and vomiting
		anxiety	paranoid psychosis
	feelings of enhanced mental capacity	insomnia	hyperthermia
		inability to concentrate	seizures
	increased sociability	visual hallucinations	death
	decreased fatigue	tactile hallucinations	
	increased energy	suspiciousness	
	anorexia	delusions	
	increased sensory awareness	paranoid psychosis	
	indifference to pain		
	dilated pupils		
Peripheral	Increased heart rate	weight loss	extreme hypertension
	increased blood pressure	personal neglect	extreme tachycardia
	increased respiratory rate	increased blood pressure	cardiac arrhythmias
	hyperactive reflexes	tachycardia	greatly exaggerated reflexes
		tremor	respiratory depression
		muscle twitching	cardiovascular collapse

tion. Users describe "snow lights," a flickering of rays of bright lights at the periphery of the visual fields.[2,7-8,11-12]

Chronic use leads to central effects that include marked cocaine craving, dysphoria, depression, sexual disinterest, impotence, anxiety, irritability, insomnia, fatigue, inability to concentrate, visual and tactile hallucinations (cocaine bugs), suspiciousness, delusions, and paranoid psychosis. Peripherally, chronic cocaine use leads to weight loss, personal neglect, increased blood pressure, tachycardia, tremor, and muscle twitching.[2,7]

Interactions with Other Drugs

Cocaine interacts synergistically with other CNS stimulant drugs, and interferes with the antihypertensive properties of guanethidine (Ismelin) and related drugs. Blood glucose levels may be difficult to control despite seemingly adequate doses of insulin or oral hypoglycemic drugs.

Toxicity

Cocaine overdose causes excessive central and peripheral stimulation (Table 13.3). Centrally, it produces acute anxiety, marked agitation, confusion, delirium, nausea and vomiting, paranoid psychosis, hyperthermia, and seizures.

Deaths do occur. Peripheral effects include extreme hypertension and tachycardia, cardiac arrhythmias, greatly exaggerated reflexes, respiratory depression, and cardiovascular collapse. Individuals with pseudocholinesterase deficiency are at particular risk of overdose effects because the enzyme is essential for metabolizing cocaine.[2,7,13]

Deaths occasionally occur from massive overdose due to "body packing" – the transport of ingested cocaine concealed in condoms or balloons. The packets can rupture spontaneously or do so when people carrying them attempt to remove them.[14]

Tolerance

Tolerance to some of cocaine's effects undoubtedly occurs with repeated use of the drug, although the literature is equivocal about this. Tolerance does not appear to develop to the ability of cocaine to produce psychosis.[1-2,14]

Dependence

Cocaine's potential for producing dependence depends on the form of the drug used and its route of administration. Chewing coca leaves produces mild stimulatory effects and, like taking cocaine orally, apparently has a low potential for dependence. Snorting cocaine has a much higher potential for dependence, but because the drug constricts blood vessels in the nose, thus limiting its absorption, its potential for producing dependence is somewhat limited. Intravenous cocaine and inhalation of crack cocaine have the highest potential for producing dependence.

Abstinence Syndrome

The cocaine abstinence syndrome consists of negativism, pessimism, lack of patience, irritability, sleepiness, hunger, fatigue, depression, and intense craving. The depression is described as "anhedonia," which is an inability to obtain pleasure in life. It may last for two to three months.[1,15]

Health Consequences of Cocaine Abuse

Many of the health consequences of cocaine abuse are the result of its route of administration. Snorting cocaine can cause rhinitis, nasal bleeding, nasal mucosa atrophy, sinusitis, hoarseness, difficulty swallowing, and nasal septum perforation. Smoking cocaine can cause chronic cough, bronchitis, hemoptysis, impaired pulmonary function, and pulmonary edema. Intravenous use can cause local infection at the site of injection, hepatitis B, bacterial endocarditis, and AIDS. Cocaine use by any of these three routes can cause vitamin deficiencies, anorexia, sexual dysfunction, hyperpyrexia, cardiac arrhythmias, myocardial infarction, seizures, subarachnoid hemorrhage, and respiratory and cardiovascular collapse. Obstetrical and neonatal consequences are discussed in Chapter 19.[8,13,15-16]

Diagnosis and Management

Intoxication

Diagnosis

The diagnosis of cocaine intoxication depends on recognizing the signs of central and peripheral nervous system stimulation. Patients may appear giddy, energetic, talkative, anxious, or agitated. They may have mild tachycardia and tachypnea and dilated pupils. A history of cocaine abuse or a positive drug screen is helpful.

Management

Management of cocaine intoxication usually consists only of placing patients in quiet rooms, reassuring them, and waiting for the effects of the drug to wear off. Some patients may require oral administration of a benzodiazepine such as diazepam, 10 to 20 mg.

Overdose

Diagnosis

The diagnosis of cocaine overdose is made based on the presence of extreme CNS and peripheral stimulation and knowledge that patients are cocaine abusers. Drug screens, if they can be obtained rapidly enough, can be very helpful. Cocaine overdose can be confused with psychotic disorders (mania, paranoid schizophrenia), thyroid storm, and other drug overdoses (amphetamines or phencyclidine).[17]

Management

Because there is no antidote for cocaine overdose, management consists of treating the symptoms. Advancing CNS stimulation and status epilepticus can be treated with diazepam, 5 mg intravenously every five minutes for four doses. Alternately, amobarbital 20 to 75 mg intravenously every five minutes for four doses can be given. Extreme hypertension, tachycardia, and premature ventricular contractions can be treated with propranolol (Inderal), 1 mg intravenously, repeated every minute up to six doses. Hyperthermia may require rapid cooling with antipyretics, ice, or a cooling blanket. If speedballing is suspected, naloxone (Narcon), 0.2 to 0.8 mg intravenously, should be given. Haldol 5 to 10 mg intramuscularly can be used for psychotic symptoms.[17]

Dependence

Diagnosis

The diagnosis of cocaine dependence is made based on the principles outlined in Chapter 2.

Management

Management of cocaine dependence is the same as that of chemical dependence described in Chapter 3. Treatment programs often state that the relapse rate of cocaine addicts is extremely high. However, at one year it may not be greater than the relapse rate of alcoholics.[18]

Abstinence Syndrome

Diagnosis

Diagnosis of cocaine abstinence syndrome is based on typical signs and symptoms of cocaine withdrawal and knowledge that patients have been abusing cocaine.

Management

Management of cocaine abstinence syndrome usually consists only of reassurance. Medication is usually not required. In recent years, several studies have suggested that pharmacological intervention may decrease the relapse rate. Dopamine precursors (tyrosine, tryptophan, levodopa, carbidopa) have been used to raise dopamine concentrations in the brain, and dopamine agonists (amantadine, bromocriptine) have been used to decrease cocaine craving. Tricyclic antidepressants (desipramine, imipramine) have been used to reduce depression. At the present time, the future role that pharmacological agents will play in managing the cocaine abstinence syndrome is uncertain.[4,17,19-22]

References

1. O'Brien, R., and S. Cohen. *The Encyclopedia of Drug Abuse*. Facts on File, New York, 1984.
2. Gottheil, E., and S.P. Weinstein. Cocaine risks: A review. *Family Practice Recertification*, 5:78–90, 1983.
3. Kleber, H.D. Cocaine abuse: Historical, epidemiological, and psychological perspectives. *Journal of Clinical Psychiatry*, 49:3–6, 1988.
4. Tennant, F.S. Cocaine withdrawal step by step. *Emergency Medicine*, April, 1987, pp. 65–68.
5. Vereby, K., and M.S. Gold. From coca leaves to crack: The effects of dose and routes of administration on abuse liability. *Psychiatric Annals*, 18:513–520, 1988.
6. Gold, M. Crack abuse: Its implications and outcomes. *Resident and Staff Physician*, 33:45–53, 1987.

7. Bouknight, L.G. Cocaine—A particularly addicting drug. *Postgraduate Medicine*, 83:115–131, 1988.

8. Cohen, S. The cocaine problems. *Vista Hill Foundation Newsletter*, vol. 17, December, 1987.

9. Dackis, C.A., and M.S. Gold. Psychopharmacology of cocaine. *Psychiatric Annals*, 18:528–530, 1988.

10. Wyatt, R.J., F. Karourn, R. Suddath, and A. Hitri. The role of dopamine in cocaine use and abuse. *Psychiatric Annals*, 18:531–534, 1988.

11. Jaffe, J.H. Drug addiction and drug abuse. In *Goodman and Gilman's The Pharmacological Basis of Therapeutics*. Ed. by A.G. Gilman, L.S. Goodman, T.W. Rall, and F. Murad. Macmillan, New York, 1985, pp. 537–581.

12. Ritchie, J.M., and N.M. Greene. Local anesthetics. In *Goodman and Gilman's Pharmacological Basis of Therapeutics*. Ed. by A.G. Gilman, L.S. Goodman, T.W. Rall, and F. Murad. Macmillan, New York, 1985, pp. 302–321.

13. Garber, M.W., and D. Flaherty. Cocaine and sudden death. *American Family Physician*, 36:227–230, 1987.

14. Wilford, B.B. (Ed.). Major drugs of abuse. In *Drug Abuse: A Guide for the Primary Care Physician*. American Medical Association, Chicago, 1981, pp. 21–84.

15. Miller, G.W. The cocaine habit. *American Family Physician*, 31:173–176, 1985.

16. Cregler, L.L., and H. Mark. Medical complications of cocaine abuse. *New England Journal of Medicine*, 345:1495–1500, 1986.

17. Dwyer, B.J. (Ed.). Cocaine: Helping patients avoid the end of the line. *Emergency Medicine Reports*, 6:17–26, 1985.

18. Strickler, H.M., C.A. Martin, R.H. Sowell, and A.J. Mooney. A comparison of alcoholics and cocaine addicts at one year following inpatient treatment. *Journal of Medical Association of Georgia*, 6:751–756, 1987.

19. Tennant, F.S. Double-blind comparison of amantadine and bromocryptine for ambulatory withdrawal from cocaine dependence. *Archives Internal Medicine*, 147:109–112, 1987.

20. Giannini, A.J., D.A. Malone, M.G. Giannini, W.A. Price, and R.H. Loiselle. Treatment of depression in chronic cocaine and phencyclidine abuse with desipramine. *Journal of Clinical Pharmacology*, 26:211–214, 1986.

21. Extein, I.L., and M.S. Gold. The treatment of cocaine addicts: Bromocryptine or desipramine? *Psychiatric Annals*, 18:535–537, 1988.

22. Garvin, F.H. Chronic neuropharmacology of cocaine: Progress in pharmacotherapy. *Journal of Clinical Psychiatry*, 49:11–16, 1988.

CHAPTER 14

CNS Stimulants: Nicotine

Introduction

Nicotine is a psychoactive agent whose continued use usually leads to addiction. The pharmacological and behavioral processes that determine nicotine addiction are similar to those that determine addiction to other drugs, such as heroin and cocaine.[1] The most common form of nicotine dependence is associated with the inhalation of cigarette smoke. Pipe and cigar smoking, the use of snuff, and the chewing of tobacco are less likely to lead to nicotine dependence.[2] This chapter, therefore, addresses cigarette smoking as the primary agent of nicotine addiction.

Despite the fact that cigarette smoking is the largest single preventable cause of death and disability in the United States, most patients report that they have not been counseled by their physicians to quit. This failure is, in part, due to the fact that physicians need to be trained in helping patients stop smoking.[3] Physicians are in an excellent position to approach stopping smoking, as well as preventing it from many vantage points.

History

Tobacco products have been used for centuries. The oldest cited evidence of tobacco use appears on a Mayan stone carving dated 600–900 A.D.[1] When Columbus landed in America in 1492, natives of the West Indies offered dried tobacco leaves as a friendly gesture. On a later voyage he observed Native Americans inhaling smoke from a hollow reed as part of their religious ceremonies. They called the reed tabacum, from which our word *tobacco* is derived. The form of tobacco use varied in different parts of the New World. Natives of the West Indies smoked rolls of dried tobacco leaves similar to today's cigars. Haitians practiced a form of snuffing, snorting tobacco through tubes into their nasal passages. South American natives smoked tobacco wrapped in palm leaves, much like modern cigarettes. They also chewed tobacco leaves. Tobacco was taken back to Europe as a novelty by Columbus's crew. The smoke from this early tobacco was harsh and irritating.[4]

Tobacco use spread throughout the rest of the world during the 16th and 17th centuries. However, its use was not uniformly accepted by everyone. In 1604, King James I condemned its use and taxed it mercilessly. The tax money was used to build extensive fleets for further exploration of the New World.[4] Opponents of tobacco attributed increased crime, nervous paralysis, loss of intellectual abilities, and visual impairment to its use.[1]

For decades tobacco poultices and extracts were used in attempts to cure virtually every known affliction, including cancer.[4] Jean Nicot, a French ambassador to Portugal, was an exponent of the medicinal values of tobacco. When the major active component was discovered in the early 1800s by Cerioli and Vaugelin, it was named nicotianine after Nicot.[1,4]

A major advancement in smoking tobacco is attributable to John Rolfe, who produced a form of tobacco with milder smoke. His marriage to Pocahontas established peace with the American Indians and allowed increased production of this new tobacco to meet increased demand. Sir Walter Raleigh experimented with planting methods and methods of curing tobacco, resulting in a more pleasant smoke. This helped popularize the use of tobacco even more.[4]

The Egyptians are credited with the development of the modern cigarette. They began rolling tobacco in paper around 1832. French and British soldiers took the paper-wrapped cylinders back to Europe in 1856, following the Crimean War. Soon after this, cigarettes made their way to the United States. They were made by hand and were expensive.[4]

James Bonsack, a young Virginia inventor, devised a machine in 1881 that could mass produce cigarettes at the rate of 100,000 a day, which reduced price and greatly increased usage.[4] Safety matches and lighters allowed people to smoke at any time or place.

A tremendous boost in cigarette consumption occurred during World War I as the result of clever marketing techniques. Smoking was associated with bravery on the front lines. Soldiers went to war with cigarettes in their C rations. About this time, too, women began to smoke.[4]

In the early part of the 20th century, cigarettes typically were unfiltered. Manufacturers began to add filters to reduce the amount of tobacco lost in the unsmoked portion of the cigarette and to increase the appeal of smoking to women, who objected to getting tobacco stains on their fingers. After the U.S. Surgeon General's 1964 report, which publicized some of the health consequences of smoking, public interest in reducing the amount of tar delivered by cigarettes increased, and the tobacco industry responded by introducing a variety of more functional filters.[4] Today, nearly 90 percent of smokers smoke filtered cigarettes.[3]

Trends in Cigarette Smoking

Despite escalating worldwide cigarette consumption, smoking rates in the United States continue to decline. Consumption reached a peak in the mid-1960s, when 42 percent of adults smoked (52 percent of men and 34 percent of women),

TABLE 14.1. Trends in cigarette smoking.

	Adults	Males	Females
1965	42%	52%	34%
1988	26.5%	29.5%	23.8%

amounting to 4,500 cigarettes per person a year. Per capita consumption began to drop after 1964, when the Surgeon General reported tobacco use to be a major health hazard. In 1988, 26.5 percent of adults smoked (29.5 percent of men and 23.8 percent of women), amounting to 2,600 cigarettes per person a year. The difference in smoking rates between the sexes for young adults is even smaller (24.4 percent of males and 21.5 percent of females).[3,5-6] During this same time period the percentage of adolescent boys who smoked showed a modest decline; however, the percentage of adolescent girls who smoked increased.[5] Because more men than women have successfully quit smoking, the percentage of women who smoke may soon surpass that of men if these trends continue (Table 14.1).[6] Smoking is more common in lower socioeconomic groups. Adults with only a high school diploma smoke at a rate of 35.4 percent, whereas those with postgraduate educations smoke at a rate of 16.5 percent.[1] An estimated 10 to 15 percent of physicians now smoke.[7] Despite the trend towards fewer and fewer smokers, there has been a considerable increase in the percentage of heavy smokers.[3]

Pharmacology

General Information

Cigarette smoke is composed of hundreds of substances. These can be divided into cigarette constituents (organic matter, nicotine alkaloids, additives) and pyrolysis products (CO_2, CO, tar).[8] Carcinogens are found primarily in particulate smoke.[9] The smoke itself consists of *mainstream smoke*, which smokers inhale directly from cigarettes, and *sidestream smoke*, which enters the atmosphere from the lit ends of cigarettes. Smokers inhale both mainstream and sidestream smoke, and others, including nonsmokers, in the vicinity inhale sidestream smoke. Of environmental tobacco smoke, 80 percent is sidestream smoke. It contains greater concentrations of various toxic and carcinogenic compounds than does mainstream smoke. Aldehydes, phenol, ammonia, and sulfur dioxide are surface irritants in cigarette smoke that cause some of its uncomfortable effects—such as eye and nasal mucosa irritation.[9]

As smokers inhale, they pull air into cigarettes through the porous paper, diluting and cooling mainstream smoke. Filters trap some of the particulate matter. The amount of nicotine absorbed in the lungs depends on how much is inhaled, how deeply it is inhaled and for how long, and the pH of the smoke.[8]

Pharmacokinetics

The average cigarette contains about 10 mg of nicotine. A variable amount, probably between 1 to 2 mg, is actually delivered to the lungs when the cigarette is smoked. A puff of smoke results in a measurable nicotine level in the brain in seconds.[5] With regular use, nicotine accumulates in the body during the day and persists overnight. Thus, smokers are exposed to the effects of nicotine 24 hours a day. It readily crosses the blood-brain barrier, where it acts as an agonist on specific cholinergic receptors in the central nervous system.[10]

Nicotine is metabolized primarily in the liver. The major metabolites are continine and nicotine-1-N-oxide; these are rapidly eliminated by the kidneys. The half-life of nicotine after inhalation is 30 to 60 minutes.[10] Continine, the major metabolite, has a half-life of between 19 and 40 hours.[9]

Pharmacological Actions

Through its direct effects on the medulla, nicotine causes a decrease in the strength of stomach contractions and nausea and vomiting. In the respiratory system, it causes local irritation and a decrease in ciliary motion. Acute cardiovascular effects include increased blood pressure, cutaneous vasoconstriction, increased strength of heart contractions, and increased platelet adherence. In the endocrine system it causes release of epinephrine and norepinephrine from the adrenals and adrenergic axons. It also causes reductions in growth hormone, cortisol, and antidiuretic hormone. It has a direct effect on the brain, causing a generalized stimulating EEG pattern, with low-voltage fast waves predominating. Peripherally it causes a decrease in muscle tone and decreased deep tendon reflexes.[5]

Interactions with Other Drugs

Nicotine can alter the activity of many drugs, usually by induction of liver microsomal enzymes. Enzyme activity may remain elevated up to six months after patients stop smoking. Smokers may have reduced blood levels of theophylline, pentazocine, propranolol, proproxyphene, phenothiazines, benzodiazepines, insulin, and some antidepressants.[10] The rate of metabolism of coumadin may also be increased.[5] Smokers, especially heavy smokers, may need to have the dosages of these drugs increased. Also, smoking increases the potential for serious adverse effects in women taking birth control pills.[10]

Toxicity

Nicotine is a potentially lethal poison at high exposure levels. Overdose occurs primarily as a result of accidental ingestion or skin exposure to nicotine-containing pesticides or, in children, after ingesting tobacco or tobacco juice. Mild nicotine intoxication occurs in first-time smokers, in nonsmoking workers who harvest tobacco, and in people who chew excessive amounts of gum that contains nicotine. Mild overdose causes nausea, salivation, abdominal pain, diarrhea, vomiting, headache, dizziness, decreased heart rate, and weakness. In higher doses these are followed by feelings of faintness, precipitous drops in blood pressure, decreases in respiration, convulsions, and death.[10]

Tolerance

Smokers develop acute and chronic tolerance to many of the effects of nicotine. However, they do not develop tolerance uniformly to all aspects of nicotine's actions. Most prominently they develop tolerance for nausea, dizziness, and vomiting.[5]

Dependence

A recent Surgeon General's report stated that cigarettes and other forms of tobacco are addicting, nicotine is the drug in tobacco that causes addiction, and the pharmacological and behavioral processes that determine tobacco addiction are similar to those that determine addiction to drugs such as heroin and cocaine.[1] In research where nicotine has been given to subjects intravenously, it has been found to be more addicting than cocaine.[3]

In all forms of drug addiction, the user's behavior is largely controlled by a psychoactive substance. People use drugs compulsively, often despite damage to themselves or to society. Drug-seeking and drug-taking behavior is driven by strong, often irresistible urges. It often takes precedence over other important priorities and can persist despite a desire to quit or even repeated attempts to quit.[1] This is certainly true of cigarette smoking. Most smokers who have heart attacks for example, resume smoking after leaving the hospital.[5] In fact, fewer than two in ten smokers who try to quit succeed in their first efforts. After seven or more attempts, fewer than half succeed.[8]

Addicting drugs are reinforcing; that is, the pharmacological actions of the drugs are sufficiently rewarding for people to keep using them.[1] This is true of nicotine. In fact, smoking patterns of nonhuman primates resemble those of stimulant self-administration.[11]

Tolerance develops to nicotine just as it does to most addicting drugs.[1] People do not just wake up one day smoking 30 cigarettes; they build up to such a point over a period of time, usually years.[12]

In addition, addictive behavior often involves regular and temporal patterns of use. Environmental factors, including drug-associated stimuli and social pressures, influence how people start smoking and their patterns of smoking. Deprivation increases people's desire for the drug, which can commonly be seen during theater intermissions, when people have not been able to smoke for a period of time.

Paired stimuli are known to increase drug use. In the case of nicotine, the sight, smell, or taste of tobacco or smoke increases a person's desire to smoke. Nicotine intake appears to remain remarkably stable from day to day. Evidence exists that

TABLE 14.2. Addictive characteristics of nicotine.

1. Drug causes psychoactive effects (euphoria, stimulation, relaxation)
2. Compulsive use occurs
3. Use continues despite known harmful effects
4. Effects reinforce use
5. Regular and temporal patterns of use exist
6. Deprivation increases desire to use drug
7. Paired stimuli increase use
8. Tolerance develops
9. Physical dependence occurs
10. Withdrawal symptoms occur
11. Has high relapse rate

From H.T. Milhorn, Jr., Nicotine dependence, *American Family Physician*, 39:214–224, 1989.

smokers tend to adjust their intake to some extent to maintain stable plasma nicotine levels.[8]

The addictive properties of nicotine are summarized in Table 14.2.

Other effects of nicotine that may promote dependence include the facts that smokers tend to perform better on some cognitive tasks involving sustained and selective attention when smoking than when deprived of cigarettes; they smoke more when their stress levels increase, indicating that smoking may have a tranquilizing effect; and they weigh less than nonsmokers (stopping smoking is associated with weight gain).[1]

The critical factor for developing nicotine dependence is exposure. A variety of factors contribute to this, including cigarettes' greater social acceptability than other drugs, their relatively low cost, and their ready availability. The tobacco industry is a $20 billion business that provides tax revenues annually in excess of $10 billion to state and federal governments.[8] It makes a considerable effort to promote tobacco, not only as an acceptable form of drug abuse but as a highly desirable form as well.[1] Its expenditures to advertise and market tobacco products total approximately $2.5 billion a year in the United States alone.[8]

Leading national and international organizations, including the American Psychiatric Association and the World Health Organization, have recognized chronic tobacco use to be a drug addiction.[1] The United States Public Health Service now considers cigarette smoking to be a form of drug abuse in which nicotine is the abuse-producing drug.[13] In 1980 the American Psychiatric Association, in the third edition of its *Diagnostic and Statistical Manual of Mental Disorders* (DSM-III), included tobacco dependence as a substance use disorder.[14] The 1987 revised edition (DSM-III-R), in recognition of the role of nicotine, changed "tobacco dependence" to "nicotine dependence."[2]

Abstinence Syndrome

Physical dependence can develop to addicting drugs and is characterized by a withdrawal syndrome. Nicotine is no exception.[1] Withdrawal from nicotine,

TABLE 14.3. Nicotine abstinence syndrome.

Decreased heart rate
Restlessness
Dullness or sleepiness
Inability to concentrate
Irritability
Feelings of hostility
Sleep disturbances
Altered rapid eye movement (REM) during sleep
Slowing of electrocardiogram with decreased arousal pattern
Constipation or diarrhea
Weight gain
Nicotine craving

From H.T. Milhorn, Jr., Nicotine dependence, *American Family Physician*, 39:214–224, 1989. Published by the American Academy of Family Physicians.

however, is not as dramatic or as life-threatening, as that from alcohol.[5] It more resembles withdrawal from central nervous system stimulants such as cocaine and amphetamines (Table 14.3). After suddenly stopping smoking or attempts to cut down, withdrawal symptoms occur within hours and tend to be disturbing. Their intensity varies greatly from person to person. The syndrome consists of decreased heart rate, slowing of the EEG with a decreased arousal pattern, restlessness, dullness or drowsiness, inability to concentrate, irritability, feelings of hostility, sleep problems characterized by altered rapid eye movement (REM) pattern, and nicotine craving. Constipation and/or diarrhea may occur early. People may also gain a significant amount of weight, frequently up to eleven pounds or more.[5] Most symptoms, which are most pronounced during the first week, decrease significantly over three weeks. During the second week they tend to decline gradually or even increase slightly. They continue to decline during the third week. Few subjects have withdrawal symptoms, other than occasional craving, after three weeks. Heavy smokers generally have more severe withdrawal symptoms than light smokers, probably because of their greater physical dependence on nicotine. Tapering may result in more intense craving than sudden cessation.[15]

Health Consequences of Nicotine Abuse

The health complications of smoking may be divided into those resulting from mainstream smoke (active smoking) and those resulting from sidestream smoke (passive smoking), as shown in Table 14.4.

Active Smoking

It is estimated that as many as 350,000 deaths a year in the United States may be attributed to cigarette smoking. This would represent 18 percent of all deaths.[3] Total smoking-related healthcare costs and lost productivity costs amount to approximately $65 billion each year.[7]

TABLE 14.4. Diseases/conditions associated with smoking.

Active smoking

Cancer—oral cavity, pharynx, larynx, esophagus, lung, pancreas, kidney, bladder

Cardiovascular—aggravation of exercise-induced angina, coronary artery disease, myocardial infarction, cardiac arrhythmias, sudden cardiac death, stroke, aortic aneurysm, arteriosclerotic peripheral vascular disease, thromboangiitis obliterans (Buerger's disease)

Pulmonary—impaired pulmonary function, emphysema, acute and chronic bronchitis, chronic cough and hoarseness due to vocal cord irritation

Perinatal effects from maternal smoking—increased mortality, reduced birth weight, spontaneous abortion, sudden infant death syndrome, congenital abnormalities, hyperactivity in childhood, risk of cancer in later life

Miscellaneous—peptic ulcer, erythrocytosis, peripheral blood leukocytosis, smoker's skin, decreased taste and smell, abnormal sperm counts and evidence of chromosomal damage, decreased fertility, increased accident rate, altered drug metabolism, adverse health consequences in women on oral contraceptives

Passive smoking

Cancer—lung

Cardiovascular—aggravation of exercise-induced angina, premature ventricular contractions

Pulmonary—impaired pulmonary function in adults, asthma attacks, pulmonary infections, bronchiolitis, decreased growth rate of lungs, impaired pulmonary function in children

Perinatal effects—decreased birth weight (maternal or paternal smoking)

Miscellaneous—increased hospital admissions of infants, middle ear effusions and sinusitis in children, decreased growth rate

From H.T. Milhorn, Jr., Nicotine dependence, *American Family Physician*, 39:214–224, 1989. Published by the American Academy of Family Physicians.

Cigarette smoking is associated with elevated rates of cancer of the lung, oral cavity, pharynx, larynx, esophagus, pancreas, bladder, and kidney.[3,5] Elevated levels of morbidity and mortality are associated with cardiovascular problems, including strokes, coronary artery disease, heart attacks, and angina.[5] Thromboangiitis obliterans and peptic ulcer disease are influenced adversely by smoking.[3,5] The role of smoking in causing lung infections and chronic obstructive pulmonary disease (COPD) is well documented.[5] Although pulmonary change in any one individual is progressive with chronic smoking, the severity of the damage depends on individual susceptibility.[6] Abstinence of five to ten years returns the risk of developing most smoking-related diseases to that of the nonsmoking population.[5]

Smoking causes a decrease in the functions of smell and taste in the nasopharynx and tongue. This allows smokers to avoid the unpleasant taste and odors associated with smoking. Vocal cord irritation causes chronic cough and hoarseness.[6]

Nicotine easily crosses the placenta. An increase in fetal heart rate can be seen for 90 minutes after a pregnant woman smokes a cigarette. Heavy smokers have an increased risk of spontaneous abortion, are more likely to deliver babies small for gestational age, and have an increased risk of giving birth to children with congenital abnormalities, including patent ductus arteriosus, tetrology of Fallot, and cleft palate and lip. Children of mothers who smoked heavily during pregnancy may be hyperactive through adolescence and may have higher risks of cancer in later life.[5] Cigarette smoking has a harmful effect on a woman's chance of becoming pregnant: Fertility rate decreases as the number of cigarettes smoked per day increases.[16]

Smoking is associated with abnormal sperm forms and evidence of chromosomal damage.[5]

Smokers drink and drive more, fail to use automobile safety belts more often, and have more accidents at work than nonsmokers do.[6]

Passive Smoking

Urinary continine and carboxyhemoglobin levels in nonsmokers have been shown to increase directly with the number of cigarettes smoked in their local environment.[3,9] Passive exposure leads to significant morbidity and mortality. It has been estimated that as many as 5,000 deaths a year in the United States may be related to passive smoking.[3]

Passive exposure causes increased heart rate, elevated systolic and diastolic blood pressure, and increased carboxyhemoglobin levels. As a result, it can further compromise the cardiovascular systems of people with heart disease, producing premature ventricular contractions and earlier onset of angina with activity.[9]

Adult nonsmokers exposed to smoke in the workplace demonstrate impaired pulmonary function equivalent to those who smoke half a pack of cigarettes a day.[6] Passive smoking can provoke acute asthma attacks.[3] The risk of developing lung cancer increases directly with the level of passive smoking.[9]

Children exposed to smoke in the home suffer a variety of consequences. Their risk of developing middle ear effusions and sinusitis increases directly with the amount of smoke exposure.[9] Children of smoking parents have higher rates of pulmonary infection[6] and of bronchiolitis (the frequency of this latter condition decreases as a child ages).[3] Passive smoking may decrease the FEV_1 of children by 7 percent in five years over those children of nonsmoking mothers.[3,9] The lungs of children exposed to passive smoking may grow more slowly.[9] Decreased infant birth weight is a well-known effect of maternal smoking, and birth weight has now been shown to be adversely affected by paternal smoking.[17] The number of hospital admissions of infants in the first year of life are increased directly with the level of maternal smoking. Infants are most often hospitalized with lower respiratory tract infections.[9]

Attempts to Control Adverse Effects

One strategy to help control the adverse health consequences of smoking has been to try to develop safer cigarettes. One approach has been to put less tobacco in each cigarette; another has been to develop filter-tip cigarettes, which have been shown to produce less tar and nicotine when measured by the Federal Trade Commission's smoking machine. However, smokers tend to compensate for reduced nicotine by taking more puffs, inhaling deeper, and smoking each cigarette longer. Furthermore, they tend to smoke more cigarettes. Physicians who advise their patients to switch to low-tar and low-nicotine cigarettes should be aware of the limitations of this approach.[3,6]

It may seem obvious that tobacco is dangerous, but individuals with a wide variety of vested interests, including long-term heavy smokers and industries that produce and distribute tobacco products deny this contention.[13]

Management

Management may involve the rare case of overdose or, most commonly, nicotine dependence.

Overdose

Management of nicotine overdose is symptomatic—that is, it involves general support of respiration and blood pressure. Gastric lavage followed by activated charcoal may be helpful. Excretion of nicotine is probably enhanced by acidification of the urine.[1,17]

Nicotine Dependence

Patients make a conscious decision to stop smoking when they perceive risks from continued smoking, when they have a net value in stopping, and when they believe they can stop. Physicians can make extremely important contributions to patients' health by helping them arrive at this point and by taking advantage of it to help patients stop smoking.

Reasons for Quitting

One single crucial motive for quitting smoking has not been identified. Several reasons are often reported. For example, patients become aware of their general health, making decisions to lead healthier lives. They may also have specific health reasons for quitting, such as genetic, occupational, or metabolic risk factors. Other smokers may decide to quit after they develop symptoms of a smoking-related disease. Parents may want to provide positive role models for their children or become aware of the health risks to their children from passive smoking. Pregnant women may want to stop smoking because of health risks to the fetus. For some people, smoking may simply become too expensive, and many simply want to gain better control of their lives. Others become aware that smoking no longer fills the function it once did: They may have smoked initially because smokers were advertised as sexy, accomplished, or independent. They may no longer need smoking for social acceptance or feel pressure to conform. Finally, some choose to quit smoking because it is now more socially acceptable to be a nonsmoker in some circles than to be a smoker.[12]

Stages of Quitting

Five stages of quitting smoking have been identified.

1. *Precontemplation.* In this stage patients are unlikely to be responsive to direct intervention. They have little concern about the negative aspects of smoking, and heavy-handed messages to this group may increase their resistance to quitting. If pushed hard they will simply find another physician. Calm, factual presentation of the risks in a low-key and matter-of-fact manner is the best approach.
2. *Contemplation.* In this stage patients are much more open to receive information about smoking and its dangers. In fact, they will often ask for help.
3. *Action.* Smokers quit.
4. *Maintenance.* This is the most difficult stage of all. It involves remaining abstinent from cigarettes.
5. *Relapse.* Relapse occurs so frequently in patients attempting to give up cigarettes that it has to be considered part of quitting.[12]

Methods of Treatment

Social, psychological, and pharmacological factors encourage people to continue smoking. Effective treatment must address all of these.[1] Ideally, it should consist of alleviating withdrawal symptoms and teaching new behaviors. It is not enough to advise patients to switch to pipes or cigars, because they will probably continue to inhale. Tapering smoking has been shown to be inferior to sudden stopping as a method of quitting.[5] However, patients who are unwilling to set dates and quit may benefit from tapering. If they are successful at this they may have the confidence to try to stop. Approaches with multiple components have been shown to be more effective than those with single components.[3]

Quitting Smoking Materials/Groups

A variety of resources are available to those who wish to stop smoking.[7] Self-help material can be obtained from local divisions of the American Cancer Society, local offices of the American Lung Association, and local offices of the American Heart Association.

Physicians and other health professionals can get kits to help patients stop smoking from local divisions of the American Cancer Society, the National Cancer Institute, the National Heart, Lung and Blood Institute, the American Academy of Family Physicians, the National Audio Visual Center, and local offices of the American Lung Association. Videotape programs to help people stop smoking can be obtained from local offices of the American Lung Association, the National Audiovisual Center, and the American Academy of Family Physicians. Group programs are sponsored locally by the American Cancer Society and the American Lung Association. Local universities and hospitals often offer programs, and local private practitioners, such as health psychologists, can be helpful.

Behavioral Techniques

Behavioral techniques used to help people quit smoking that may be useful to physicians include self-control strategies, stimulus-control strategies, coping skills, and contingency management.

Self-control strategies consist of having smokers continuously remind themselves of why they want to stop and having them smoke in the least pleasurable way possible. For instance, they can be told never to smoke after meals, always to smoke alone, or to use their least favorite brand of cigarettes.[5]

Stimulus control strategies involve limiting the number of cues for smoking and reducing the ability of cues to evoke the desire for a cigarette (cue extinction). In the first step, smokers monitor themselves to identify cues. A cue may be a specific time, place, emotion, or social setting. One approach to cue extinction is for smokers, about seven to ten days before quitting, to select three cues they have identified as being the most difficult to endure without a cigarette. During this time they continue to smoke but do not smoke while experiencing selected cues. This usually involves waiting at least ten minutes after a cue has passed before lighting a cigarette.[12]

Coping skills include learning to reduce stress and learning relaxation techniques, setting up rewards for success, and seeking out nonsmoking environments and social support. Useful techniques involve such things as thinking of the negative aspects of smoking and the positive aspects of not smoking, self-encouragement, avoiding situations where the temptation to smoke will be the greatest, and substituting other activities, such as having something low in calories to eat or drink, for a cigarette.[7]

Contingency management involves arranging for some reward or punishment that is contingent on not smoking during a specified time period after quitting smoking. This is best done by making a written contract with friends, family, or physician. Reward is usually more effective than punishment. The reward does not have to be large, but it should be frequent; for example, have the kids agree to clean the table each night a mother or father does not smoke.[12]

Pharmacological Approaches

Pharmacological approaches to quitting smoking that have been studied include nicotine fading, gum that contains nicotine, clonidine, mecamylamine, and various anticholinergic agents.

Nicotine fading consists of gradually reducing nicotine consumption by changing to brands with less tar and nicotine and progressively smoking fewer and fewer cigarettes. As already discussed, smokers tend to compensate for the reduced nicotine in each cigarette by taking more puffs, inhaling deeper, and smoking each cigarette longer. For practical purposes, telling smokers to gradually cut down and then quit is like telling heroin addicts to use less and less heroin. For obvious reasons, this approach, when used by itself, has a limited impact. A variant of this approach makes use of a series of dilution filters that progressively mix more air with the smoke in hopes that smokers can gradually decrease their nicotine intake to zero. This approach suffers from similar shortcomings.[3]

Gum that contains nicotine (Nicorette) consists of 2 mg of nicotine and a polycrilex exchange resin. It should be started only after smoking has stopped. The rapid nicotine blood levels obtained from smoking are not achieved from chewing the gum. The average daily dose is eight to ten pieces, but more can be, and probably should be, used. Smokers tend to underutilize the gum, thus limiting its effectiveness. Heavy smokers with signs of physical dependence are the best candidates for it.[18] As many as 3 to 10 percent of gum users may become dependent on it. To minimize this, prescriptions should be given on a restricted basis.[3] Ideally, tapering should occur over three to four weeks, and the gum should not be prescribed for more than six months. It reduces the desire to smoke, although it does not eliminate it, and lessens withdrawal symptoms.[19] The gum is most effective when combined with a clear-cut treatment plan.[20-21] It is the only medication approved by the Food and Drug Administration for helping people quit smoking.

Clonidine, an α-2-adrenergic agonist, has been investigated as a possible medication for use in quitting smoking. It appears to suppress anxiety, tension, irritability, restlessness, and cigarette craving. The mechanism of this is not known. At present, although it looks promising, there is insufficient information on its use to justify routine prescription for smokers.[22]

Mecamylamine, a centrally acting nicotine blocking agent, has been shown to extinguish nicotine dependence in animals and to stop smoking in some people. It works similar to the concept of opiate blockade by naltrexone. It may prove to be useful not only for stopping smoking but for long-term maintenance as well. It warrants further study.[11,23]

Anticholinergic agents (atropine, scopolomine, chlorpromazine) are currently being investigated as tools for helping people stop smoking. They are thought to prevent the acetylcholine rebound that occurs after people quit smoking and that is thought to be responsible for withdrawal symptoms. These agents too require further study.[24]

Maintenance

For people to maintain programs that help them abstain from smoking requires at least as much attention as quitting itself. Like addiction to other drugs (alcohol, heroin, cocaine), recovering nicotine addicts must treat their addiction one day at a time the rest of their lives.[12]

Maintenance, for practical purposes, can be viewed as relapse prevention. A maintenance program should consist of:

1. *Social support*: Ongoing support from family, friends, and coworkers is needed to help ex-smokers maintain their altered behavior. Quitters who have few friends or relatives who smoke are more likely to have continued success.

2. *Coping skills*: Ex-smokers must avoid social and environmental cues and situations that can stimulate their desire to smoke or must develop effective behaviors to deal with them. They should remove environmental cues (cigarette lighters, ashtrays, pipes, and other smoking paraphernalia) from their environment and should continually guard against stimuli that trigger smoking (finishing a meal, having a cocktail, talking on the phone). They need to recognize situations that may provoke relapse (social pressures, stress, conflicts, anger, frustration, depression) and deal with them in a healthy manner.

3. *Changes in knowledge, attitudes, and self perception*: Smokers need to be educated about cigarettes and nicotine and their harmful effects and must continually work on their attitude toward smoking. Through education and change in attitude they will begin to think of themselves as nonsmokers.[3]

Relapse

Because it occurs so often in those attempting to quit smoking, relapse must be considered part of a program to stop smoking. Circumstances leading to relapse generally vary with time from the moment of quitting. The most common reason given for relapse in the first week is withdrawal symptoms. After the first week, coping with crisis situations and exposure to smoking triggers, such as other smokers or drinking alcohol or coffee, are prominent reasons. The majority of crises occur at work or involve family situations, most commonly arguments with spouses or other family members or serious illnesses of family members. Inactivity and boredom are also dangerous. Relapses during the first week are more apt to occur in the home and in the evening; after the second week they are more apt to occur outside the home.[25-26] In one study, over half of relapses occurred in the home, about a fourth occurred in the workplace, and another fourth occurred in other places, such as bars, restaurants, or friends' homes.[26]

Patients should not view relapse as a failure but should learn from the reason for the relapse. They should set another quit date and include the reason for relapse in their revised maintenance program. They should receive continued support and encouragement. The best predictor of relapse may be the quality of support from family, friends, and coworkers.[12]

Prevention

Because most cigarette smokers begin smoking in their early teens (between the ages of 12 and 16) and because people who do not become regular smokers in adolescence rarely begin later in life, prevention is ultimately a pediatric problem. Many environmental factors influence the onset of smoking. Among these, peer pressure and parental smoking are the greatest predictors of adolescent smoking—peer pressure being the most potent factor. Over half of adolescent smokers report smoking their first cigarette with a friend.[27]

A social environment that tolerates smoking facilitates smoking. As the total number of smokers in a child's environment increases, the risk of his or her becoming a smoker escalates. Mass media contributes to the acceptance of smoking by portraying smokers as attractive, outgoing, popular, and sexy. The success of advertising companies is evident. Adolescents believe that 83 percent of people their age are smokers, whereas only 15 to 30 percent actually are; they also believe that 70 percent of teachers smoke when only 20 percent do. Thus, adolescents tend to exaggerate the prevalence of smoking, believing smoking is the norm.[27]

Adolescent girls, adolescents from lower socioeconomics backgrounds, and those from single-parent households are all more likely to smoke. Intervention with these high-risk adolescents should be a priority.[27]

Nicotine is a gateway drug. Few young people begin using marijuana or other substances unless they smoke cigarettes first.[5,7]

Physicians must counterbalance factors that encourage tobacco use. Children generally accept their statements as fact. Six strategies are useful:

1. Provide information about the harmful health consequences of smoking, including those from passive smoking. Don't dwell on the long-term adverse effects of smoking. Adolescents are considerably more motivated by concern for the immediate consequences of smoking, such as greater and earlier skin wrinkling, tobacco-stained teeth and fingers, and the stale odor of breath and clothes.
2. Discuss societal changes in attitude towards smoking.
3. Correct mistaken notions about the percentage of adults who smoke.
4. Emphasize the fact that smoking is addicting and that not starting to smoke is the best way to avoid becoming a regular smoker.
5. Teach children to see the falsity of smoking advertisements in magazines that appeal to adolescents.
6. Provide a nonsmoking environment in the office.[7,26]

Role of the Physician

General Information

In the United States 75 percent of adults make at least one visit to a physician each year, with the mean yearly number of visits being five. Thus, for the majority of physicians, the opportunity for helping people stop smoking will come in the office.[3] The majority of smokers say they want to quit.[3]

A history of smoking should be part of every medical history. It should include questions such as does the patient smoke; if so, how much does he or she smoke; how long has he or she smoked; how early each day does he or she smoke; what type of cigarettes does he or she smoke; has he or she ever tried to quit; reasons for success or failure; whether he or she smokes in public or in restricted places; whether he or she smokes when ill; and why does he or she smoke. These questions are aimed at determining the degree of nicotine addiction as well as building on past successes and failures.[3]

During the physical examination, abnormalities related to smoking should be emphasized as they are found. These might include cigarette-stained fingers, smoker's lines and crows feet on the face, pulmonary rales or rhonchi, and increased resonance on percussion.[3]

Patients who are ready to quit sign contracts to do so. These can be preprinted or handwritten. Patients who are unwilling to sign probably are not ready to quit.[3]

A major obstacle to getting people to quit smoking is that they fear they will or actually do gain weight. This must be addressed. Exercise and good nutrition for maintaining weight are essential.[28]

Some of the immediate consequences of quitting smoking include improved breathing, less coughing, better taste and smell, saved money, fresh breath, no burn holes, no ashtrays to empty, no more tobacco stains on teeth and fingers, better insurance risk, decreased risk of passive smoking on family and coworkers, and improved tolerance for exercise. Physicians can take advantage of these and use them as early positive reinforcement.

Physicians should encourage patients to call them if they relapse to identify a reason for the relapse and to use it in revising their maintenance programs after they set new quit dates.[3]

If physicians choose not to counsel patients, their minimum intervention should be to explain the health risks to patients and to advise them to quit smoking. Between 5 and 10 percent of smoking patients will quit simply on the advice of their physician.[7]

Finally, physicians should play a major role in preventing adolescents from beginning to smoke.[26]

Five-Step Program for Quitting Smoking

A useful, five-step program for quitting smoking is summarized in Table 14.5.

Step 1. The first step is to discuss a patient's smoking. It is always appropriate to review smoking status and take a brief smoking history whether a patient has been in your care for years or is being seen for the first time. Providing health risk information on continued smoking is an integral part of this step. Medical findings should be personalized whenever possible. The health effects of involuntary smoking on a patient's spouse and children should be included in this discussion.[7,29]

Step 2. Assess a patient's interest in quitting, whether he or she is ready to make a commitment to stopping, and the patient's level of motivation and confidence in succeeding. If a patient is not ready to make an attempt, supply recommendations and materials that may orient him or her toward stopping at a later date. Encourage the person to cut down. If a patient is contemplating quitting, determine why he or she is thinking of doing so. This can be used to reinforce quitting. Physicians can then move on to the next step.[7,29]

Table 14.5. Five-step program to quit smoking.

Step 1: Discuss patient's smoking
   Review smoking history
   Provide health risk information
      Personalize when possible
      Include effects of passive smoking

Step 2: Assess interest in smoking cessation
   Determine patient's readiness to quit in terms of motivation and confidence
   If in precontemplation stage, encourage to cut down
   If in contemplation stage, determine the reason patient is thinking about quitting, advise to quit, and go to Step 3

Step 3: Set a target quit date
   Pick a realistic quit date
   Have the patient sign a contract agreeing to quit on that date
   Prescribe nicotine gum if indicated

Step 4: Suggest smoking cessation strategies
   Furnish self-help material
   Arrange to work with the patient using material available to physicians
   Refer to a smoking cessation group/clinic
   Describe preparatory techniques to be used by patient
      List reasons for quitting
      Become aware of smoking-related situations
      Seek social support
      Reduce number of cigarettes to 10 to 15 a day
      Plan to replace cigarettes with low-calorie food or gum or to use Nicorette
      Plan to deal with weight gain
      Plan to eliminate environmental cues
   Discuss withdrawal symptoms
   Review strategies to be used in high-risk situations
   Schedule follow-up

Step 5: Follow-up
   Encourage maintenance of abstinence
   Discuss slips and relapse
   Taper nicotine gum
   If slips or relapse occur, encourage the patient to resume abstinence
   Schedule follow-up appointments

From H.T. Milhorn, Jr., Nicotine dependence, *American Family Physician*, 39:214–224, 1989. Published by the American Academy of Family Physicians.

Step 3. Set a target quit date. Ask a patient to sign a contract acknowledging such a date and to commit to stop smoking entirely on it.[7]

Physicians may wish to prescribe nicotine gum once patients stop smoking. If they plan to refer patients to community programs, they should be sure the gum is compatible with those programs. The gum should be prescribed in a tapering dose over three to four weeks and should not be prescribed for more than six months. The risk of addiction to the gum is real and significant. Simply prescribing it as if it were a magic bullet is ineffective and is to be discouraged.[7,29-31] Package inserts have directions for its use, contraindications, and side effects.

Step 4. Suggest strategies for stopping smoking. This is the step that is usually the most difficult for physicians, probably because they have so many options to choose from. They may choose to furnish patients with self-help material, work with patients using material supplied specifically for this purpose by several organizations, or refer patients to community programs. Like many other things in medicine, physicians should decide which one of these approaches they are most comfortable with and use it regularly. In brief, strategies to stop smoking may include preparing for quitting, discussing withdrawal symptoms and their time course, reviewing strategies for dealing with high-risk situations for relapse, and scheduling follow-up appointments or telephone calls. Preparatory techniques patients can use prior to their quit dates include listing reasons for wanting to quit, becoming more aware of the situations (when, where, why) in which they smoke, seeking social support, reducing tobacco intake to 10 to 15 cigarettes a day, planning to substitute sugar-free chewing gum or low-calorie food for cigarettes or to use Nicorette, developing a plan to deal with weight gain, and eliminating from sight cues for smoking, such as ashtrays and matches.[7,29]

Step 5. Follow-up visits or telephone calls should be initially scheduled weekly to provide support as well to see how well patients stick to their programs. Follow-up visits or phone calls can also be used to taper nicotine gum. Successful abstinence requires continued coping, not instant mastery. It takes at least six months before ex-smokers are at relatively low risks of relapse. Occasional brief slips may occur, or patients may totally relapse. Patients and physicians should view relapses as part of quitting. Patients should be urged to use the reason for a slip or relapse to prevent reoccurrence in a continued or renewed program.[7,29]

Utilization of Office Staff

Both a physician's office staff and office environment can be used effectively to promote nonsmoking. The office itself can be smoke-free, both for staff and patients. Magazines can be selected that do not accept cigarette advertisements, or such advertisements could be torn out of magazines. Recent articles describing the adverse effects of smoking, declining trends in smoking rates, or methods of dealing with the behavioral and addictive aspects of smoking can be clipped from newspapers and magazines and photocopied for patients to take home. The office staff could review plans for quitting smoking and strategies with patients, help them find outside referral sources when desired, explain self-help material, and schedule follow-up contacts.[3,7]

Other Forms of Tobacco Use

Other forms of tobacco use (cigars, pipes, snuff, chewing tobacco) also have deleterious health effects. The mortality rates for these other forms of tobacco use are between those of cigarette smokers and nonsmokers. Cigar and pipe smoking usually involve less exposure to carbon monoxide and less exposure of lung tissues to smoke constituents. However, some cigar and pipe smokers, especially those who used to be cigarette smokers, continue to inhale. Use of snuff or chewing tobacco eliminates both of these exposures. However, with all of these tobacco products (cigar, pipe, snuff, chewing tobacco), nicotine is absorbed through mucous membranes, and people are exposed topically to tobacco or smoke in the oral-nasal cavity and throat. Site-specific cancer rates in these areas are five times as great as in people who do not use tobacco. In addition, patients have slightly higher risks of getting cardiovascular disease. Treatment for these other varieties of tobacco dependence are the same as those described for cigarette smoking.[32-33]

References

1. U.S. Public Health Service. *Report of the Surgeon General: Nicotine Addiction.* U.S. Department of Health and Human Services, Rockville, Maryland, 1988.
2. *Diagnostic and Statistical Manual of Mental Disorders, Revised (DSM-III-R).* American Psychiatric Association, Washington, D.C., 1987, pp. 181–182.
3. Greene, H.L., R.J. Goldberg, and J.K. Ockene. Cigarette smoking: The physician's role in cessation and maintenance. *Journal of General Internal Medicine,* 3:75–87, 1988.
4. McCusker, K. Landmarks of tobacco use in the United States. *Chest* (Supplement), 93:34–36, 1988.
5. Shuckit, M.A. *Drug and Alcohol Abuse.* Plenum Press, New York, 1984, pp. 189–197.
6. Brown, R., R. Pinkerton, and M. Tuttle. Respiratory infections in smokers. *American Family Physician,* 36:133–140, 1987.
7. Gritz, E.R. Cigarette smoking: The need for action by health professionals. *Ca-A Cancer Journal for Clinicians,* 38:194–212, 1988.
8. Henningfield, J.E., and R. Nemeth-Coslett. Nicotine dependence: Interface between tobacco and tobacco-related disease. *Chest* (Supplement), 93:37–55, 1988.
9. Cheseboro, M.J. Passive Smoking. *American Family Physician,* 37:212–218, 1988.
10. *AMA Drug Evaluations.* W.B. Saunders, Philadelphia, 1986, pp. 157–160.
11. Henningfield, J.E. Pharmacological basis and treatment of cigarette smoking. *Journal of Clinical Psychiatry,* 45:14–34, 1984.
12. Fisher, E.B., Jr., D.B. Bishop, J. Goldmunz, and A. Jacobs. Implications for the practicing physician of the psychosocial dimensions of smoking. *Chest* (Supplement) 93:69–78, 1988.
13. Smith, D.E. *Addictions Alert,* 2:13–16, 1988.
14. *Diagnostic and Statistical Manual of Mental Disorders, 3rd ed. (DSM-III).* American Psychiatric Association, Washington, D.C., 1980, p. 176.
15. Hughes, J.R., D.K. Hatsukami, R.W. Pickens, and D.S. Svikis. Consistency of the tobacco withdrawal syndrome. *Addictive Behaviors,* 9:409–412, 1984.
16. Howe, G., C. Westhoff, M. Vessey, and D. Yeates. Effects of age, cigarette smoking, and other factors on fertility: Findings in a large prospective study. *British Medical Journal,* 290:1697–1700, 1985.
17. Katzung, B.G. (Ed.). *Basic Clinical Pharmacology.* Appleton and Lange, Norwalk, 1987, pp. 73–74.

18. Jarvik, M.E., and N.G. Sneider. Degree of addiction and effectiveness of nicotine gum therapy for smoking. *American Journal of Psychiatry*, 141:790–791, 1984.

19. West, R.J., and M.A.H. Russell. Effects of withdrawal from long-term nicotine gum use. *Psychological Medicine*, 15:891–893, 1985.

20. Rubin, D.H., J.M. Leventhall, P.A. Krasilnikoff, and B. Weile. Effect of passive smoking on birth weight. *Lancet*, 2:415–417, 1986.

21. Schneider, N.G., and M.E. Jarvik. Nicotine gum versus placebo gum: Comparison of withdrawal symptoms and success rates. National Institute on Drug Abuse Research Monogram Series, 53:83–101, 1988.

22. Glassman, A.H., W.K. Jackson, B.T. Walsh, S.P. Roose, and B. Rosenfeld. Cigarette craving, smoking withdrawal and clonidine. *Science*, 226:864–866, 1984.

23. Tennant, F.S., and A.L. Tarver. Withdrawal from nicotine dependence using mecamylamine: Comparison of three-week and six-week dosage schedules. National Institute on Drug Abuse Research Monogram Series, 55:291–297, 1984.

24. Bachnysky, N. The use of anticholinergic drugs for smoking cessation: A pilot study. *International Journal of the Addictions*, 21:789–805, 1986.

25. Shiffman, S., L. Read, and M.E. Jarvik. Smoking relapse situations; a preliminary topology. *International Journal of the Addictions*, 20:311–318, 1985.

26. Cummings, K.M., C.R. Jaen, and G. Giovino. Circumstances surrounding relapse in a group of recent smokers. *Preventive Medicine*, 14:195–202, 1985.

27. Silvis, G.L., and C.L. Perry. Understanding and deterring tobacco use among adolescents. *Pediatric Clinics of North America*, 34:363–378, 1987.

28. Fagerstrom, K.O. Reducing weight gain after stopping smoking. *Addictive Behaviors*, 12:91–93, 1987.

29. McCusker, K. Notes from a smoking cessation clinic. *Chest* (Supplement), 93:66–68, 1988.

30. Hughes, J.R., D.K. Hatsukami, and K.P. Skoog. Physical dependence on nicotine in gum. *Journal of the American Medical Association*, 255:3277–3279, 1986.

31. Hjalmarson, A.I. Effect of nicotine chewing gum on smoking cessation. *Journal of the American Medical Association*, 252:2835–2838, 1984.

32. Bigelow, G.E., C.S. Haines, and M.L. Stitzer. Tobacco use and dependence. In *Principles of Ambulatory Medicine*. Ed. by L.R. Barker, J.R. Burton, and P.D. Zieve. Williams and Wilkins, Baltimore, 1986, pp. 234–244.

33. Milhorn, H.T., Jr. Nicotine dependence. *American Family Physician*, 39:214–224, 1989.

CHAPTER 15

Cannabinoids

Introduction

Cannabinoids (cannabinols) are derivatives of the Indian hemp plant, *Cannabis sativa*. The plant contains more than 60 cannabinoids, of which delta-9-tetrahydrocannabinol (THC) is the major psychoactive substance. The plant grows wild practically everywhere but flourishes in temperate and tropical climates. Plants grown in hot, dry climates are the most potent.[1]

Marijuana is the dried flowering tops, leaves, and stems of the plant, which are chopped up and smoked in cigarettes (joints) or pipes. The chopped marijuana resembles grass clippings from which the name "grass" comes. The marijuana smoked today is three to four times as potent as the marijuana available 10 years ago.[1-2]

Hashish, the resinous extract of the hemp plant, is obtained by boiling the parts of the plant that are covered with the resin in a solvent or by scraping it off. It is a very potent form of cannabis, with a THC content of 5 to 12 percent. An even more potent form of cannabis is known as hash oil. Its THC content may be as high as 20 to 50 percent. Hashish is usually smoked in a water pipe (bong) to regulate the intake and cool the smoke. Hashish is classified as a Schedule I drug. Common street/slang names for the cannabinoids are given in Table 15.1.[1]

Because marijuana is by far the most frequently used form of cannabis in the United States, we will restrict the remainder of our discussion to it.

History

Cannabis use has been recorded for thousands of years. Marijuana was referred to in a Chinese pharmacology treatise in 2737 B.C., and a reference to its use in 2000 B.C. was found in India. It is not known when cannabis was introduced to Western Europe, but it must have been very early. An urn containing marijuana found in Germany dated from 500 B.C. In 1545 the Spaniards introduced the hemp plant to South America. Around 1611 early colonists in Virginia cultivated it for its fibers, from which they made cloth. Around 1850 it was recognized for

TABLE 15.1. Street/slang names for cannabis.

Marijuana	
A-bomb (marijuana + heroin)	Maryann
AMP (marijuana + formalde-hyde)	Maryjane
	Mexican Brown
Doobie	Mexican locoweed
Ganga	M.J.
Giggleweed	Pot
Grass	Ragweed
Hay	Reefer (marijuana cigarette)
Hemp	Roach (butt end of marijuana cigarette)
Indian hay	Root (marijuana cigarette)
J	Rope
Jane	Stick (marijuana cigarette)
Joint (marijuana cigarette)	Supergrass (high potency marijuana,
Joy stick (marijuana cigarette)	marijuana + PCP)
Kiff (tobacco + marijuana)	Tea
Killer weed	Texas tea
Mary	Weed
Hashish	
Bhang	Charas (Far East)
Black hash	Hash
Black Russian	Lebanese
Blond hash	Mahjuema
Canned satira	Soles

its medical use. During the latter half of the 19th century physicians used it to treat pain, convulsive disorders, hysteria, asthma, rheumatism, and labor pains. In 1875 "hasheesh houses" modeled after opium dens began to appear. From the 1920s to the 1930s, during Prohibition, marijuana use increased; it was linked to a crime wave in the 1930s. Cannabis preparations were on the shelf of every pharmacy and were widely prescribed until medical use was prohibited in 1937 by the Marijuana Tax Act. During the 1950s, marijuana use spread widely among middle-class people. In the 1960s it gained even more widespread popularity in high schools and on college campuses. It was placed in Schedule I by the Controlled Substance Act of 1970 because it had no medical use. The Act made possession a misdemeanor and the intent to sell or transfer the drug a felony.[1-2]

Pharmacology

Pharmacokinetics

In the United States, the THC content of most marijuana is 1 to 2 percent. Selective breeding, however, yields marijuana with much higher THC concentrations. The most potent marijuana is known as sinsemilla, with a THC concentration that averages 7 percent but may be as high as 14 percent. No more than 60 percent of THC in a marijuana cigarette is actually absorbed when smoked. To obtain maximal effect from marijuana, users must master a smoking technique that is different from that used to smoke regular cigarettes. Users inhale smoke as deeply into their lungs as possible and hold their breath for 20 to 30 seconds or more to extract as much THC from the smoke as possible.[3]

With smoking, plasma concentrations reach their peak in seven to ten minutes, and psychoactive effects peak in 20 to 30 minutes. The effects seldom last longer than two to three hours. After oral administration, the effects begin in 30 to 60 minutes, but peak effects may not occur until the second or third hour. Effects may persist for three to five hours. Although gastrointestinal absorption is largely complete, THC is extensively metabolized as it passes through the liver. THC is only about a half to a third as effective when eaten as when it is when smoked.[1,3-5]

THC is rapidly converted into an active metabolite, 11-hydroxy-detla-9-tetra-hydrocannabinol, which produces effects identical to the parent compound. The metabolite is then converted to inactive metabolites and excreted in the feces (65 percent) and urine (35 percent). Very little unmetabolized THC is found in the urine. After reaching its peak, the plasma THC level falls rapidly at first due to the distribution of this lipid-soluble drug to lipid-rich tissues, including the brain. This is followed by a much slower decline (a half-life of 30 minutes) reflecting the gradual metabolism and elimination of the drug from the body.[1-2,5-6]

Traces of THC can be detected in the urine for two to three days after isolated smoking of the drug. With heavy daily smoking, a urine drug screen may be positive for up to four weeks.[4,7]

Drugs that might be mixed with marijuana to increase its effects include phencyclidine, opium, formaldehyde, and Raid insect spray.[4]

Pharmacological Actions

The mechanism of action of THC is unknown. To date, no specific receptor for THC has been identified. It is likely that its mode of action is on the cell membrane itself. THC exerts its most prominent effects on the CNS and cardiovascular system. Smoking marijuana affects mood, memory, motor coordination, cognitive ability, sensorium, time sense, and self-perception (Table 15.2). Most commonly, smokers have an increased sense of well-being or euphoria and feelings of relaxation and sleepiness. Anxiety reaching panic proportions may replace euphoria, often as a result of the feeling that the drug-induced state will never end. Short-term memory is impaired, and smokers have trouble doing tasks requiring multiple mental steps to reach a specific goal. Depersonalization—a sense of strangeness and unreality about oneself—may occur. Balance is affected, and perception, attention, and information processing are impaired. Psychomotor performance is impaired for four to eight hours. Marijuana smokers report more vivid visual imagery and a keener sense of hearing. Subtle visual and auditory stimuli may take on a novel character. The senses of touch, taste, and smell seem to be enhanced; time seems to pass more slowly, hunger usually increases (marijuana munches). Marijuana use may precipitate flashbacks in previous users of D-lysergic acid diethylamide (LSD).[5-6]

TABLE 15.2. Pharmacological effects of marijuana.

Central nervous system effects
    increased sense of well-being
    euphoria
    sense of detachment
    feelings of relaxation and sleepiness
    short-term memory impairment
    difficulty carrying out tasks requiring multiple mental steps to
        reach a goal
    depersonalization
    balance difficulty
    impaired perception, attention, and information processing
    vivid visual imagery
    impaired psychomotor function
    keener sense of hearing
    subtle visual and auditory stimuli may take on a novel character
    senses of touch, taste, and smell seem to be enhanced
    altered perception of time (time seems to pass more slowly)
    increased hunger
    antiemetic effect
Peripheral effects
    increased heart rate
    increased systolic pressure in the supine position
    decreased blood pressure in the erect position
    marked reddening of conjunctiva
    plasma volume expansion
    increased body temperature due to impaired sweating
    decreased intraocular pressure
    dry mouth and throat
    muscle weakness
    tremors
    unsteadiness
    increased deep tendon reflexes

Cardiovascular effects include increased heart rate, increased systolic pressure while supine, decreased blood pressure while erect, and a marked reddening of the conjunctiva due to blood vessel dilation. Sodium retention and expanded plasma volume occur, as do muscle weakness, tremors, unsteadiness, and increased deep tendon reflexes.[2,5]

Cannabis inhibits sweating, which leads to an increase in body temperature if users are in a hot environment. Marijuana smoking causes dry mouth and throat, although it does not affect respiratory rate and pupillary diameter. Intraocular pressure is decreased, and THC exerts an antiemetic effect.[5]

Interactions with Other Drugs

Cannabis acts synergistically with alcohol and other CNS depressants to cause intoxication. It can also potentiate the stimulatory effects of amphetamines, cocaine, and phencyclidine. It alters the metabolism of barbiturates and ethanol.[5]

Toxicity

High concentrations of THC can induce delusions, hallucinations, and paranoia. Thinking becomes confused and disorganized, and depersonalization and altered time sense are accentuated. A toxic psychosis may occur. Deaths from marijuana overdose have not been reported.

Tolerance

Chronic use of marijuana does increase the rate of metabolism of THC. However, most of the tolerance that develops to marijuana is pharmacodynamic in nature —developing to changes in mood, tachycardia, decreased skin temperature, increased body temperature, decreased intraocular pressure, and psychomotor impairment. Regular marijuana smokers may require more potent cannabis or larger amounts of the drug to achieve the desired effects.[3,5,8]

Dependence

Dependence on THC occurs with regular, heavy use.

Abstinence Syndrome

People who stop smoking marijuana after chronic use of high doses become irritable, restless, and nervous. They have decreased appetite, insomnia, and increased REM sleep. They may suffer tremor, increased body temperature, and chills. Symptoms are relatively mild, begin with a few hours after drug use is stopped, and last four to five days. It is unclear if a postacute withdrawal syndrome occurs with marijuana use.

Therapeutic Uses

THC has several potential therapeutic applications, including use as an antiemetic, especially against nausea and vomiting produced by cancer chemotherapy, and to lower intraocular pressure. Nabilone (Cesamet) and dronabinol (Marinol) are synthetic analogs that are effective against nausea and vomiting; they also lower intraocular presssure.[5,9]

Health Consequences of Marijuana Abuse

Over the years, marijuana has caused concern about adverse health effects on users, probably because so many of them are young. Inhaling marijuana smoke normally causes bronchodilation; however, for some individuals the particles in the inhalant act as irritants and cause bronchoconstriction. In some chronic users, airway resistance increases. Pharyngitis, sinusitis, and bronchitis may also occur, particularly in hashish users. The presence of carcinogens in marijuana smoke and the development of epithelial abnormalities, which are precursors to lung cancer, suggest an increased risk of lung cancer in marijuana smokers. Men who are heavy marijuana smokers may have decreased sperm counts and sperm mobility, both of which are reversible with abstinence. Marijuana may also temporarily disrupt the menstrual cycle. Teratogenicity has not been linked to marijuana use. Angina pectoris may be aggravated by the increased heart rate and increased carboxyhemoglobin concentration that marijuana causes. Whether marijuana use suppresses cell-mediated immunity is uncertain.[2,9-12]

Some heavy marijuana smokers develop an *amotivational syndrome*, which consists of loss of energy, apathy, absence of ambition, loss of effectiveness, inability to carry out long-term plans, problems with impaired memory, and marked decline in school or work performance. Whether or not the amotivational syndrome is the result of marijuana abuse is controversial. In some individuals marijuana use could be one of the results of preexisting behavioral problems rather than the cause.[2,5-6]

Diagnosis and Management

Intoxication

Diagnosis

The diagnosis of marijuana intoxication is made based on signs of intoxication when patients do not have alcohol on their breath. Red conjunctiva and increased pulse rate in an adolescent or young adult should arouse suspicion.

Management

Management of marijuana intoxication usually consists of allowing patients to sleep until symptoms abate. If patients panic or are anxious, talking down is usually sufficient. Sedatives, such as benzodiazepines, are seldom needed.

Overdose

Diagnosis

Diagnosis of marijuana overdose can be difficult. Delusions, hallucinations, and paranoia can wrongfully be attributed to nonchemical psychosis, phencyclidine toxicity, or CNS stimulant overdose. A history of heavy marijuana use or a positive toxicology screen is extremely helpful.

Management

Deaths from marijuana overdose have not been reported. Therefore, managing marijuana toxicity consists of symptomatic treatment.

Dependence

Diagnosis

Diagnosis of marijuana dependence is based on the principles outlined in Chapter 2.

Management

Management of marijuana dependence is the same as for chemical dependence, outlined in Chapter 3.

Abstinence Syndrome

Diagnosis

The diagnosis of marijuana abstinence syndrome is based on typical signs and symptoms and the knowledge that patients have been using marijuana heavily.

Management

Because of its relatively mild nature, the marijuana abstinence syndrome does not require treatment.

References

1. O'Brien, R., and S. Cohen. *The Encyclopedia of Drug Abuse.* Facts on File, New York, 1984.
2. Katzung, B. G. (Ed.). Drugs of abuse. In *Basic and Clinical Pharmacology.* Appleton and Lange, Norwalk, Connecticut, 1987, pp. 350–361.
3. Spector, I. AMP: A new form of marijuana. *Journal of Clinical Psychiatry,* 46:498–499, 1985.
4. Schwartz, R. H. Marijuana: An overview. *Pediatric Clinics of North America,* 34:305–317, 1987.
5. Jaffe, J. H. Drug addiction and drug abuse. In *Goodman and Gilman's Pharmacological Basis of Therapeutics.* Ed. by A. G. Gilman, L. S. Goodman, T. W. Rall, and F. Murad. Macmillan, New York, 1985, pp. 532–581.
6. Wilford, B. B. (Ed.). Major drugs of abuse. In *Drug Abuse: A Guide for Primary Care Physician.* American Medical Association, Chicago, 1981, pp. 21–84.
7. Schwartz, R. H., and R. L. Hawks. Laboratory detection of marijuana use. *Journal of the American Medical Association,* 254:788–792, 1981.
8. Hunt, A., and R. T. Jones. Tolerance and disposition of tetrahydrocannabinol in man. *Journal of Pharmacology and Experimental Therapeutics,* 215:35–44, 1980.
9. American Medical Association Council on Scientific Affairs. Marijuana: Its health hazards and therapeutic potentials. *Journal of the American Medical Association,* 246:1823–1827, 1981.
10. Schonberg, S. K. (Ed.). Specific drugs. In *Substance Abuse: A Guide for Health Professionals.* American Academy of Pediatrics, Elk Grove Village, Illinois, 1988, pp. 115–182.

11. Wu, T. C., D. P. Tashkin, B. Djahed, et al. Pulmonary hazards of smoking marijuana as compared with tobacco. *New England Journal of Medicine*, 318:347–351, 1988.
12. Morris, R. R. Human pulmonary pathophysiology changes from marijuana smoking. *Journal of Forensic Science*, 30:345–349, 1985.

CHAPTER 16

Hallucinogens

The Hallucinogens

People throughout the world have used hallucinogenic drugs in religious ceremonies for thousands of years. Native American Church members use peyote, a cactus plant that contains mescaline, believing that it allows them to communicate easily with God. In a similar fashion, native populations of Mexico use mushrooms that contain psilocybin in their religious rites. In 1986, 12 percent of high school seniors had tried a hallucinogenic drug, and about 4 percent had used a hallucinogen in the past month. The illicit hallucinogens are classified by the DEA as Schedule I drugs.[1-3]

The hallucinogens include the indolealkylamines (LSD, psilocyn, psilocybin, DET, DMT), the phenylethylamines (mescaline), the phenylisopropylamines (DOM, MDA, MMDA, MDMA, MDEA), and a miscellaneous group (nutmeg, mace, morning glory seeds, mappine, ibogaine) as shown in Table 16.1. They are often referred to as psychedelic drugs. The feature that separates them from other classes of drugs is their capacity to induce states of altered perception, thought, and feeling that are not experienced otherwise except in dreams or in religious experiences. Users call hallucinogens by a variety of names (Table 16.2). LSD (D-lysergic acid diethylamide) is the prototype of the hallucinogens.[4-5]

LSD

LSD is a semisynthetic drug derived from the alkaloid lysergic acid, which is found in ergot, a parasitic fungus that grows on rye and other grains. It is also known as lysergide and LSD-25.[1]

History

LSD was synthesized in 1938 during experimentation with ergot fungus. Accidental ingestion in 1943 led to discovery of the drug's psychedelic properties. From 1949 to 1954, LSD was widely studied. The U.S. Army tested it for use as

TABLE 16.1. The hallucinogens.

Drug group	Drug name
indolealkylamines	LSD (D-lysergic acid diethylamide) psilocyn, psilocybin DMT (dimethyltryptamine) DET (diethyltryptamine)
phenylethylamines	mescaline (peyote)
phenylisopropanolamines	DOM (4-methyl-2,5-dimethoxyamphetamine) MDA (3,4-methylenedioxyamphetamine) MMDA (3-methoxy-4,5-methylenedioxyamphetamine) MDMA (3,4-methylenedioxymethamphetamine) MDEA (3,4-methylenedioxyethamphetamine)
others	nutmeg, mace morning glory seeds mappine ibogaine

a brainwashing agent and as a way of making prisoners talk more readily. Psychiatrists believed that its effects mimicked a psychotic state and used it in an attempt to better understand mental disorders. It came into widespread use as an adjunct to psychotherapy. Until the 1960s, LSD use was restricted to a small number of intellectuals. Its illicit use on a broad scale began in the United States around 1962, encouraged by Dr. Timothy Leary of Harvard University, who recommended that people should "turn on, tune in, and drop out." Chronic LSD users became known as acid heads. LSD is classified as a Schedule I drug.[1,5]

Pharmacology

Pharmacokinetics

LSD is a tartrate salt that is soluble in water. In its pure form, it is a white odorless crystalline material, but street preparations are usually mixed with colored substances. It may be manufactured as a capsule, tablet, or liquid and is always taken orally. It is extremely potent, with an average dose being 25 to 150 micrograms. Because such small amounts produce the desired effects, it is often put on sugar cubes, blotter paper, or small gelatin squares. LSD is 200 times as potent as psilocybin and 5,000 times as potent as mescaline.[1]

When they take it orally, users usually feel the effects of LSD within an hour. The effects peak in three to five hours and last six to twelve hours. The drug is rapidly distributed to the brain and throughout the body, is metabolized in the liver and kidneys, and is excreted mostly in the feces, but also in the urine.[1]

TABLE 16.2. Street/slang names for hallucinogenic drugs.

Drug	Street/slang names	
LSD	Acid	L
	Big D	Lysergide
	Blotter	Mellow Yellows
	Blotter acid	Microdots
	Blue acid	Orange cubes
	Blue heaven	Paper acid
	Blue mist	Pellets
	Brown dots	Sugar
	Cubes	Sugar cubes
	D	Tabs
	Deeda	Wedges
	Dots	Window panes
	Haze	
psilocybin/psilocyn	Magic mushrooms	Shrooms
	Mushrooms	Silly putty
	Sacred mushrooms	
DMT	Businessman's lunch	Businessman's LSD
mescaline/peyote	Bad seed	Mesc
	Beans	Mescal
	Big chief	Moon
	Buttons	P
	Cactus	Peyoti
	Cactus buttons	Topi
DOM	STP	Serenity-tranquility-peace
MDA	Love drug	
MDMA	Adam	M & M
	Ecstasy	X
	Love Drug	XTC
MDEA	Eve	
morning glory seeds	Bindweed	Heavenly Blue
	Blue Star	Pearly Gates
	Flying Saucers	Wedding Bells
mappine	Yopo	Cohoba

Pharmacological Actions

The hallucinogens probably exert their effects by modifying neurotransmitter pathways in the brain. The chemical structure of serotonin is similar to that of LSD. Other hallucinogens are similar in structure to norepinepherine and dopamine.[2]

The effects of LSD depend on the quantity of the drug taken and the user's psychological and emotional state, as well as the setting in which the drug is used. The most striking effect of LSD is that it causes dramatic alterations in perceptions. Colors seem brighter and often split into the full spectrum, so that objects appear to have rainbows around them. The shapes and sizes of objects are distorted, and their boundaries seem to shift and dissolve. Synesthesia, a mixing of senses, is common, and users often say they can see music as a series of colors and shapes. Time seems to pass very slowly. Hallucinogens are often described as mind-expanding because of their psychological effects.[1-2]

Sympathetic effects of LSD include pupillary dilation, increased body temperature, increased blood pressure and body temperature, tachycardia, hyperreflexia, piloerection, muscle weakness, and tremor.[3-4]

Interactions with Other Drugs

LSD acts synergistically with other hallucinogenic drugs to produce psychedelic effects. Because of its stimulatory effects, it also acts synergistically with amphetamines, cocaine, marijuana, and PCP to increase pulse rate and blood pressure.

Toxicity

LSD in high doses may cause panic (bad trips) more often than usual doses. Confusion, depression, and paranoia may occur. Some individuals experience toxic psychosis with hallucinations after taking very high doses. Deaths due to LSD overdose have not been reported, although deaths from suicides and accidents have occurred.[1-2,4]

Tolerance

A high degree of tolerance to the behavioral effects of LSD develops after three or four doses, although tolerance to the cardiovascular effects is less pronounced. Sensitivity returns after a few drug-free days. There is considerable cross-tolerance between LSD, mescaline, and psilocybin.[4-5]

Dependence

Physical dependence does not occur with repetitive use of hallucinogens; psychological dependence does.

Abstinence Syndrome

Hallucinogens do not cause an abstinence syndrome.

Health Consequences of LSD Abuse

One disturbing effect of LSD is the flashback, a reexperiencing of the effects of the drug weeks or even months after taking it. The etiology is uncertain. Flashbacks seem to occur most frequently in people who have used LSD repeatedly. There is no evidence that even long-term, high-dose use of LSD results in any permanent damage to the body or brain.[1-2,6]

Diagnosis and Management

Intoxication

The diagnosis of LSD intoxication is based on typical signs and symptoms and knowledge that patients have used the drug. Treatment consists only of reassuring and monitoring patients to prevent harm until the effects of the drug wear off.

Overdose

The diagnosis of LSD overdose is difficult without knowing that patients have taken the drug. Overdose can be confused with psychiatric or other drug-induced states in which panic reactions or psychosis predominate. A toxicology screen may be required to make the diagnosis. Management consists of simple talking down when possible. Alternatively, a benzodiazepine, such as diazepam (10 to 15 mg orally) or aprazolam (2 mg intramuscularly), may be required.

Dependence

Diagnosis of LSD dependence is based on the principles discussed in Chapter 2. Treatment is that of chemical dependence discussed in Chapter 3.

Abstinence Syndrome

LSD does not cause an abstinence syndrome so no treatment is required.

Other Hallucinogenic Drugs

Other Indolealkylamines

In addition to LSD, indolealkylamines include psilocybin, psilocyn, dimethyl-tryptamine (DMT), and diethyltryptamine (DET).

Psilocybin and Psilocyn

Psilocybin is the active hallucinogenic ingredient of the *Psilocybe mexicana* mushroom and of a few other species. Ritual use of psilocybin by Mexican and Central American cultures dates back at least to 1500 B.C. The mushrooms were considered sacred and were named *teonanacatl*, or "flesh of the gods." In 1958 psilocybin and its active cogener, psilocyn, were isolated. In pure form psilocybin is a white crystalline material; in other forms it may consist of crude mushroom preparations, intact dried mushrooms, or capsules. The usual dose of psilocybin is 4 to 5 mg, although larger doses are not unusual. The drug's potency is between that of mescaline and LSD. Although psilocybin and psilocyn can be manufactured synthetically, most of what is sold illicitly as psilocybin consists of other chemical compounds such as phencyclidine.[1,4,7]

When users take the drugs orally, they feel their initial effects in 10 to 15 minutes. Reactions reach maximum intensity in about 90 minutes and may not begin to subside for two to three hours. The effects usually last five to six hours.

The effects, both physiological and psychological, are similar to those of LSD. In large doses, numbness of the tongue, lips, or mouth may occur.[1,8]

Tolerance and psychological dependence to psilocybin and psilocyn do develop, as does cross-tolerance to the effects of LSD and mescaline. Physical dependence has not been reported.[1,7]

DMT

A fast-acting hallucinogen somewhat similar in structure to psilcocyn, DMT (dimethyltryptamine) is found in the seeds of the *Piptadenia* shrub, in the climbing vine *Banisteriopsis caapi*, and in the roots of *Mimosa hostilis*. It can also be synthesized. Within five to ten minutes after ingestion, DMT produces an LSD-like experience that lasts from 30 to 60 minutes. Unlike LSD, it affects only visual perceptions. It can cause lack of coordination and spasticity, which LSD does not cause. Because of its short duration of action, it is known as the businessman's lunchtime high. Tolerance and psychological dependence do develop with repeated use of the drug; physical dependence does not occur.[1]

DET

A synthetic hallucinogen similar to DMT, DET (diethyltryptamine) produces a psychedelic experience similar to that of DMT except that it is milder and of shorter duration. It can easily be manufactured in home laboratories.[1]

Mescaline

A phenylethylamine and the principle alkaloid in the peyote cactus (*Lophophora williamsii*), mescaline is found in northern Mexico and Texas. It has been used in religious rites from the earliest recorded times and is now used legally by the Native American Church, although this may change as the result of a recent court decision. Mescaline was isolated in 1897, and its chemical structure was determined in 1918. It is considerably less potent than LSD. The drug is usually ingested, but it can be inhaled by smoking ground up peyote buttons. The average hallucinogenic dose is three to eight buttons, which contain 300 to 500 mg of mescaline. More rarely, it is injected. At low doses the effects appear in one to three hours and last for four to twelve hours. They are fairly similar to the effects of LSD. At higher doses the drug may cause fever, headache, hypotension, and depressed cardiac and respiratory activity. Tolerance and psychological dependence develop with repeated doses, as does cross-tolerance to LSD. Physical dependence does not develop. Most of what is sold on the street as mescaline is actually LSD or phencyclidine.[1,4,9]

Phenylisopropylamines

DOM

First synthesized in 1963, DOM (4-methyl-2,5-dimethoxyamphetamine) was quickly renamed STP by the drug culture after a commercial motor oil additive.

STP was said to stand for serenity-tranquility-peace. It has a structural resemblance to both amphetamine and mescaline. It is less potent than LSD, but its effects last longer. They begin about an hour after ingestion, reach their highest intensity in three to five hours, and subside in seven to eight hours. Physiological effects include increased heart rate and systolic blood pressure, dilation of the pupils, and a slight rise in body temperature. Nausea, tremor, and perspiration may occur. The effects vary with the dose. Doses of about 3 mg produce euphoria and enhanced self-awareness; doses above 5 mg produce hallucinations and changes in perception. Tolerance and psychological dependence to the effects of DOM probably develop with repeated doses; physical dependence probably does not. STP, for the most part, is now relegated to history.[1,4]

MDA

A semisynthetic drug produced by modifying the major psychoactive components of nutmeg and mace, MDA (3,4-methylenedioxyamphetamine) can also be produced from safrole, the oil of sassafras. It was first synthesized in 1910. Its effects are similar to those of mescaline and amphetamine. Physiological responses to low doses include pupillary dilation and increased blood pressure and pulse rate. Higher doses may cause increased body temperature, profuse sweating, and muscle rigidity. Low doses may cause a sense of well-being with heightened tactile sensations, while high doses cause illusions and hallucinations. Because it produces warm, loving feelings, it is known in the drug culture as the love drug. The average dose of MDA is 50 to 150 mg. Its effects set in 30 to 60 minutes after ingestion and peak in 1.5 to 2 hours and last about 8 hours. Mental and physical exhaustion may follow the use of MDA. It can be highly toxic, and deaths have occurred from overdose. Tolerance and physical dependence probably do not occur.[1,4]

MMDA

A derivative of the alkaloid myristicin found in nutmeg, MMDA (3-methoxy-4,5-methylenedioxyamphetamine) has psychedelic properties and is said to intensify present experiences, as opposed to MDA, which is said to intensify past experiences.[1,4]

MDMA

Most commonly known in the drug culture as ecstasy, other common names for MDMA (3,4-methylenedioxymethamphetamine) are X, M and M, XTC, Adam, and love drug. It is a derivative of methamphetamine and was used legally by psychiatrists in the 1970s to facilitate psychotherapy. Since 1983 it has been a popular drug among adolescents and young adults. In 1985 the DEA placed it in Schedule I. However, it is still readily available on the illicit market. In oral doses of 100 mg, it produces euphoria and enhanced self-awareness; in higher doses, it acts as a CNS stimulant. It probably does not produce true hallucinations.

Animal studies suggest that the drug may destroy the nerve cell endings in the brain that release serotonin. Deaths have occurred from its use.[2,10-13]

MDEA

Known in the drug culture as Eve, MDEA (3,4-methylenedioxyethamphet-amine) is a designer drug and appeared as a legal street drug in 1985. It has effects similar to MDMA but milder. It was placed in Schedule I in 1987. Deaths have occurred from its use.[2,11,14]

Other Hallucinogens

Other hallucinogens include nutmeg, mace, morning glory seeds, mappine, and ibogaine.

Nutmeg and Mace

Nutmeg is the dried seed of *Myristica fragrans*, an evergreen tree indigenous to East India. Mace, its seed root, has similar properties. Both are common cooking spices. Nutmeg contains two hallucinogenic substances, myristicin and elemicin, that are closely related to mescaline. Because of their unpleasant side effects, nutmeg and mace have limited popularity, being used primarily by adolescents as substitutes for illegal drugs. The usual dose is one to two tablespoons (less than 20 gm) in tea, hot chocolate, or orange juice. Nutmeg and mace produce euphoria similar to mescaline. In doses greater than 20 gm, they can produce visual hallucinations, fear, anxiety, and sometimes panic. They may cause vomiting, rapid heartbeat, excessive thirst, bloodshot eyes, temporary constipation, and difficulty urinating. Physical effects begin about 45 minutes after ingestion, and psychological effects after one to two hours. The effects usually last two to four hours and then begin to subside. The sale of nutmeg and mace is not regulated by law.[1,12]

Morning Glory Seeds

The seeds of certain members of the bindweed family convolvulaceae contain hallucinogenic substances similar to LSD. The active ingredients in morning glory seeds have about one-tenth the potency of LSD. Native Americans have long used these seeds in religious ceremonies. The Aztecs were the first to discover the hallucinogenic properties of morning glory seeds, whose effects in doses of 200 to 300 seeds are somewhat like those of LSD. Perceptual disturbances and mood changes occur. Physiological effects include nausea, vomiting, intense headache, drowsiness, diarrhea, chills, impaired vision, decreased blood pressure, and even shock. Effects occur in 25 to 40 minutes after ingestion and last up to six hours. The seeds are first pulverized and soaked in water, then the liquid is strained and drank. The sale of morning glory seeds is not regulated by law.[1,4]

Mappine

Mappine (bufotenine) is dimethyl-serotonin. It can be extracted from the skin of the *Bufo marinus* toad, the *Amanita mappa* toadstool, or the South American shrub *Piptadenia peregrina*. The Vikings used it, as did natives of Siberia and the Caribbean, where it is called cohoba snuff. When administered intravenously, it produces altered perceptions of time and space.[4]

Ibogaine

A complex compound that is derived from the African shrub *Tabernanthe iboga*, ibogaine has hallucinogenic properties similar to those of LSD and also acts as a stimulant. It was isolated in 1901 and synthesized in 1966. It is sold in Europe in tonics. Indian tribes in South America used iboga in a rite of passage into adulthood and call it the Ordeal Bean. Hunters stalking game use it in Africa. It allows users to remain motionless for long periods of time while remaining conscious and mentally alert.[1,4]

References

1. O'Brien, R., and S. Cohen. *The Encyclopedia of Drug Abuse.* Facts on File, New York, 1984.
2. Schonberg, S. K. (Ed.). Specific drugs. In *Substance Abuse: A Guide for Health Professionals.* American Academy of Pediatrics, Elk Grove Village, Illinois, 1988, pp. 115–182.
3. Johnston, L. D., P. M. O'Malley, and J. M. Bachman. Drug use in high school seniors: The class of 1986. U.S. Department of Health and Human Services publication number (ADM)87-1535. Rockville, Maryland, 1987.
4. Wilford, B. B. (Ed.). Major drugs of abuse. In *Drug Abuse: A Guide for the Primary Care Physician.* American Medical Association, Chicago, 1981, pp. 21–84.
5. Jaffe, J. H. Drug addiction and drug abuse. In *Goodman and Gilman's The Pharmacological Basis of Therapeutics.* Ed. by A. G. Gilman, L. S. Goodman, T. W. Rall, and F. Murad. Macmillan, New York, 1985, pp. 532–581.
6. Strassman, R. J. Adverse reaction to psychedelic drugs: A review of the literature. *Journal of Nervous & Mental Disease*, 172:572–578, 1984.
7. Beck, J. E., and D. V. Gordon. Psilocybin mushrooms. *Pharm. Chem. Newsletter*, 4:1–4, 1982.
8. Schwartz, R. H., and D. E. Smith. Hallucinogenic mushrooms. *Clinical Pediatrics*, 27:70–73, 1988.
9. Schwartz, R. H. Mescaline: A survey. *American Family Physician*, 37:122–124, 1988.
10. Clinko, R. P., H. Roehtich, D. R. Sweeney, et al. Ecstasy: A review of MDMA and MDA. *International Journal of Psychiatry Medicine*, 16:359–372, 1987.
11. Dawling, D. G., E. T. McDonough III, and R. O. Bost. Eve and ecstasy: A report of five deaths associated with MDEA and MDMA. *Journal of the American Medical Association*, 257:1615–1617, 1987.
12. Seymour, M. A., D. Smith, D. Inaba, and M. Landry. MDMA. In *New Drugs: Look-Alikes, Drugs of Deception, and Designer Drugs.* Hazelden, Center City, Minnesota, 1989, pp. 117–132.

13. Barnes, D. M. New data intensify the agony over ecstasy. *Science*, 239:864–866, 1988.
14. Brown, R. T., and N. J. Braden. Hallucinogens. *Pediatric Clinics of North America*, 34:341–347, 1987.

CHAPTER 17

Phencyclidines

History

Phencyclidine (PCP) was synthesized in 1957 by Parke-Davis Laboratories and shortly afterwards was entered into clinical trials under the brand name of Sernyl. It was originally intended to be the perfect intravenous, surgical anesthetic and did not, in fact, depress respiratory and cardiovascular functions. However, 10 to 20 percent of the patients to which it was administered exhibited bizarre postoperative behavior, including extreme agitation, delirium, muscle rigidity and seizures.[1-3] Because of this, PCP was removed from the market for use as a human anesthetic in 1965. Ketamine (Ketalar), a shorter-acting homolog with fewer side effects, replaced PCP as a dissociative anesthetic for humans and is still used today.[4] PCP continued to be manufactured and marketed from 1965 to 1978 as a veterinary anesthetic, Sernylan. In 1979 all legal manufacture of PCP ceased. It was placed in Class II by the Drug Enforcement Administration (DEA) in 1970.[2,5-6]

The first illicit PCP appeared on the streets of San Francisco in a pill known as the "PeaCe Pill" in 1967. It rapidly developed a bad reputation because it was regularly associated with bad trips that resulted in dangerous behavior. It subsequently fell in disfavor as a street drug, only to resurface a few years later when smoking the drug, which allowed titration of its effects, became popular.[2] Within a few years its use spread throughout the United States. It is produced inexpensively in clandestine laboratories set up in kitchens, garages, and basements. In addition to being used for its own properties, it is frequently misrepresented by dealers as some other drug, most often as LSD, mescaline, psilocybin (mushrooms), THC (the major psychoactive component of marijuana), or synthetic cocaine.[3-6] Because of its low cost and ease of manufacture, it is also used to adulterate other drugs.[4]

Pharmacology

PCP is most commonly mixed with dried leaf materials, such as marijuana, tobacco, oregano, or parsley, and smoked. It can also be snorted through the nose. It is sometimes taken orally as a pill or liquid; less often, it is injected intravenously.[1,3,7] It is used for its euphoric effects, ability to decrease inhibitions, ability to instill feelings of power and eliminate pain, and for a dissociative state in which altered perceptions of time, space, and body image occur.[3-4]

The Phencyclidines

PCP, in its hydrochloride form, exists as a white to off-white powder that is easily and inexpensively synthesized from readily available chemicals. It is a member of the arylhexylamine class. At least 60 precursors, derivatives, and analogs of PCP have been prepared. Nearly all cause pharmacological effects similar to those of PCP.[2]

Pharmacokinetics

The onset of action of PCP depends on the route of administration. When taken orally, users begin to feel the drug's effects in 15 minutes. Effects occur in about 2.5 minutes when it is smoked, with peak effects occurring in 15 to 30 minutes. With usual street doses, the major effects generally last four to six hours with return to normalcy in 24 to 48 hours.[5]

The most prominent pharmacological actions of PCP are depression of the central nervous system and sympathomimetic effects. Variable cholinergic and anticholinergic effects may also occur. Effects on the cerebellum, including dizziness, ataxia, slurred speech, and nystagmus, may be prominent.[2,6]

PCP is a basic substance. As a result, it is better absorbed in the small intestines than in the acidic medium of the stomach. It is metabolized by the liver, and a small amount is excreted unchanged in the urine. Acidification of the urine increases the rate of excretion.[1,5,8] PCP that is excreted into the stomach from the blood is rapidly ionized by stomach acid and trapped there because of the impermeability of membranes to ions. It again passes into the small intestine, where it is reabsorbed. Thus, it is recirculated in the body, regardless of its route of administration. PCP's gastric concentration may be several times its serum concentration.[6,8-9]

PCP is lipophilic and, as a consequence, is rapidly removed from the blood and concentrated in adipose tissue and the brain. It remains in these storage sites for days to weeks. Blood and urine levels may, therefore, be low while the effects of the drug persist.[2,8]

Pharmacological Actions

PCP appears to affect several neurotransmitters in the brain. It inhibits the reuptake of dopamine, increases the releases of dopamine, and competitively inhibits norepinephrine and serotonin. Depending on the dosage, it can either excite or depress different areas of the brain to produce psychiatric and physical manifestations.[10]

Toxicity

PCP overdose results in a stuporous to comatose state. Classically, patients' eyes are open and their muscles are extremely contracted. They are largely unaware of pain and may have a hypertensive crisis. They may suffer temporary periods of excitement, as well as seizures.

Tolerance

Continued use of PCP leads to tolerance.

Dependence

Dependence occurs in humans. Experimental animals will administer PCP to themselves.[11-12]

Abstinence Syndrome

Acute withdrawal symptoms consisting of nervousness, anxiety, and depression can occur. Chronic users may experience a postacute withdrawal syndrome consisting of depression and loss of recent memory, which may last for months or years.[1]

Health Consequences of PCP Abuse

Medical consequences of PCP intoxication include acute tubular necrosis secondary to rhabdomyolysis, acute hepatic necrosis secondary to hyperpyrexia, aspiration pneumonia, high output cardiac failure, pulmonary edema, hypertensive encephalopathy, intracranial hemorrhage, and death.[8,13-18]

Diagnosis

Physicians must develop an accepting, noncritical attitude when attempting to gain drug information from patients or those accompanying them. Patients should be searched; any drugs found, such as partially smoked joints, should be sent to a laboratory for analysis.[5] Knowledge of slang associated with PCP can be helpful in interpreting information obtained from patients, friends, or family (Table 17.1).[7]

The signs and symptoms of PCP intoxication are related to its dose, route of administration, and an individual's response to it. Because the signs and symptoms of PCP intoxication vary greatly, classification according to dosage is confusing and difficult. Dosage is rarely known or is impossible to determine. In many cases, patients are not even aware that PCP is the drug they took. Even when PCP blood levels can be measured, results are rarely available quickly enough to be of diagnostic or therapeutic value.[5,13] For this reason, it is more helpful to divide PCP intoxication into stages based on patients' signs and symp-

Table 17.1. Street/slang names for phencyclidine.

Angel dust	Mint Weed
Angel hair	Mist
Angel mist	Monkey dust
Animal tranquilizer	PCP
Cadillac	Peace
C.J.	PeaCe Pill
Crystal	Rocket fuel
Crystal Joints	Scuffle
Cyclones	Selma
Dust	Sherman
Elephant tranquilizer	Snorts
Embalming fluid	Soma
Goon	Supercools
Gorilla biscuits	Superweed
Hog	Surfer
Horse tranquilizer	T
Jet fuel	TAC
Kay jay	TIC
K.J.	Tranks
Killer Weed	Whacky weed
Krystal joint	Wooble Weed
K.W.	Zombie dust
Lovely	

PCP + marijuana = supergrass

From H.T. Milhorn, Jr., Diagnosis and management of phencyclidine intoxication, *American Family Physician*, in press. Published by the American Academy of Family Physicians.

toms. If patients are conscious, their level of intoxication is said to be Stage I. If they are stuporous or mildly comatose, with active response to deep pain, their level of intoxication is Stage II. Comatose patients with no response to deep pain are classified as Stage III.[19]

Behavioral Manifestations

Stage I intoxication generally corresponds to about 2 to 5 mg of ingested or smoked PCP and a serum concentration of 25 to 90 ng/ml. The major manifestations of Stage I intoxication are behavioral. Patients' behavior may be unpredictable. They may appear drunken and euphoric or may be disoriented, with alternating periods of lethargy and fearful agitation. They may be negative, hostile, and have disorganized thoughts. They are sometimes combative and violent and may display sudden rage. They misperceive distance and time and may feel dissociated from parts of their body. They may be catatonic and/or have stereotyped behavior (sucking, picking, repetitive motor movements). They may stare blankly at their surroundings, appear to be unable to speak, or talk to themselves, and may demonstrate echolalia (involuntary repetition of a word or sentence just spoken by another person) or hyperacusis (increased sense of hearing). They are usually unconcerned about their grooming. They may be socially uninhibited, obscene, and exhibit nudity.[2,7,9,19]

PCP users' perception of imminent danger is impaired, and they may not flee from fires or avoid obvious danger. They have decreased perception of pain and may harm themselves with apparent lack of concern. They may have delusions of invulnerability, may seem to possess inordinate strength, and may be without fear. They are capable of violent or self-destructive behavior. They have been known to set fire to themselves and stab or assault others. Patients have been described as trying to stop a train by standing in front of it.[7,19]

Symptomology may be indistinguishable from functional psychosis (paranoid schizophrenia, catatonia, mania). Although visual, auditory, and tactile delusions may occur, patients seldom admit to true hallucinations.[2,12,19]

State II intoxication usually results from 5 to 25 mg of ingested or inhaled PCP and a serum concentration of 90 to 300 ng/ml. Stage III intoxication results from greater than 25 mg ingested or injected PCP and a serum level of greater than 300 ng/ml.[7,19] Because the prominent features of Stages II and III intoxication are stupors or comas, psychological manifestations are generally not associated with these stages.

Physical Signs and Symptoms

Physical signs and symptoms of PCP intoxication generally depend on the stage of intoxication (Table 17.2). They consist of central nervous system signs—dysarthria, agitation, and loss of concentration at lower doses, progressing to tonic-clonic seizures and deep coma at higher doses. Patients have little or no response to pain. Motor system impairment consists of ataxia, muscle rigidity, grimacing, and bruxism, progressing to generalized myoclonus, opisthotonus or decerebrate posture, and extreme muscle rigidity. Eye signs range from horizontal nystagmus with lost lid reflex to nystagmus in any direction, hippus, disconjugate gaze, absent corneal reflex, and ptosis. Body temperature may be mildly elevated (98–101°F) or very high (103–108°F). Pulse rate and blood pressure may be mildly increased or could be as much as twice normal. High cardiac output failure can occur. Respiration may range from mildly increased to only periodic breathing or apnea, and patients may suffer aspiration pneumonia. Deep tendon reflexes may range from being increased with clonus on stimulation to absent. Laryngeal/pharyngeal reflexes may range from being hyperactive to absent. Autonomic signs (nausea, vomiting, diaphoresis, flushing, lacrimation, hypersalivation) may increase in intensity with the dose.[2,9,12,19]

Summary of Patient Presentation

Physicians should be aware that patients who are conscious, behave bizarrely, giddily, or drunkenly, have little awareness of pain, have blank stares, nystagmus on stimulation, ataxia, elevated pulse rate and blood pressure, increased deep

TABLE 17.2. Physical signs and symptoms of phencyclidine intoxication.

	Stage I	Stage II	Stage III
Central nervous system	conscious loss of concentration illogical speech dysarthria agitation	stupor to mild coma tonic-clonic seizures on stimulation	deep coma tonic-clonic seizures to status epilepticus possible stroke
Response to pain	blunted decreased pin prick response	deep pain intact	deep pain absent
Motor system	ataxia impaired tandem gait muscle rigidity masseter and neck muscle spasms repetitive purposeless movements grimacing bruxism	generalized muscle rigidity muscle twitching	generalized myoclonus opisthotonic or decerebrate posturing muscle rigidity
Eye signs	horizontal nystagmus late vertical nystagmus lid reflex lost blank stare	nystagmus (any direction) corneal reflex lost roving eyes or fixed stare disconjugate gaze pupils midposition possible ptosis	nystagmus (any direction) eyes opened or closed hippus increasing pupillary size absent corneal reflex disconjugate gaze ptosis
Temperature	normal to mildly elevated (98–101°F)	moderately elevated (101–103°F)	hyperpyrexia (103–108°F) possible malignant hyperthermia
Pulse rate and blood pressure	mildly increased	further increased (25% above normal)	greatly increased (100% above normal) spikes in blood pressure high output failure
Respiration	mildly increased respiratory rate, tidal volume and minute volume	further increased respiratory rate (25% above normal)	periodic breathing apnea possible apiration pneumonia or pulmonary edema
Deep tendon reflexes	increased clonus on stimulation	further increased cross limb reflexes	absent
Laryngeal/ pharyngeal reflexes	hyperactive	diminished	absent
Autonomic signs	nausea vomiting diaphoresis flushing lacrimation hypersalivation	protracted vomiting diaphoresis flushing lacrimation hypersalivation	diaphoresis flushing hypersalivation

From H.T. Milhorn, Jr., Diagnosis and management of phencyclidine intoxication, *American Family Physician*, in press. Published by the American Academy of Family Physicians.

tendon reflexes, and increased temperature may be in Stage I of PCP intoxication. By far the vast majority of patients on PCP will be in this stage of intoxication.[2,9,12,19]

Signs and symptoms that should alert physicians to the possibility of a Stage II PCP intoxication include stupor to mild coma with eyes open, response to deep pain stimuli, spontaneous nystagmus, muscle rigidity (sometimes extreme), increased blood pressure and pulse rate, and increased deep tendon reflexes.[2,11,12,19]

Stage III PCP intoxication usually results from an intentional oral overdose. These patients are in deep comas, with their eyes opened or closed, have no response to deep pain, suffer extreme muscle rigidity, opisthotonic or decerebrate posturing, hypoventilation, periodic breathing or apnea, and increased blood pressure and pulse rate. They may have tonic-clonic seizures, which may progress to status epilepticus, and malignant hyperthermia. Their comas may last for several days. Not uncommonly patients wax and wane between stages of intoxication as their serum levels fluctuate, probably due to enteric recirculation.[2,9,12,19]

In addition to overdose, deaths occur from drownings (some in shallow water), falls, automobile accidents, failure to flee fires and other imminent dangers, or self-inflicted injuries.[2]

Laboratory Data

Other than drug screens, if they can be rapidly obtained, laboratory data are usually not helpful. White blood cell counts may be increased. When rhabdomyolysis occurs, CPK, AST, and uric acid are elevated and a urine analysis may indicate myoglobinuria. Liver enzymes may be elevated in the presence of acute liver necrosis. An EEG may be of diagnostic significance, showing diffuse theta activity with periodic slow wave complexes.[4,7]

Polydrug Use

Patients often use several drugs, and this always poses problems. Drugs taken together do not always act in the same fashion as each drug does when taken alone. Some drugs may enhance one another's effects, while others may partially cancel some effects. For example, when drugs that depress the central nervous system (alcohol, barbiturates, narcotics) are combined with PCP, vital signs that may be increased by PCP alone may be somewhat lower than expected. Also, some symptoms of PCP intoxication, such as increases in vital signs, ataxia, vomiting, and seizures, may be misinterpreted as part of an alcohol or solid sedative withdrawal syndrome.[5]

Differential Diagnosis

PCP intoxication can easily be confused with stimulant (amphetamines, cocaine) or hallucinogen (LSD, psilocybin, mescaline) abuse and with psychotic states (paranoid schizophrenia, catatonia, mania). A drug screen may be the only way distinctions can be made.[4,7]

Stimulants often cause severe tachycardia, hypertension, tremulousness, and hyperthermia but are not associated with the increased muscle tone PCP produces. Also, the presence of nystagmus or ataxia rules out stimulants. Frank hallucinations are more characteristic of hallucinogenic drugs. Fear (panic reactions) can occur with stimulant, hallucinogen, and marijuana abuse as well as with PCP abuse.[4,7]

Coma can result from a variety of central nervous system insults, including trauma, metabolic disturbances, and drug overdoses. The characteristic muscle rigidity of PCP overdose, coupled with tachycardia and hypertension, may be helpful in diagnosis. Depressant drugs tend to lower pulse rate and blood pressure.[7]

Management

Management of PCP intoxication includes the use of general principles of drug overdose, controlling agitation or psychotic reactions, eliminating PCP from the body, treating muscle rigidity, managing medical complications, and treating hypertension, seizures, and hyperpyrexia. There is no antidote for PCP poisoning.[2,11,20]

General Principles

Level of consciousness should be assessed continually and vital signs monitored closely in all stages of PCP intoxication. Blood and urine specimens should be obtained.[5] If a patient is in a coma with a respiratory rate less than 12 breaths a minute, a physician should suspect a concomitant opiate overdose and should give the patient naloxone (Narcan) 0.4 mg intravenously. Also, physicians should consider 50 ml of 50 percent dextrose in water (D50W) to rule out the possibility of hypoglycemia.[13]

Stage I Intoxication

Treatment of Stage I PCP intoxication consists primarily of managing behavioral manifestations. External stimuli should be reduced whenever possible. Patients should be placed in quiet rooms with minimal visual, auditory, and tactile stimuli. They may have hyperacusis, so treatment personnel should speak softly. If a talking down strategy does not appear to be effective or if patients seem to become more agitated, sometimes just leaving them alone may quiet them. If not, diazepam (Valium) in incremental, intravenous doses of 2.5 mg at ten-minute intervals, up to 25 mgs total, may be helpful. Cooperative patients can take diazepam orally.[5,19] If intramuscular injection is necessary, lorazepam (Ativan) in a 2 to 4 mg dose can be used as necessary. Benzodiazepines should be used with caution, because they may delay the metabolism of PCP. Cholinergic agents, such as physostigmine (Antilirium), should be avoided, because they may increase secretions.[19] Psychosis is best treated with haloperidol (Haldol) 5 to 10 mg intramuscularly.[14,21]

Activated charcoal is usually not used in Stage I intoxication. Urinary catheters, nasogastric tubes, and orotracheal intubations should be avoided. Attempts to suction airways may precipitate laryngospasms and so should be avoided. Secretions can be removed from the corners of the mouth and inner posterior cheek walls. Because PCP-intoxicated patients are prone to seizures, Ipecac to induce vomiting is contraindicated in all stages. Diphenhydramine (Benadryl) 50 mg intravenously may be given for localized dystonic reactions.[5,9,13,19]

If symptoms continue to diminish with no cognitive impairment after 12 hours, patients may be discharged.[5]

Stage II Intoxication

Patients' clothes should be loosened, and sponging, ice, and fans should be used as necessary to encourage heat dissipation to try to avoid possible hyperthermic crises. Because of the possibility of laryngospasm, deep oropharyngeal suctioning should be avoided when possible, but secretions should be gently suctioned orally as needed. Nasogastric and orotracheal tubes should be inserted only if necessary.[5] Wheezing due to bronchospasm can be treated with an intravenous aminophylline infusion (250 mg over 20 minutes). Some evidence suggests that restraint may contribute to rhabdomyolysis[14-15] and so should be used only when absolutely necessary. If restraints are needed, totally immobilizing patients by rolling their bodies in sheets is probably the best method.[12] A continuous infusion of 5 percent dextrose in lactated Ringer's solution (D5LR) should be started. Propranolol (Inderal) can be given intravenously in 1.0 mg increments every 30 minutes to control hypertension and tachycardia.[5] Propranolol should be avoided if patients are wheezing. Hydralazine (Apresoline) 5-10 mg intravenously may also be used to control blood pressure.

Since acute urinary retention may occur, a urinary catheter should be placed. A urine sample should be sent to a laboratory for analysis for myoglobin. Blood for blood gases, electrolytes, CPK, AST, ALT, BUN, creatinine, and uric acid should be obtained and sent for analysis.[5,13]

Although the magnitude of its effectiveness is somewhat controversial, urinary excretion of PCP may be increased by acidification of the urine to a pH of 5.0 to 5.5.[20] This can be done by intravenous infusion of ascorbic acid 0.5 to 1.5 gm every four to six hours as required.[5] Ammonium chloride is avoided because the ammonia breakdown products might place a burden on the oftentimes damaged liver.[19] Furosemide (Lasix), 20 to 40 mg intravenously, at six-hour intervals can increase urinary output and hasten PCP excretion. Acidification of the urine is contraindicated in two situations: the presence of myoglobinuria and concomitant abuse of large doses of long-acting barbiturates or salicylates for which the treatment is alkalinization of the urine.[5,19] Extreme muscle rigidity, not respon-

TABLE 17.3. Procedures for acute phencyclidine intoxication.

	Stage I	Stage II	Stage III
Check level of consciousness	assess continually	assess continually	assess continually
Vital signs (T,P,R,BP)	closely monitor	closely monitor	closely monitor
Collection of specimen (blood, urine)	yes	yes	yes
Urinary bladder catheterization	no	yes	yes
Nasogastric tube insertion	no	only if necessary	yes
Orotracheal intubation	no	only if necessary	yes
Oral suctioning	only if necessary	gently as needed	yes
Tracheobronchial suctioning	no	only if necessary	yes, frequently as needed
Cooling procedures	no	loosen clothing, sponge, use ice and fans	sponge and use ice when necessary
Gastric lavage	no	if necessary	yes
Neuromuscular blockage and mechanical ventilation	no	if necessary	if necessary

From H.T. Milhorn, Jr., Diagnosis and management of phencyclidine intoxication, *American Family Physician,* in press. Published by the American Academy of Family Physicians.

sive to diazepam, especially in the face of rhabdomyolysis, may require neuromuscular blockage and mechanical ventilation.[19]

Stage III Intoxication

Intravenous fluids should be initiated, a urinary catheter inserted, and urinary output monitored as in Stage II intoxication. Orotracheal intubation should be performed. Vigorous tracheobronchial suctioning is indicated. A large bore gastric tube should be placed and gastric contents suctioned and saved for analysis. Activated charcoal, 50 to 150 gm, should be instilled into the stomach following gastric lavage with normal saline. A nasogastric tube can be placed and connected to continuous suction to remove the PCP secreted into the stomach. Because of the possibility of electrolyte abnormalities with continuous suction, some prefer an alternate approach—putting 30 to 40 gm of activated charcoal in the stomach every six to eight hours to bind the PCP.[5,9,13,19]

In the absence of contraindications, urinary acidification should be instituted and furosemide should be given as in Stage II treatment. Some authors recommend acidification of arterial blood to slightly less than 7.3 for up to 72 hours to facilitate movement of PCP out of the central nervous system.[2,8-9] Strict attention should be paid to a patient's core temperature, and measures should be instituted to control it when necessary. Hypertension and tachycardia can be controlled by titration of intravenous propranolol, 1.0 mg every 30 minutes, as necessary to a maximum of 8 mg. Alternately, hypertension can be controlled with hydralazine 10-20 mg or diazoxide (Hyperstat) 300 mg intravenously.[5,19,21] Status epilepticus, should it occur, can usually be effectively treated with diazepam, 5 to 10 mg

TABLE 17.4. Medications for phencyclidine intoxication.

	Stage I	Stage II	Stage III
Ipecac	none	none	none
Activated charcoal	none	if necessary	50–150 gm initially followed by 30–40 gm every 6–8 hours
Diazepam	for agitation: 10–30 mg P.O. or 2.5 mg IV up to 25 mg total	for muscle rigidity— same IV dosage as Stage I for agitation	for muscle rigidity— same as Stage II for status epilepticus— 5–10 mg IV every 5 min up to 30 mg total
Lorazepam	for agitation 2–4 mg I.M. PRN		
Haldol	5–10 mg I.M.	none	none
D5LR	none	1.5 times maintenance	1.5–2.5 times maintenance
Ascorbic acid	none	0.5–1.5 gm IV every 4–6 hours as needed to reduce urine pH < 5.5	same as Stage II
Hydralazine	none	5–10 mg IV	10–20 mg IV
Propranolol	none	1.0 mg IV every 30 min. as needed up to 8 mg total	1.0 mg IV every 30 min. as needed up to 8 mg total
Diazoxide	none	none	300 mg IV
Furosemide	none	20–40 mg IV every 6 hours	20–40 mg IV every 6 hours
Aminophylline	none	250 mg IV	250 mg IV
Naloxone	none	0.4 mg respiratory rate < 12/min	0.4 mg respiratory rate < 12/min
D50W	none	50 cc IV	50 cc IV
Diphenhydramine	50 mg IV	none	none

From H.T. Milhorn, Jr., Diagnosis and management of phencyclidine intoxication, *American Family Physician,* in press. Published by the American Academy of Family Physicians.

intravenously, every five minutes, up to a total of 30 mg. Neuromuscular blockage and mechanical ventilation may be required for refractory cases.[9,13] Similarly, extreme muscle rigidity not responsive to diazepam may also require neuromuscular blockage and mechanical ventilation. Dialysis has been shown to be ineffective in removing PCP from the body.[19]

Not only may PCP overdose be life-threatening, but PCP itself tends to be the longest acting of any drug of abuse. The entire picture may take up to six weeks to clear.[21-22] Procedures that may be required for PCP intoxication are summarized in Table 17.3; medications that may be needed are summarized in Table 17.4

Emergence Phenomenon

One should remember that when patients emerge from one level of intoxication to the next lightest level, they will exhibit the signs and symptoms of that stage. For example, patients emerging from Stage II may become violent or self-destructive as they enter Stage I if appropriate measures are not taken.[19,23]

References

1. Miller, N.S., M.S. Gold, and R. Millman. PCP: A dangerous drug. *American Family Physician*, 38:215–218, 1988.
2. Aniline, O., and F.N. Pitts, Jr. Phencyclidine (PCP): A review and perspectives. *CRC Critical Reviews in Toxicology*. 10:145–177, 1982.
3. Robinson, B., and A. Yates. Angel dust: Medical and psychiatric aspects of phencyclidine intoxication. *Arizona Medicine*, 41:808–811, 1984.
4. Young, T., G.W. Lawson, and C.B. Gacono. Clinical aspects of phencyclidine (PCP). *The International Journal of the Addictions*, 22:1–15, 1987.
5. Woolf, D.S., C. Vourakis, and G. Bennett. Guidelines for management of acute phencyclidine intoxication. *Critical Care Update*, 7:16–24, 1980.
6. Davis, B.L. The PCP epidemic: A critical review. *International Journal of the Addictions*, 17:1137–55, 1982.
7. Gibson, M.S. Phencyclidine intoxication. *Ear Nose and Throat Journal*, 62:75–80, 1983.
8. Done, A.K., R. Aronow, and J.N. Miceli. Pharmacokinetic bases for the diagnosis and treatment of acute PCP intoxication. *Journal of Psychedelic Drugs*, 12:253–258, 1980.
9. Aronow, J.N., J.N. Miceli, and A.K. Done. A therapeutic approach to the acutely overdosed PCP patient. *Journal of Psychedelic Drugs*, 12:259–267, 1980.
10. Johnson, K.M., Jr. Neurochemistry and neurophysiology of phencyclidine. In *Psychopharmacology: The Third Edition*. Ed. by H.Y. Meltzer, Raven Press, New York, 1987, pp. 1581–1587.
11. Balster, R.L. The behavioral pharmacology of phencyclidine. In *Psychopharmacology: The Third Generation of Progress*. Ed. by H.Y. Meltzer, Raven Press, New York, 1987, pp. 1573–1579.
12. Pearlson, G.D. Psychiatric and medical syndromes associated with phencyclidine (PCP) abuse. *Johns Hopkins Medical Journal*, 148:25–33, 1981.
13. McCarron, M.M., B.W. Schulze, G.A. Thompson, M.C. Condor, and W.A. Goetz. Acute phencyclidine intoxication: Clinical patterns, complications, and treatment. *Annals of Emergency Medicine*, 10:290–297, 1981.
14. Giannini, A.J., C. Nageotte, R.H. Loiselle, and D.A. Malone. Comparison of chlorpromazine, haloperidol, and pimozide in the treatment of phencyclidine psychosis: DA-2 receptor specificity. *Clinical Toxicology*, 22:573–579, 1984–85.
15. Patel, R., G. Connor, and C.R. Drew. A review of thirty cases of rhabdomyolysis associated acute renal failure among phencyclidine users. *Clinical Toxicology*, 23:547–556, 1986.
16. Giannini, A.J., M.S. Eighan, R.H. Loiselle, and M.C. Giannini. Comparison of haloperidol and chlorpromazine in the treatment of phencyclidine psychosis. *Journal of Clinical Pharmacology*, 24:202–204, 1984.

17. Bessen, H.A. Intracranial hemorrhage associated with phencyclidine abuse. *Journal of the American Medical Association*, 248:585–586, 1982.

18. Armen, R., G. Kanel, and T. Reynolds. Phencyclidine-induced malignant hyperthermia causing submassive liver necrosis. *American Journal of Medicine*, 77:167–172, 1984.

19. Rappolt, R.T., G.R. Gay, and R.D. Farris. Phencyclidine (PCP) intoxication: Diagnosis in stages and algorithms of treatment. *Clinical Toxicology*, 16:509–529, 1980.

20. Rumack, B. Phencyclidine overdose: An overview. *Annals of Emergency Medicine*, 9:595, 1980.

21. Schuckit, M.A. *Drug and Alcohol Abuse: A Clinical Guide to Diagnosis and Treatment*. Plenum Press, New York, 1984, pp. 152–160.

22. Milhorn, H.T., Jr. Diagnosis and management of phencyclidine intoxication. *American Family Physician*, in press.

23. Milhorn, H.T., Jr. Phencyclidine overdose: A case report. *Journal of the Mississippi State Medical Association*, 31:37–40, 1990.

CHAPTER 18

Inhalants

History

Inhaling substances for their euphoric and intoxicating effects has a long history. Thousands of years ago people inhaled vapors from burning spices and herbs, particularly during religious ceremonies. Nitrous oxide and other anesthetics were used recreationally long before they were used medically. Discovered in the 1700s, anesthetics were most often abused by students and physicians, and "inhalant parties" were popular in the 1800s. Gasoline sniffing began to be reported as recreational behavior in the early 1950s. In the 1960s glue sniffing became a nationwide concern when several deaths were reported. In the 1970s and 1980s, volatile substances and aerosols came into widespread use as inhalants. The alkyl nitrites (amyl, butyl) became popular in the 1970s as enhancers of sexual experience, especially among male homosexuals. Amyl nitrite was originally the major nitrite of abuse. When it was classified as a prescription drug in 1960, butyl nitrite to a large extent replaced it in the drug culture. In 1986, 20 percent of high school seniors reported having abused inhalants; however, only 3 percent reported having used them in the 30 days prior to the survey. Local and state governments now prohibit minors from purchasing certain substances, particularly plastic model glues.[1-5]

The Inhalants

The inhalants abused today include solvents, aerosols, alkyl nitrites, and nitrous oxide.

Solvents and Aerosols

Types of Drugs

The solvents and aerosols are complex compounds of distilled petroleum and natural gas and include benzene, toluene, acetone, and related chemicals. Varnish, varnish remover, paint thinners and lacquers, lighter fluid, nail polish remover, cleaning solutions, spot removers, glues, and cements are common household products containing solvents and aerosols (Table 18.1). Solvents and aerosols are liquids at room temperature but evaporate readily.[1-2,6-7]

Adolescent boys most commonly use solvents and aerosols recreationally because they have access to many common household products and do not have access to more conventional drugs. Most users inhale either directly from a bottle or from a solvent-soaked rag. Another method, known as "bagging," involves placing a piece of cotton or a rag soaked with solvent in the bottom of a paper bag

TABLE 18.1. The major solvents and aerosols.

Class	Substance	Product
alcohols	ethanol	aerosol sprays, model cement, paint thinners
	isopropanol	aerosol sprays, antifreeze, degreasers, model cement, paint thinner, spray shoe polish
	methanol	antifreeze, paint thinner, windshield washing fluids
aliphatic hydrocarbons	n-heptane	adhesives, rubber cement, gasoline, paint thinner
	n-hexane	adhesives, rubber cement, gasoline, model cement
anesthetics	methylene chloride	degreasers, paint thinner
	tetrachloroethylene	degreasers
aromatic hydrocarbons	benzene	adhesives, rubber cement, degreasers, gasoline, cleaning fluids, tube repair kits
	naphthalene	adhesives, rubber cement, gasoline, paint thinner, lighter fluid
	styrene	adhesives, rubber cement, model cement
	toluene	adhesives, rubber cement, aerosol sprays, degreasers, gasoline, model cement, paint thinners, spray shoe polish
	xylene	adhesives, rubber cement, aerosol sprays, degreasers, gasoline, model cement, paint thinner
chlorinated hydrocarbons	carbontetrachloride	spot remover, dry cleaner
	trichlorethylene	degreaser, dry cleaner, liquid paper typewriter correction fluid, refrigerant
esters	ethylacetate	paint thinner
	n-butyl acetate	degreasers
	n-propylacetate	paint thinner
freons	trichlormonofluoromethane	aerosols, refrigerant
	dichlordifluoromethane	aerosols, refrigerant
gasoline	—	motor fuel
ketones	acetone	model cement, paint thinner, finger nail polish remover
	methyl butyl ketone	paint thinner
	methyl ethyl ketone	degreasers, paint thinner

Based on Inhalants: The deliberate inhalation of volatile substances. National Institute of Drug Abuse, Rockville, Maryland, Report Series 30 (No. 2), 1978 that is then placed over the mouth and nose and inhaled from. Solvent and aerosol inhalation is known as "huffing."[1,6,8]

Pharmacology

Absorbed by the lungs, solvent and aerosol vapors rapidly enter the bloodstream and are then distributed throughout the body. Because most solvents and aerosols are fat-soluble, they are rapidly absorbed into the central nervous system. The kidneys metabolize and excrete some solvents and aerosols. Others are eliminated unchanged, primarily through the lungs. The lipid solubility of solvents and aerosols apparently causes their CNS effects by impairing membrane permeability and neural transmission.[1,4]

After a quick onset, effects last a few minutes to an hour, depending on the substance and the dosage. Among the effects generally felt are excitement, lowering of inhibitions, restlessness, uncoordination, confusion, and disorientation. The effects are similar to alcohol intoxication. In larger doses, solvents and aerosols can produce sedation, changes in perception, impaired judgment, fright, and panic, which sometimes result in accidental death.[1,4]

Prolonged exposure can result in nausea, vomiting, muscular weakness, fatigue, and weight loss. Overdose produces delirium, delusions, hallucinations, seizures, coma, respiratory depression, and death.[1,4]

Health Consequences of Solvent and Aerosol Abuse

A variety of adverse health consequences can result from solvent and aerosol abuse. In addition to those listed in Table 18.2, death from suffocation can occur when a user loses consciousness and falls on a cloth containing evaporating material or suffocates in a plastic bag placed over the head to concentrate the vapors.[4,9-12]

Acute hazards associated with aerosol inhalation include laryngospasm or airway freezing as a result of rapid vaporization. In addition, freon can block oxygen diffusion at the pulmonary membrane. The most prominent health hazard associated with aerosol inhalation is sudden sniffing death (SSD) syndrome, which results from inhalation of the flurocarbons contained in aerosols. The flurocarbons sensitize the heart to the stimulant effects of epinephrine, leading to cardiac arrhythmias and cardiac arrest. Deaths have also occurred from inhaling the fumes from typewriter correction fluid (liquid paper).[4,13]

Alkyl Nitrites

Types of Drugs

The alkyl nitrites include amyl and butyl nitrite. Amyl nitrite was discovered in 1857, and its use in medicine began in 1867 as an antianginal drug. It is supplied in glass ampules, which are broken open and inhaled. It became prized by drug abusers because of its purported ability to slow the passage of time and prolong

TABLE 18.2. Some probable health consequences of solvent and aerosol abuse.

Chemical	Consequence
benzene	leukocytosis, anemia, pancytopenia, myeloid leukemia fatty degeneration and necrosis of the liver anorexia, dyspepsia, chronic gastritis headache, drowsiness, irritability
carbon tetrachloride	anemia seizures renal failure hepatic failure nausea, vomiting, anorexia, abdominal pain, weight loss
gasoline	confusion, tremor, ataxia, paresthesias, neuritis, paralysis of peripheral and cranial nerves lead poisoning nausea, vomiting, anorexia, abdominal pain, weight loss, hepatic damage myopathy anemia fatigue
hexane	anemia muscle weakness, hypoesthesias, paresthesias, muscle atrophy, slowed nerve conduction
toluene	nausea, epigastric discomfort, anorexia, jaundice, hepatomegally pyuria, hematuria, renal tubular necrosis hepatic damage anemia mental dullness, tremors, emotional lability, nystagmus, cerebellar ataxia, polyneuropathies, seizures, permanent encephalopathy
trichlorethylene	centrilobular necrosis of the liver optic and other cranial nerve damage renal tubular necrosis cardiac arrhythmias hepatic toxicity sudden death (SSD)

Based on S. Cohen, Inhalants and solvents, in *Youth Drug Abuse*, edited by G.M. Beschner and A.S. Friedman, Lexington Books, Lexington, Massachusetts, 1979.

orgasm. It is favored by male homosexuals because it helps relax the anal sphincter. The street name—"poppers"—came from the popping sound the ampule makes when it is crushed. Its medical use, for the most part, has been replaced by trinitroglycerin (TNG).[1,4]

Butyl nitrite first appeared on the drug scene in 1969 when amyl nitrite was classified as a prescription drug. Its properties are very similar to those of amyl nitrite. It is sold as a room odorizer and liquid incense and is widely and legally available in liquid form in novelty stores, record and tape stores, and drug paraphernalia shops (head shops) or by mail order. It is often used in discotheques to promote a sense of abandon while dancing.[1,4,14–15]

TABLE 18.3. Street/slang names for alkyl nitrites.

Drug	Street/slang name
amyl nitrite	amies, amys, pearls, poppers, snappers
butyl nitrite	banaple gas, joc aroma, kick, locker popper, locker room, rush, Satan's scent, thrust, toilet water

In 1986, 5 percent of high school seniors reported nitrite use in the previous 12 months, 1.6 percent had used them in the previous 30 days and 0.5 percent used them daily.[5]

The nitrites are known in the drug culture by a variety of names, some of which are listed in Table 18.3.[1,4–5]

Pharmacology

The nitrites are decomposed by gastric secretions, so they are ineffective when taken orally. When inhaled, their effects begin in 15 to 30 seconds and last a few minutes. They rapidly cross the pulmonary membrane to reach the bloodstream, where they relax vascular smooth muscle. The antianginal effect results from dilation of peripheral vessels and reduced venous return, resulting in decreased cardiac preload. Direct coronary artery dilation may contribute as well. The alkyl nitrites produce a brief euphoria.[8,16]

In toxic doses, the alkyl nitrites produce nausea, dizziness, and weakness, probably due to drop in blood pressure and increase in heart rate. Fainting, especially when patients are erect, can occur.[16]

Health Consequences of Alkyl Nitrite Abuse

Dilation of cerebral vessels and stretching of the meninges produces a pulsating headache. A deep flush spreads over the head and neck, and methemoglobinemia may also occur. Prolonged exposure to the vapors can cause irritation of the eyes and tracheobronchial tree and development of crusty lesions around the nose. The use of alkyl nitrites can be dangerous in people with recent head injury, cardiac disease other than angina pectoris, and glaucoma. At least one death from massive hemolysis has been reported in a patient with G6PD deficiency. Deaths have also been reported as a result of accidental burns while using a nitrite near an open flame.[3,8,15,17–18]

Nitrite inhalation induces changes in the immune system, initially suppressing it, then nonspecifically stimulating it. It has been postulated that through this mechanism the nitrites activate HIV replication and, thereby, contribute to the progression of AIDS.[19]

Nitrous Oxide

Despite a detailed description of the effects of nitrous oxide in 1800, in which its analgesic and euphorogenic properties were noted, its potential for abuse was not fully recognized until the latter part of the 1960s. The nonmedical use of nitrous oxide appears to be on the increase, possibly because of its ease of availability to the general public. It is a commonly used industrial agent, particularly in the food industry, where it is used as a propellant in whipped cream dispensers, which are known in the drug culture as "whippets." It is also available as an additive for automobile engines and is used as an anesthetic. Furthermore, it can be made in illicit laboratories with relative ease. Whippits, balloons for inhaling gas, and pipes for smoking it (buzz bombs) are readily available in drug paraphernalia shops.[4,20]

Pharmacology

Nitrous oxide is a colorless gas without appreciable odor or taste. It has been used as an anesthetic since 1844 and is currently used as an adjuvant during most procedures in which general anesthesia is used. When used with an inhalation anesthetic, it allows smaller doses of that drug to be given, thus reducing possible side effects of the anesthetic. It is a popular anesthetic among dentists and is referred to as "laughing gas."[21]

A normal adult breathing 70 percent nitrous oxide will achieve 90 percent saturation of nitrous oxide in about 15 minutes. During this time, approximately 10 liters of nitrous oxide will have been absorbed from the alveoli into the body. The drug is relatively insoluble in blood and fat, so that the blood and the brain become rapidly saturated with it. It is excreted unchanged by the lungs; little or none is metabolized.[21-22]

Nitrous oxide has little effect on the respiratory, gastrointestinal, muscular, and renal systems. It has mixed effects on the cardiovascular system. It is a mild myocardial depressant and an indirect sympathomimetic agent. Little change in blood pressure occurs because the cardiac depressant effect is offset by a mild increase in peripheral resistance. It is abused for its euphoric effect.[1,22]

Health Consequences of Nitrous Oxide Abuse

A variety of adverse health consequences from chronic nitrite use have been reported. Psychological effects include depression, recent memory loss, confusion, delirium, paranoid delusions, and visual hallucinations. Neurological effects include distal limb weakness, mild loss of vibratory sensation, parasthesias, decreased ankle and knee reflexes, and gait abnormalities. Impotence and bladder and bowel dysfunction have also been reported. The neurological dysfunction may be due to the drug's inactivation of vitamin B_{12}.[19,28]

In patients with coronary artery disease and myocardial dysfunction, nitrous oxide can produce significant degrees of cardiac depression. Death can occur from hypoxia when sufficient oxygen is not mixed with the nitrous oxide. At least one death has occurred from pneumomediastinum when an attempt was made to inhale nitrous oxide directly from the tank without a pressure reduction value.[20,22]

Tolerance

Development of tolerance to all of the inhalants is known to occur.

Dependence

Although physical dependence has been reported with heavy chronic abuse of solvents, it is rare. Physical dependence has not been reported to develop with nitrite and nitrous oxide abuse. Psychological dependence does occur to all three groups of drugs.

Abstinence Syndrome

An abstinence syndrome consisting of hallucinations, abdominal cramps, chills, and delirium tremens has been reported with heavy chronic abuse of solvents. However, if an abstinence syndrome does occur, it is extremely rare. An abstinence syndrome for nitrites and nitrous oxide has not been reported.

Diagnosis

The diagnosis of intoxication and overdose of aerosols, solvents, nitrites, and nitrous oxide depends on recognition of typical signs and symptoms, along with a history of inhalant abuse. Solvent abuse may cause a rash around the mouth and nose; nitrite abuse may cause crusty lesions around the nose. The odor of the abused solvent may be present on patients' breath. For gasoline sniffers, a serum lead level should be obtained. Inhalants are not detected on routine drug screens. Diagnosis of dependence is based on the principles outlined in Chapter 2.[3]

Management

The management of inhalant intoxication and overdose is symptomatic. It should include reassurance, elimination of unnecessary stimuli, protecting patients from injury, and providing a generally supportive environment. Chelation therapy is effective for lead toxicity resulting from gasoline inhalation. Management of dependence is based on the principles outlined in Chapter 3.[3,23]

References

1. O'Brien, R., and S. Cohen. *The Encyclopedia of Drug Abuse*. Facts on File, New York, 1984.
2. Cohen, S. Solvent and aerosol intoxication. In *The Substance Abuse Problems: Volume One*. Haworth Press, New York, 1981, pp. 40–45.
3. Schonberg, S.K. (Ed.). Specific drugs. In *Substance Abuse: A Guide for Health Professionals*. American Academy of Pediatrics, Elk Grove Village, Illinois, 1988, pp. 115–182.
4. Wilford, B.B. (Ed.). Major drugs of abuse. In *Drug Abuse: A Guide for the Primary Care Physician*. American Medical Association, Chicago, 1981, pp. 21–84.
5. Johnston, L.D., P.M. O'Malley, and J.G. Bachman. Drug use by high school seniors: The Class of 1986. U.S. Department of Health and Human Services Publication No (ADM) 87-1535, Rockville, Maryland, 1987.
6. Cohen, S. Inhalant abuse. In *The Substance Abuse Problems: Volume One*. Haworth Press, New York, 1981, pp. 46–50.
7. Inhalants: The deliberate inhalation of volatile substances. National Institute of Drug Abuse, Rockville, Maryland, Report Series 30 (No. 2), 1978.
8. Schuckit, M.A. Glues, solvents, and aerosols. *Drug Abuse and Alcoholism Newsletter*, Vista Hill Foundation, July, 1989.
9. Cohen, S. Amyl nitrite rediscovered. In *The Substance Abuse Problems: Volume One*. Haworth Press, New York, 1981, pp. 51–55.
10. Fortenberry, D.J. Gasoline sniffing. *American Journal of Medicine*, 8:36–51, 1985.
11. Edminister, S.C., and M.J. Bayer. Recreational gasoline sniffing: Acute gasoline intoxication and latent organolead poisoning. *Journal of Emergency Medicine*, 3:365–370, 1985.
12. Cohen, S. Inhalants and solvents. In *Youth Drug Abuse*. Edited by G.M. Bescher and A.S. Friedman. Lexington Books, Lexington, Massachusetts, 1979.
13. King, G.S., J.E. Smialek, and W.G. Troutman. Sudden death in adolescents from the inhalation of typewriter correction fluid. *Journal of the American Medical Association*, 253:1604–1606, 1985.
14. Lange, W.R., E.M. Dex, C.A. Haertzen, F.R. Snyder, and J.H. Jaffe. Nitrite inhalants: Contemporary patterns of abuse. *National Institute of Drug Abuse Research Monograph Series*, 83:86–95, 1988.
15. Schwartz, R.H. Deliberate inhalation of isobutyl nitrite during adolescence: A descriptive study. *National Institute of Drug Abuse Research Monograph Series*, 83:81–85, 1988.
16. Cohen, S. The volatile nitrites. *Journal of the American Medical Association*, 241:2077–2078, 1979.
17. Bogart, L., J. Bonsignore, and A. Carvalho. Massive hemolysis following inhalation of volatile nitrites. *American Journal of Hematology*, 22:327–329, 1986.
18. Wood, R.W. The acute toxicity of nitrite inhalants. *National Institute of Drug Abuse Research Monograph Series*, 83:23–38, 1988.
19. Lange, R.W., and J. Fralich. Nitrite inhalants: Promising and discouraging news. *British Journal of Addiction*, 84:121–123, 1989.

20. Gillman, M.A. Nitrous oxide, an opioid addictive agent. *The American Journal of Medicine*, 81:97–102, 1986.
21. Marshall, B.E., and H. Woolman. General anesthetics. In *Goodman and Gilman's The Pharmacological Basis of Therapeutics*. Edited by A.G. Gilman, L.S. Goodman, T.W. Rall, and F. Murad. Macmillan, New York, 1985, pp. 276–301.
22. Shlafer, M., and E.N. Marieb. General anesthetic agents. In *The Nurse, Pharmacology, and Drug Therapy*. Addison-Wesley, Redwood City, California, 1989, pp. 314–331.

Part III   Special Groups

CHAPTER 19

Women

Women, like men, are at risk for developing alcoholism, prescription drug addiction, and addiction to illicit drugs. Women, however, can directly affect other human beings (their unborn fetuses) by their drug use.

Alcohol

In recent years equality for women has included greater freedom to drink. As a result, heavy drinking is on the rise among young, employed women. In the United States the number who drink alcohol has increased from 45 percent to 66 percent over the past 40 years, and community surveys indicate that 5 percent of women are heavy drinkers. Because society considers it less acceptable for a woman to be a heavy drinker than a man, family, friends, and employers often hide or ignore a woman's drinking problem. This attitude delays or prevents women from receiving treatment.[1-2]

Alcohol-related ulcer surgery, gastrointestinal hemorrhage, fatty liver, hypertension, anemia, and malnutrition occur at significantly higher rates in women, who also seem to be more susceptible to the hypertensive and cirrhotic effects of alcohol. For comparative ages, death rate for alcoholic women is greater than the death rate for nonalcoholic women. Their unique physiology (menopause, postpartum depression, premenstrual mood changes) have been mentioned as possible contributors to alcohol abuse in women, but there is no clear documentation of this.[1-2]

In the early days of ancient Rome, drinking wine for women was an offense punishable by death. This law, which prohibited women from drinking alcohol, was linked to the prohibition against adultery by women. Thus, drinking women were considered to be "loose" early in Western culture. In contemporary U.S. society, women who drink excessively are triply stigmatized. First, they are included in society's negative attitude towards all alcoholics. Secondly, they are subjected to the special disgust focused on intoxicated women. And third, the idea that drunkenness and sexual promiscuity are linked add to the burden of disapproval. As a result, alcoholic women drink alone more commonly than alcoholic men, so that female alcoholics are often referred to as "hidden alco-holics." The negative attitude of society in general influences not only the behav-ior of the alcoholic woman herself, her family, and her friends, but also affects the attitudes and expectations of those in the helping professions (physicians, nurses, psychologists, social workers).[3] Rather than diagnosing alcoholism, a physician all-too-often prescribes tranquilizers, with the result that many alco-holic women are cross-addicted to prescription drugs.[2]

Divorce rates for alcoholic women are much higher than for alcoholic men. Nonalcoholic wives are far more likely to remain with their alcoholic husbands than nonalcoholic husbands with their alcoholic wives.[2,4]

When women drink at a rate comparable to that of men, their smaller size and higher proportion of body fat causes higher blood alcohol levels. Whereas men are inclined to snack while drinking, women often diet, so they drink on empty stomachs, which results in quick absorption of alcohol into the bloodstream.[2] Women taking oral contraceptives metabolize ethanol significantly more slowly than women who do not. Furthermore, in the premenstrual phase, women absorb alcohol more quickly and completely than in the postmenstrual phase. Women tend to begin using alcohol at a later age than men and to progress more rapidly into middle- and late-stage alcoholism, a phenomenon known as *telescoping*.[1-2]

Other Drugs

Women are particularly at risk for becoming dependent on prescription drugs. They make visits to physicians more frequently than men and tend to complain of nonspecific anxiety. As a result, physicians often prescribe them minor tran-quilizers, such as diazepam (Valium), alprazolam (Xanax), or lorazepam (Ativan). They thus learn that the use of chemicals is a quick and easy way to cope with stress. It is not as easy for many women to unwind with a few drinks in a bar as it is for men, so they are more likely to seek medical relief from stress.[5-6]

Women are at risk for addiction to the same illicit drugs as men. However, some differences do exist. Female cocaine addicts, for example, have a greater incidence of major depression than men. Furthermore, abstinent women do not appear to recover from their depression as rapidly as men. Women also tend to become addicted to cocaine more rapidly than men.[7]

Fertility

Psychoactive substances disrupt neuroendocrine and gonadal function with suffi-cient magnitude to cause infertility in some patients. Normal individuals may only experience subtle changes in sexual function. However, women with com-promised reproductive function may have major problems. The disruptive effects of these drugs are usually completely reversible after patients stop taking them. Most protocols for evaluating unexplained infertility now include drug abuse history.[8]

Diagnosis

The information required to confirm a diagnosis of chemical dependence in women is basically the same as that for men (Chapter 2). Women complain more often of a wide range of symptoms, including depression, anxiety, sleeplessness, lethargy, stomach problems, and injuries from accidents or physical abuse. Compared with controls, chemically dependent women report a higher incidence of infertility, postpartum depression, irregular menstrual cycles, and amenorrhea. Women addicts are less likely than men to have problems at work or with the law or to behave violently. They are more inclined than men to report problems with their relationships and children as a result of substance abuse.[1]

In taking a drug history, additional questions specifically appropriate for women include: Do you ever carry an alcoholic beverage in your purse? Does your drug use vary with your menstrual cycle? Has your drinking or drug taking had any effect on the regularity or quantity of your menstrual periods? What effect do you think your drug abuse has had on your children? Has there been physical violence in your home (spouse abuse or child abuse)?[9]

Treatment

Women are a minority in most treatment programs, averaging about 20 percent of patients. As a result, many chemically dependent women find themselves in treatment programs designed for men. They need to feel comfortable with themselves and are reluctant to discuss many of their problems, such as rape or spouse abuse, in mixed company. Hence, attending all-women groups is important for most women addicts, especially in early recovery.[2,4]

Alcoholic women are more likely than nonalcoholic women to have alcoholic husbands or lovers and are at increased risk for domestic violence. Frequently, women addicts are victims of incest, child or spouse abuse or rape, or are daughters of alcoholic parents. To be most effective, a treatment program for chemically dependent women must address their practical needs, such as child care and job training. Unfortunately, because of their low socioeconomic status in our society, many women addicts are unable to afford treatment.[1,4]

Low self-esteem seems to be an important feature of all addiction, but particularly for female addicts. How a woman feels about herself depends on developmental, psychological, and societal factors. Self-esteem for many depends on occupation. The lesser value assigned to tasks normally identified as women's work and the lower salaries women earn are important factors in their self-esteem. Housekeeping and child care in the United States are assigned little or no economic value. Most married women in the work force still carry the major responsibility for family cleaning, shopping, cooking, laundry, and child care in addition to their outside employment. Both as a factor in her illness and her recovery, the importance of occupation should be explored individually with each chemically dependent woman. Vocational rehabilitation, more adequate child care, and changes in family attitudes and behavior will be indicated in many cases.[4,9]

Because women are usually responsible for the care of children in the United States and because chemically dependent women are frequently separated or divorced, female addicts entering treatment are far more often the heads of single-parent families than are the chemically dependent men.[9] As a result, child care is a major need in the treatment of chemically dependent women. Women cannot benefit maximally from treatment if they are concerned about the welfare of their children. Guilt for being a failure as a mother may be a major problem.[2,4]

The most useful categorization of alcoholism is the distinction between primary alcoholism (no preexisting emotional disorder) and secondary alcoholism (preexisting emotional disorder). Most patients who undergo treatment are of the primary type. Among men, the most common form of secondary alcoholism is associated with antisocial personality disorder. This is true of other drug addictions as well. In women the most common secondary type is associated with depression. Diagnosis of primary depression must be based on a careful life history, since the presence of depressive symptoms early in treatment will not differentiate between primary and secondary alcoholism. Once a woman is identified as a secondary alcoholic, long-term treatment should include, in addition to alcoholism treatment, attention to possible recurrence of depression. Early treatment of such recurrence may help women maintain sobriety. Women alcoholics attempt suicide or make suicide gestures more frequently than alcoholic men.[2,9]

A woman is often defined through her relationship to others. She is someone's daughter, someone's wife, someone's mother, or even someone's ex-wife. Women's dependence on men may be a treatment issue. Helping alcoholic women confront their feelings about themselves as independent individuals is an important part of treatment.[9]

It is important for all female addicts to structure their lives. If they go back to the unstructured world of housework and child care they run a greater risk of relapse, especially if they do not prefer those roles. Women should explore edu-

TABLE 19.1. Female treatment issues.

ACOA issues	incest
assertiveness	job training
child abuse	life structuring
child care	premenstrual drinking or
depression	drug using
divorce or separation	relationship with spouse or
eating disorders	significant other
feelings about being an inde-	self-esteem
pendent individual	spouse abuse
fetal concerns	unhealthy dependence on
guilt	male relationships

cational goals, whether that means getting a high school equivalency diploma, a college degree, or a postgraduate degree. Trade schools should be used as resources.[10]

Some alcoholic women relate drinking episodes to their menstrual cycle, particularly in the premenstrual period. Strategies for relief or prevention of dysmenorrhea, such as taking ibuprofen (Motrin), attending extra AA meetings, and calls from AA sponsors should be planned with patients to help them negotiate this difficult period.[10]

Female treatment issues are summarized in Table 19.1.

The Pregnant Addict

Although drug use of all types, including drinking alcohol, appears to be increasing in this country, it appears to be increasing faster in women than in men, and the overwhelming majority of drug-using women are reproductively active. It is now abundantly clear that gestational abuse of any mood-altering substance can cause serious maternal and perinatal problems. Many women addicts use more than one drug, commonly combining, for instance, alcohol, marijuana, cocaine, and nicotine. Evaluating risk factors for pregnant addicts and their newborns must take into consideration all of these drugs. Identifying pregnant addicts, however, is difficult. They often attempt to conceal their addiction by obtaining medical treatment for an array of somatic complaints, such as headaches, anxiety, or low back pain. Although they usually deny illicit drug use, most chemically dependent pregnant women will admit to using legal drugs (caffeine, nicotine, alcohol).[11-12]

Medical Problems

A 40 to 50 percent incidence of medical complications among illicit drug-dependent women has been reported. The most frequently reported ones include anemia, endocarditis, phlebitis, cellulitis, hepatitis, hypertension, urinary tract infection, and venereal disease. In addition, pregnant intravenous drug users are at increased risk for contracting AIDS. Regardless of the route of drug administration, the economic necessities of supporting drug addiction by illegal means (theft, prostitution), secondary malnutrition, and the associated unhealthy personal and family psychosocial environment further complicate maternal well-being and prenatal care.[11]

Obstetrical Concerns

The obstetrical concerns of pregnant addicts include low birth weight, preterm labor and birth, intrauterine infection, fetal distress in labor, and congenital abnormalities.[11] Opioid withdrawal symptoms in adults include abdominal cramps, which may be confused with premature contractions or abruptio placenta.[13]

Maternal Detoxification

Detoxification of pregnant women should be individualized according to the primary drug of abuse and the stage of gestation. Detoxification before 14 weeks of gestation is not advocated because of the risk of inducing abortion. Likewise, during the last trimester of pregnancy, detoxification is not advised because of the risk of provoking preterm labor or fetal distress.[11]

CNS Depressants

Detoxification from alcohol can be accomplished with hospitalization and a tapering dose of a benzodiazepine, as can withdrawal from barbiturates and benzodiazepines themselves. Withdrawal from benzodiazepines may be prolonged, and delayed seizures sometimes occur.[11]

Opioids

Whether to detoxify for opioid dependence at any time during pregnancy remains controversial. Currently, most patients are switched from their abused opioids to methadone to avoid the danger of relapse and repeated intoxication and withdrawal cycles. Mother and baby are individually detoxified from methadone after birth. Methadone maintenance for opioid-addicted pregnant women removes them from the drug-seeking environment, eliminates the illicit behavior associated with it, prevents vacillations in maternal (and fetal) drug levels, improves maternal nutrition, and involves them in prenatal care and psychological/social rehabilitation.[10]

When it is absolutely essential for pregnant opioid addicts to be detoxified from methadone during pregnancy, it should be done by decreasing the dose by 5 mg every other week between the 14th and 28th week of gestation.[14]

Other Drugs

Detoxification of pregnant women from other drugs of abuse (CNS stimulants, cannabinoids, hallucinogens, phencyclidines, inhalants) is associated with few or no withdrawal symptoms and does not present any special maternal concerns.

The Fetus

Because approximately 85 percent of drug-addicted women are of child-bearing age, there is a corresponding increase in the number of infants at risk for a complicated prenatal and postnatal course, including congenital defects and withdrawal symptoms.[15]

Congenital Defects

During the embryonic period (second to eighth week after conception) each organ system in the body undergoes a sensitive stage in its development during which adverse influences can cause congenital anomalies. During the fetal period (nine weeks after conception to delivery), the fetus has concluded new organ development and is, therefore, less likely to develop congenital malformations. Instead, after that point, it may suffer altered skeletal growth, growth retardation, alteration of external genitalia, and central nervous system defects. The affected child may have behavioral and psychological disturbances later in life.[11]

Alcohol

In 1748 a British physician noted that when gin became cheap, more mothers gave birth to babies that were physically defective or mentally retarded. In 1759 the London College of Physicians petitioned the British Parliament to reinstate taxes on gin, so that it would be less available and constitute less of a risk to pregnant women and their offspring. Fetal alcohol syndrome (FAS), identified in 1973,[2,16] consists of a combination of birth defects, including both prenatal and postnatal growth retardation, small head circumference, mild to moderate mental retardation (average IQ 68), small eyes (often with strabismus and/or ptosis), hypoplasia of the maxilla, a long upper lip with a flattened philtrum and thinned vermilion, and a small upturned nose. In addition, infants may have skeletal, joint, genital, rectal, renal, skin, or cardiac defects. To date, full-blown FAS has been seen only in children of women who were very heavy drinkers during pregnancy.[9,17]

Fetal alcohol syndrome is the leading preventable congenital birth defect and occurs in 1.9 in 1,000 births. Among all birth defects, it ranks third behind Downs syndrome and spina bifida. Raising a physically and mentally handicapped child presents problems, particularly to a mother who cannot cope with her own problems.[10,18]

Less severe, but significant birth defects, including some that are subtle, may occur in offspring of women who drink lesser amounts of alcohol (including social drinkers). Neuropsychological testing of children of drinking mothers have found IQ scores lower than controls, as well as retarded development of concept formation and practical reasoning. Emotional instability, hyperactivity, distractibility, and short attention span were also significantly more prevalent in children of drinking mothers.[16,18] For every child born with FAS, as many as ten others may be born with *fetal alcohol effects* (FAE). In addition, the risk of spontaneous abortion is increased.[18]

A safe level of alcohol consumption has not been established. The best advice for pregnant women is to abstain from alcohol.[16]

Benzodiazepines

Maternal benzodiazepine addiction may result in teratogenic effects on fetuses, including dysmorphic features, growth aberrations, and central nervous system abnormalities. The dysmorphic features resemble those of FAS, although greater focal involvement of cranial nerves may occur. The infants at birth may appear to have a sullen and expressionless face and to have little vitality.[19]

Phenobarbital

Phenobarbital abuse has been associated with fetal facial dysmorphia and congenital malformations.

Opioids

Common metabolic disturbances in opioid-addicted neonates include hyperbilirubinemia, hypoglycemia, hypocalcemia, and hypomagnesemia. Convulsions may occur, and even with prompt and early attention the mortality rate may be increased. Most deaths are associated with low birth weight. Respiratory problems such as aspiration pneumonia, in particular from meconium aspiration, are commonly reported. Thrombocytosis and increased circulating platelet aggregation can occur and may persist for over 16 weeks, causing local infarcts and subarachnoid hemorrhage. Prolonged exposure to opioid drugs may cause irreversible damage to an infant's central nervous system, resulting in mental retardation.[13] Intrauterine growth retardation appears to be highest for pentazocine (Talwin) abuse.[6]

Cocaine

Cocaine abuse can produce a variety of neonatal effects, including growth retardation in utero, smaller head circumference, and premature rupture of membranes. There is an increased incidence of abruptio placenta, prematurity, stillbirth, and spontaneous abortion in cocaine-abusing pregnant women. Infants may have depressed interactive behavior and impaired organizational abilities after birth, as well as increased tremulousness and startle response. Infants born to cocaine-abusing mothers may suffer meconium aspiration leading to neurological damage or death. They also tend to have low birth weight and heart defects, and they may have seizures.[20] Although the mechanism for cocaine teratogenicity is not known, it is hypothesized that cocaine-induced vasoconstriction, acute hypertension, and cardiac arrhythmias interrupt the interoplacental blood supply causing fetal hypoxia.[21-22]

Nicotine

Nicotine causes a dose-related decrease in birth weight and head circumference. Congenital defects may occur. A permanent long-term effect on linear growth of infants born to mothers who smoke has been documented. Early in life, infants of smoking mothers appear to be less alert and by age seven may be hyperactive. By age eleven, children suffer decreases in general abilities, most evident in reading comprehension and mathematics.[6,23]

Marijuana

Marijuana appears to cause less fetal harm than many other drugs. No clear-cut visible birth defects have been demonstrated. Signs of nervous system excitation, including increased tremors, startles, hand-to-mouth activity, knee resistance, and reflexes may occur in cannabinoid-addicted neonates. Poor response to visual stimuli may also occur. A dose-related decrease in birth weight and head circumference has been documented. It is not clear if any effects persist in the long term.[6,20]

Phencyclidines

Virtually all phencyclidine abusers are multiple drug users. Hence, it has been difficult to determine fetal effects of phencyclidine alone. Phencyclidine-addicted infants have sudden outbursts of agitation, rapid changes in level of consciousness, increased lability, poor consolability, course arm flapping, tremors, nystagmus, and roving eye movements. They may have respiratory depression at birth. There does not seem to be an effect on weight or length.[6]

Inhalants

Sniffing of volatile hydrocarbons containing toluene during pregnancy may result in a syndrome of prenatal and postnatal growth retardation, microcephaly, CNS dysfunction, and cranial, facial, limb, and renal anomalies. The facial features consist of short palpebral fissures, deep-set eyes, narrow midface, ear anomalies, and narrow forehead.[6]

Abstinence Syndromes

Dependence can develop in the fetus as well as the mother. Symptoms of neonatal withdrawal are often present at birth but may not reach a peak for three to four days of life. They may peak as late as 10 to 14 days after birth for some drugs.[15]

Opioids

Neonatal opioid abstinence syndrome consists of central nervous system, gastrointestinal, autonomic, and respiratory effects (Table 19.2).[7,17,24-25] Withdrawal from narcotics can persist in a subacute form for four to six months after birth, with a peak in symptoms around six weeks of age.[15,26]

High doses of maternal methadone (80–120 mg per day) produce a severe and prolonged abstinence syndrome in newborns. This complication is avoided when the pregnant woman is placed on low-dose methadone maintenance, especially if the third trimester dose is less than 20 mg per day.[15]

Other Drugs

Abstinence syndromes in neonates exposed to nonnarcotic drugs in utero have been described for a variety of drugs. Withdrawal from these drugs does not appear to result in symptoms as severe as for withdrawal from narcotics. In general, these infants are irritable, restless, feed poorly, cry, and have impaired neurobehavioral abilities (Table 19.3).[6,15,22]

TABLE 19.2. Neonatal opioid abstinence syndrome.

Central nervous system	Autonomic system
tremor	sneezing
irritability	fever
hyperactivity	sweating
high-pitched cry	nasal congestion
sleep disturbances	salivation
hypertonicity	frequent yawning
hyperactive reflexes	
frantic fist sucking	*Respiratory*
	tachypnea
Gastrointetinal	respiratory distress
vomiting	
poor feeding	
diarrhea	

Neonatal Detoxification

Opioids

The mainstay of therapy for opioid-addicted newborns is sedation and gradual reduction of the dose and lengthening the intervals between administrations according to response. Elixir paregoric (camphorated tincture of opium), initially 4 to 6 drops with each feeding, usually controls symptoms. Phenobarbital, starting with 5–10 mg/kg daily in four divided doses is also usually effective. Chlorpromazine, diazepam, and methadone have also been used for neonatal detoxification.[13]

TABLE 19.3. Signs and symptoms of infants born to mothers addicted to nonnarcotic psychoactive drugs.

Drug	Signs/symptoms
alcohol	hyperactivity, crying, irritability, poor suck, tremors, convulsions, poor sleeping pattern, hyperphagia, diaphoresis; onset at birth
barbiturates	irritability, severe tremors, hyperacusis, excessive crying, vasomotor instability, diarrhea, restlessness, increased tone, hyperphagia, vomiting, disturbed sleep; onset 24 hours to 14 days
chlordiazepoxide and diazepam	irritability, tremors, hypotonia, poor suck, hyperreflexia, vomiting, hyperactivity, tachycardia; onset up to 21 days
ethchlorvynol and glutethimide	jitteriness, hyperphagia, irritability, poor suck, hypotonia or increased tone, opisthotonos, high pitched cry, hyperactivity
meprobamate	irritability, tremors, poor sleep patterns, abdominal pain
phencyclidine	jitteriness, hypertonia, vomiting, lethargy, vertical nystagmus
cocaine	abnormal sleep patterns, poor feeding, tremors, hypertonia, tachycardia, irritability

Other Drugs

Neonatal abstinence syndromes also occur with other drugs, with most intensity being from CNS depressant drugs (including alcohol). Gradually tapered doses of phenobarbital are usually effective.

The Role of the Physician

Physicians should be aware that women, like men, are at risk for addiction to alcohol, nicotine, and illicit drugs, and that they are especially at risk for iatrogenic prescription drug dependence. The rate of alcoholism is increasing in women, especially among younger employed ones. Also, drug abuse can have an adverse effect on fertility. Certain areas of women's lives are more apt to be affected than men's, and women have specific treatment issues different from those of men. By their drug abuse, women can adversely affect other beings (their fetuses). In addition, physicians should, once they make diagnoses of chemical dependence, refer pregnant addicts for obstetrical and neonatal care. They should also have a general knowledge of the teratogenic effects of drugs on the fetus and have a general knowledge of neonatal withdrawal symptoms and detoxification.

References

1. Holliday, A., and B. Bush. Women and alcohol abuse. In *Alcoholism: A Guide for the Primary Care Physician*. Ed. by H.N. Barnes, M.D. Aronson, and T.L. Delbanco. Springer-Verlag, New York, 1987, pp. 176–180.
2. Royce, J.E. Alcoholism problems and alcoholism: A comprehensive survey. Free Press, New York, 1981, pp. 65–68.
3. Cohen, S. Alcoholism and women. In *The Substance Abuse Problems: Volume One*. Haworth Press, New York, 1981, pp. 341–346.
4. Reed, B.G. Drug misuse and dependency in women: The meaning and implications of being considered a special population. *International Journal of Addictions*, 20:13–62, 1985.
5. Phillips, K. Neonatal drug addicts. *Nursing Times*, March, 1986, pp. 36–38.
6. Hill, R.M., and L.M. Tennyson. Maternal drug therapy: Effect on fetal and neonatal growth and neurobehavior. *Neurotoxicology*, 7:121–140, 1986.
7. Griffe, M.L., R.D. Weiss, S.M. Mirin, and V. Lange. A comparison of male and female cocaine abusers. *Archives of General Psychiatry*, 46:122–126, 1989.
8. Smith, C.G., and R.H. Asch. Drug abuse and reproduction. *Fertility and Sterility*, 48:355–373, 1987.
9. Blume, S. Women and alcohol. In *Alcoholism and Substance Abuse: Strategies for Clinical Intervention*. Ed. by T.E. Bratter and G.G. Forrest. Free Press, New York, 1985, pp. 623–638.
10. Hennecke, L., and V. Fox. The woman with alcoholism. In *Alcoholism: A Practical Treatment Guide*. Ed. by S.E. Gitlow and H.S. Peyser, Grune and Stratton, Orlando, Florida, 1980, pp. 181–191.

11. Martin, J.N., R.W. Martin, L.W. Hess, S.W. McColgin, J.F. McCall, and J.C. Morrison. Pregnancy-associated substance abuse and addiction: Current concepts and management. *Journal of the Mississippi State Medical Association*, 29:369–374, 1988.

12. Matteo, S. The risk of multiple addictions: Guidelines for assessing a woman's alcohol and drug abuse. *Western Journal of Medicine*, 149:941–945, 1988.

13. Wolman, I., D. Niv, I. Yovel, D. Pausner, E. Geller, and M. David. Opioid-addicted parturient, labor, and outcome: A reappraisal. *Obstetrical and Gynecological Survey*, 44:592–597, 1989.

14. Williams, A. When the client is pregnant: Information for counselors. *Journal of Substance Abuse Treatment*, 2:27–34, 1985.

15. Chesnoff, I., Jr. Drug use in pregnancy: Parameters of risk. *Pediatrics Clinics of North America*. 35:1403–1412, 1988.

16. Fetal alcohol syndrome. In *Alcohol and Health*. U.S. Department of Health and Human Services, Rockville, Maryland, 1987, pp. 80–96.

17. Cohen, S. The fetal alcohol syndrome: Alcohol as a teratogen. In *The Substance Abuse Problems: Volume One*. Haworth Press, New York, 1981, pp. 245–250.

18. The effects of alcohol on pregnancy outcome. In *Fifth Special Report to the U.S. Congress on Alcohol and Health*. U.S. Department of Health and Human Services, 1983, pp. 69–82.

19. Laegreid, L., R. Olegard, J. Walstrom, and N. Conradi. Teratogenic effects of benzodiazepine use during pregnancy. *Journal of Pediatrics*, 114:126–131, 1989.

20. Silverman, S. Interaction of drug-abusing mother, fetus, types of drugs examined in numerous studies. *Journal of the American Medical Association*, 26:1689–1690, 1989.

21. Bingol, N., F. Magdalena, V. Diaz, R.K. Stone, and D.S. Gromisch. Teratogenicity of cocaine in humans. *Journal of Pediatrics*, 110:93–96, 1987.

22. Oro, A., and S.D. Dixon. Perinatal cocaine and methamphetamine exposure: Maternal and neonatal correlates. *Journal of Pediatrics*, 111:571–578, 1987.

23. Milhorn, H.T., Jr. Nicotine dependence. *American Family Physician*, 39:214–224, 1989.

24. Niv, D. Protracted treatment with narcotics in pregnancy: Placenta filtration. Effects on the newborn and treatment. In *Pain Therapy*. Ed. by R. Rizzi and M. Visentin. Elsevier Biomedical Press, New York, 1983, p. 127.

25. Caviston, P. Pregnancy and opiate addiction. *British Medical Journal*, 195:285–286, 1987.

26. Rivers, R.P.A. Neonatal opiate withdrawal. *Archives of Disease of Childhood*, 61:1236–1239, 1986.

CHAPTER 20

Adolescents

The Normal Adolescent

We define adolescence as the period between the ages of 13 and 18. During this period, physical and psychological development is in transition. Hormonal changes accelerate physical growth and sexual maturation, and, as a result, adolescents may feel awkward and insecure. They frequently feel inadequate about their physical appearance, popularity with peers, school achievement, and ultimate prospects of functioning as independent adults. Because adolescence is a time of frustration, it is also a time of anger and rebellion.[1]

Peer affiliation and peer acceptance are hallmarks of adolescence. Young people have intense needs for acceptance, praise, and approval, needs that are more profound during adolescence than at any other time in life. Adolescents test limits and manipulate others; they tend to experiment with extremes of values and behaviors and are often confused and scared. One minute they demand total independence, and the next they cry out for protection from themselves and the world they live in. They often experience free-floating anxiety and identity crises. They commonly act out, expressing unacknowledged internal conflicts.[2-3] Adolescence is a period of exploratory, risk-taking, sensation-seeking behavior. Experimenting with chemicals is now a part of this world.[4]

The Substance Abuse Problem

Drug Use

In this country, on average, boys first use psychoactive substances at 11.9 years of age; girls at 12.7 years of age. Drug use has become an integral part of coming of age in American culture (Table 20.1).[3-4]

Among high school seniors, 91 percent have used alcohol at least once, 66 percent use it during any one month, and 5 percent use it daily. Of the daily users, 6.7 percent are boys and 2.8 percent are girls.[5-6]

Among high school seniors, 51 percent have smoked marijuana at least once, 23 percent use it during any one month, and 4 percent use it daily.[6]

TABLE 20.1. Drug abuse by high school seniors (1986).

	Percent ever used	Percent past month	Percent daily use
alcohol	91	66	5
nicotine (cigarettes)	67.5	30.1	19.5
marijuana	51	23	4
stimulants	23	6	0.3
inhalants	20	3	0.4
cocaine	17	5	0.2
hallucinogens	12	4	0.3
tranquilizers	11	2	0.0
sedatives	10	2	0.1
heroin	1	<0.5	0.0

Based on L.D. Johnston, P.M. O'Malley, and J.G. Bachman, Drug use by high school seniors—Class of 1986, U.S. Department of Health and Human Services, Rockville, Maryland, 1987.

Of high school seniors, 17 percent have used cocaine at least once, 5 percent use it during any one month, and 0.2 percent use it daily. Cocaine use by teenagers is on the rise. As for other stimulants, 23 percent of high school seniors have used them at least once, 6 percent use them during any one month, and 0.3 percent use them daily.[6]

As for inhalants, 20 percent of high school seniors have used them at least once, 3 percent use them during any one month, and 0.4 percent use them daily.[6]

More than two-thirds of high school seniors have smoked cigarettes at some time, 30.1 percent have used them in the last month, and 19.5 percent smoke at least half a pack daily. Cigarette smoking has declined among teenage boys but has increased among teenage girls. However, the use of smokeless tobacco is increasing among boys.[7-8]

Of all high school seniors, 65 percent have used an illicit drug;[9-10] 30 percent report having used alcohol prior to high school; and 10 percent report having used marijuana prior to high school.[6]

These data are somewhat conservative, because students who drop out of school before their senior year are not included. Drug use among this group is expected to be higher than among their in-school peers.[3]

Alcohol and tobacco are often considered to be gateway drugs because most people who become seriously involved with illicit drugs started with them.[3]

Consequences

Accidents are the leading cause of death among adolescents. Of the 25,000 accidental deaths among them annually, approximately 40 percent (10,000) are alcohol-related. Homicide is the second leading cause of death among adolescents. Of the 5,500 adolescent homicide victims each year, 30 percent are intoxicated at the time of death. Of all teen suicides, 88 percent are the result of drug overdoses. Drug abuse is a leading, if not the leading, cause of death among adolescents.[3] Less dramatic but more insidious are the developmental, emotional, and social costs of adolescent chemical dependence.[11]

Why Adolescents Use Drugs

We live in a drug-taking society, surrounded by images of people using drugs. Television advertisements depict drug use in two ways. Some link drinking to having fun; others link drug use (medication) to getting relief. Both give viewers the message that there is a drug to alter every human feeling and mood and that it is acceptable to use drugs for this purpose. Most adolescents who experiment with drugs or use them socially do not become chemically dependent. Unfortunately, some do.[1]

Adolescents have many specific reasons for beginning to use drugs (Table 20.2)—for recreation, to help them socialize more easily, and as a rite of passage into adulthood. They try drugs because their use represents a new experience and because they produce pleasure. Adolescents use drugs to rebel, in response to an impulse, and as part of self-exploration. They use them to conform to their peers, to prove sexuality, to reduce stress, to relieve anxiety, fatigue, or boredom, and to solve their personal problems. The overwhelmingly predominant reason adolescents give for recurrent drug use is that drugs make them feel good and that they experience no adverse consequences from them.[12]

TABLE 20.2. Why adolescents use drugs.

as recreation
as a rite of passage
as a socializer
for a new experience
for pleasure
in rebellion
in response to an impulse
in self-exploration
to conform
to prove sexuality
to reduce stress
to relieve anxiety, depression, or fatigue
to relieve boredom
to solve personal problems

Based on R.G. MacKenzie and E.A. Jacobs, Recognizing the adolescent drug abuser, *Primary Care,* 14:225–235, 1987.

The Chemically Dependent Adolescent

Differences from Adult Chemical Dependence

Chemical dependence among adolescents differs in several aspects from that of adults. Adolescents lack adult coping skills, and most have not separated completely from their parents. They are developing physically and psychologically, and many feel sexually insecure. They have not yet experienced meaningful loving, bonding relationships. Most still live at home and are not responsible for their financial support or for the financial support of others. Parents seldom withdraw food and shelter, so that adolescents do not suffer the same consequences as adults.[11,13] Whereas adult alcoholics may get cited for driving under the influence, for example, adolescents may not suffer this consequence simply because they have not yet begun to drive.[14]

Unlike adults, chemically dependent adolescents in treatment must undergo habilitation rather than rehabilitation—that is, they must learn, not relearn.

Denial

The Adolescent

Most chemically dependent people, and particularly adolescents, undergo denial, which results from the chemical dependence. It leaves adolescents unable to perceive themselves or others as they really are. Because of this self-deception, adolescents begin to deceive others. They lie about their behaviors and feelings and hide them from those who might confront them about their drug use. They avoid people who might make them aware of their fear of loss of control over the chemical.[2]

Adolescents in denial lie about substance use; guard supplies of chemicals; appear in public in altered states of consciousness; hide drugs; are preoccupied with chemicals; continue to use despite punishment, warnings, or advice; self-prescribe; frequently visit emergency rooms or their physicians; have dysfunctional emotional involvements with others; feel anger, rage, and defensiveness about their drug use; blame others for problems; pity themselves; attempt to control others; intellectualize; withdraw; isolate; and are chronically irresponsible. In a vicious cycle, denial produces greater drug use that, in turn, causes greater denial.[2]

Adolescents use the same mechanisms of denial as adults (Chapter 1). These include rationalization, projection, repression, suppression, isolation, and minimization.[2]

The Parents

Unfortunately, parents are often caught up in adolescent denial and develop a denial system of their own. Typical statements parents make in denying their child's drug dependence are listed in Table 20.3.

TABLE 20.3. Typical statements made by parents in denial.

This is just a phase of rebellion. All teenagers go through this.

He or she is just shy.

My child makes poor grades because he or she does not like school.

He or she doesn't drink all the time.

They will grow out of it. All they need is more time.

It's his or her friends. My child picks the wrong friends. It's their fault.

All I need to do is spend more time with him or her and everything will be alright.

He or she only drinks beer. At least my child is not shooting heroin.

He or she has so many pressures in school and with friends.

He or she just does not have enough willpower.

Behavioral Signs and Symptoms

The behavioral signs and symptoms of adolescent chemical dependence are numerous (Table 20.4). Chemically dependent teenagers drink and use drugs to get high, to escape (not simply for the elation or euphoria they once pursued), and to block emotional pain and discomfort. They gradually change friends to include drinking and drug using peers. Blackouts occur.[2]

With the progression of chemical dependence, difficulties occur more frequently at home, and family conflict increases. Adolescents may be suspended at school, and their grades may decline. They may be verbally abusive, rebellious, fight, and be sexually promiscuous. They believe they can stop using drugs anytime they choose and that they can stop by themselves.[2]

For drug-using adolescents, life becomes centered around alcohol and other drugs. Their peer groups change dramatically, so that eventually all their friends are exclusively alcohol and drug users. They attempt to stop drinking or using other drugs, but the fact that they can cut down or stop for a limited period of time leads them mistakenly to believe they can control drug use.[2]

Drug-using adolescents may deteriorate physically—in appearance or health. They may feel increasingly lonely and isolated, feelings that may be profound and dramatic. Parents, teachers, and even friends begin to express concern. Adolescents frequently visit psychiatrists, other physicians, or emergency rooms and may make psychosomatic complaints and have a lot of accidents.[2]

Gradually, adolescents lose self-esteem, increase their denial, and become angrier and more depressed. Serious family conflicts occur.[8] Persistent chemical use in adolescents may lead to repeated institutionalization, incarceration, or even death.[2]

Progression of chemical dependence in adolescents is much more rapid than in adults, and it delays the emotional maturation of adolescents. It is not unusual to deal with an 18 year old in treatment who thinks and behaves as a 15 year old.[1,13]

TABLE 20.4. Behavioral signs and symptoms of adolescent chemical dependence.

drinking or using to get high or to escape
drinking or using to block emotional pain and discomfort
gradual change to drinking and other drug using friends
blackouts
family conflict
school suspensions
declining grades
verbal abusiveness
rebelliousness
fighting
sexual promiscuity
stating that they can quit anytime they choose
life centered around alcohol and other drugs
failed attempts to stop drinking or using
physical deterioration in appearance
increased feelings of aloneness and isolation
concern expressed by parents, teachers, or friends
frequent visits to psychiatrist, other physicians, or emergency rooms
psychosomatic complaints
increased number of accidents
loss of self-esteem
increased denial
anger
depression
suicide gestures/attempts

Diagnosis of Adolescent Chemical Dependence

Careful distinction must be made between drug abuse and dependence. During the using and abusing stages, behavior controls the drug; in the dependence stage, the drug controls behavior, and addicts no longer have a choice in using the drug. Drug use becomes controlled by deeper, more primitive, centers of the brain, and compulsion to use drugs precludes rational and logical thought.[2]

Assessment

Assessment is difficult because adolescents often deny that they have any problems related to drinking alcohol or using other drugs. They typically withhold accurate information about drinking or other drug use. Consequently, physicians must often obtain information from others who know the adolescents. The cooperation of family members is essential for this process. Open-mindedness is important in determining whether an adolescent is addicted. Chemical dependence is not the cause of every behavior disorder; the diagnosis of chemical dependence must be made on factual information.

Persistent, careful, and comprehensive investigation is the key to the difficult process of diagnosing adolescent chemical dependence. The Michigan Alcohol Screening Test (MAST), a 29-item questionnaire, has been adapted for use with adolescents, and several other screening tests for adolescent chemical dependence have been developed. None have found widespread use and acceptance.[11,15]

Psychosocial Assessment

A general psychosocial assessment of an adolescent provides the basis for addressing chemical use and the foundation for determining whether he or she behaves dysfunctionally. It should include an assessment of home and family relationships, the young person's functioning at school, peer relationships, legal difficulties, leisure activity, employment, and self-perception.[14]

Drug-Use History

The interviewer should start with the least threatening and move to increasingly sensitive subjects. Because drugs from legitimate prescriptions are necessary and socially approved, this is a good place to start. The next step is to ask about the adolescent's use of over-the-counter medicines. The interviewer can then progress to tobacco products, including cigarettes and smokeless tobacco, and then to alcohol use and marijuana use. Finally, the interviewer should ask about other illicit drugs.[14]

Physical Signs

Physical addiction and withdrawal symptoms do occur in adolescents, but with much less frequency than in adults. Alcoholic hepatitis is uncommon in adolescents, and cirrhosis of the liver is rare. Marijuana smokers may have conjunctivitis, a chronic cough, or pharyngitis. Inhalant abusers may have a chronic rash around their mouth or nose. The unusual adolescent who uses intravenous drugs may have needle tracks.[11,14]

Laboratory Tests

Laboratory evidence of chemical dependence in the adolescent is not very helpful. Elevated liver enzymes due to alcoholic hepatitis are uncommon. A drug screen, when positive, is helpful but not diagnostic. Many adolescents are aware that a urine drug screen can be made to give a falsely negative result by substituting their urine with someone's else's or by adulterating their sample. Commonly used adulterants are vinegar, lemon juice, and chlorine bleach. Ingesting large amounts of water or diuretics may dilute the drug in the urine to such a level that it is not detectable.[10]

Intervention

A useful tool for getting adolescents into treatment, intervention is described in Chapter 5.

Treatment

Today there are a variety of treatment alternatives for chemically dependent adolescents. Among these are inpatient treatment, residential treatment, and outpatient treatment.

Inpatient Treatment

Programs offering inpatient treatment are usually in hospitals. These programs offer short, intense courses of treatment, providing a structured residential stay. They consider chemical dependence to be a disease, use the twelve steps of Alcoholics Anonymous, and are committed to total abstinence from psychoactive substances as a way of life. Staffing is multidisciplinary and includes physicians, nurses, and chemical dependence counselors. Fewer than 5 percent of adolescents admitted for treatment require medication for detoxification. Healthy activities are explored to replace chemical use. Inpatient programs often have elaborate rules with some sort of behavioral privilege system.[16]

If adolescents perceive the treatment setting as one simply imposed on them by adults, they resent it and it is ineffective.[13] Preaching, lecturing, and scolding are not effective. Positive peer influence is a powerful force; when this approach is used, peers replace adults, at least in part, as authority figures.[1]

Patient government groups serve several functions. They promote responsibility and accountability. Group leaders are in charge of unit meetings and act as positive role models for other patients; unit secretaries record the minutes of meetings and post duties on the bulletin board; and other patients are elected to make coffee, clean lounges, act as buddies to new patients on the unit, and buy necessities for patients without shopping privileges. Indirectly, patient government groups build confidence and improve patient self-esteem.[3]

Adolescents have a higher energy level than most adults and are often bored. Treatment programs need to incorporate this energy into program activities and so must make sufficient recreational activities available to patients.[1]

Visits by program graduates are well received by adolescent patients. Graduates may return to a facility on regularly scheduled visits, perhaps once a month, and conduct Alcoholics Anonymous meetings or informal discussions. They are able to speak with credibility about the kinds of problems patients will face after they complete treatment. They serve as living examples of adolescents in recovery.[1]

Many authorities believe that adolescents need a longer length of stay than the usual 28 days adults spend in programs. Therefore, many adolescent programs last 46 to 60 days. Regardless of the length of inpatient treatment, most programs feel that follow-up care is extremely important. Extended care is thought to be necessary for adolescents because their age, immaturity, lack of nonchemical coping skills, and emotional and developmental lags from prolonged drug use during a period when adolescents normally mature emotionally. Some programs require six weeks of partial day-care following discharge from an inpatient stay. Following this, once-weekly aftercare, extending for six months, may be required. Continued academic training is extremely important, and maintaining academic performance may increase an adolescent's self-esteem and sense of responsibility.[16]

A program for direct family involvement is an integral part of treatment. Other details of inpatient treatment are discussed in Chapter 3.

Residential Treatment

Therapeutic communities constitute one form of residential treatment. These programs stress open and frank communication and emphasize acceptance of one's responsibility with the group. They tend to use a relatively high proportion of paraprofessional staff. A traditional therapeutic community may have only one or two professional counselors.[16]

Another type of residential treatment, half-way houses are not intended as primary treatment facilities. They are structured settings from which recovering adolescents can reenter the community before returning home from inpatient treatment. They offer places for newly recovering adolescents to give one another support.[16]

Other details of therapeutic communities and half-way houses are discussed in Chapter 3.

Outpatient Treatment

Patients in outpatient treatment do not live at treatment facilities and are free to maintain their daily school schedule. A typical outpatient program might require a patient to attend three evening sessions a week at the treatment center and two or three Alcoholics Anonymous or Narcotics Anonymous meetings a week in the community.[1]

Because of the deep-seated denial that chemically dependent adolescents develop, many authorities believe that outpatient treatment cannot be effective. Instead, it is used for adolescents who have not yet developed dependence to keep them from reaching that stage. It can also be used to support an adolescent returning home from an inpatient treatment program.[16] An adolescent should meet two criteria to be a candidate for outpatient treatment. First, the patient must come from a functionally healthy family. The family plays an important role in outpatient treatment. Second, the adolescent must be in the abuse stage, not yet having reached full-blown dependence.[1] Other details of outpatient treatment are discussed in Chapter 3.

Psychiatric Disorders

Although adolescents are subject to almost any psychiatric disorder, three occur in the treatment of chemical dependence with sufficient frequency that they deserve mention: attention deficit disorder, anorexia nervosa, and bulimia.

Attention Deficit Disorder

Characterized by inappropriate inattention and impulsivity, attention deficit disorders (ADD) include as subtypes ADD with hyperactivity, ADD without hyperactivity, and ADD residual type, which occurs in older adolescents and adults who had ADD with hyperactivity in childhood. Patients with ADD residual type lose their hyperactivity but remain impulsive and inattentive.[17]

Adolescents who have developed both chemical dependence and ADD tend to be disruptive and may pose a treatment dilemma. Stimulants are the usual pharmacological treatment for children with ADD. Two problems arise from this treatment. First, chemically dependent individuals tend to abuse mood-altering drugs; second, the goal of treatment is for individuals to live chemically free. It is clear then that physicians must explore nonchemical methods of managing adolescents with ADD.[2,17]

Anorexia Nervosa

A disorder primarily of young females, anorexia nervosa is characterized by an intense fear of becoming obese, a disturbance of body image (feeling fat in spite of obvious visual evidence to the contrary), weight loss of at least 25 percent of original body weight, and a preoccupation with losing weight. Anorexics diet, exercise, and abuse diuretics and laxatives, even while family members and their physicians try to stop them. Because death from starvation can occur from this disorder, patients should be referred to physicians or treatment programs that specialize in eating disorders.[2,17]

Bulimia

The main features of bulimia include recurrent binge episodes, awareness that the eating pattern is abnormal, fear of being unable to stop voluntarily, depressed mood following binges, use of diets, cathartics, diuretics, and self-induced vomiting, inconspicuous eating during a binge, and consumption of high-calorie foods during a binge. Recently, bulimia has become viewed as an addictive disorder, and treatment programs based on a 12-step program similar to that of Alcoholics Anonymous have evolved.[2,17]

Aftercare

A very small number of adolescent patients complete treatment with the insight, determination, and courage needed for successful recovery. Therefore, a well-developed aftercare plan is essential. Concerns to be addressed in aftercare include maintaining sobriety, continued involvement with community support groups and sponsors, educational priorities, vocational goals, and psychological counseling. Also included in the aftercare plan are goals for having fun while remaining clean and sober and a no-use contract. This is an agreement between the patient and the family that the adolescent will not use alcohol or other drugs.[1]

Role of the Physician

In general, physicians who care for adolescents have important roles in evaluating and diagnosing chemical dependence, managing physical consequences of drug use, counseling adolescents and their families, recommending appropriate treatment options, assisting families in intervention, continuing to care for acute episodic illnesses, and supporting patients and families through the long and sometimes chaotic course of habilitation and recovery.[12]

References

1. Heaslip, J., D. Van Dyke, D. Hogenson, and L. Vedders. *Young People and Drugs: Evaluation and Treatment*, Hazelden, Center City, Minnesota, 1989.
2. Morrison, M.A., and Q.T. Smith. Psychiatric issues of adolescent chemical dependence. *Insight*, 3:3–10, 1987.
3. Schonberg, S.K. (Ed.). *Substance Abuse: A Guide for Health Professionals*. American Academy of Pediatrics, Elk Grove Village, Illinois, 1988.
4. Cohen, S. Coming of age in America—with drugs: Contemporary America. In *The Substance Abuse Problems: Volume Two*. Haworth Press, New York, 1985, pp. 203–207.
5. Statistical Bulletin/Metropolitan Insurance Companies, 68:2–11, 1987.
6. Johnston, L.D., P.M. O'Malley, and J.G. Bachman. Drug use by high school seniors—Class of 1986. U.S. Department of Health and Human Services, Rockville, Maryland, 1987.
7. Sanders, J.M., Jr. Identifying substance use in adolescents. *Postgraduate Medicine*, 84:123–136, 1988.
8. Wallock, L., and K. Corbett. Alcohol, tobacco, and marijuana: An overview of epidemiological, program, and policy trends. *Health Education Quarterly*, 14:223–249, 1987.
9. Beschner, G.M., and A.S. Friedman. Treatment of adolescent drug abusers. *International Journal of the Addictions*, 20:971–993, 1985.
10. Semlitz, L., and M.S. Gold. Adolescent drug abuse: Diagnosis, treatment, and prevention. *Pediatric Clinics of North America*, 9:455–473, 1986.
11. Bean-Bayog, M. The adolescent drinker. In *Alcoholism: A Guide for the Primary Care Physician*. Ed. by H.N. Barnes, M.D. Aronson and T.L. Delbanco. Springer-Verlag, New York, 1987, pp. 181–193.
12. MacKenzie, R.G., and E.A. Jacobs. Recognizing the adolescent drug abuser. *Adolescent Medicine*, 14:225–235, 1987.
13. Royce, J.E. Special groups. In *Alcohol Problems and Alcoholism*. Free Press, New York, 1981, pp. 103–118.

14. Anglin, T.M. Interviewing guidelines for the clinical evaluation of adolescent substance abuse. *Pediatric Clinics of North America*, 4:381–399, 1987.
15. Blum, R.W. Adolescent substance abuse: Diagnosis and treatment issues. *Pediatric Clinics of North America*, 34:523–537, 1987.
16. Wheeler, K., and J. Malinquist. Treatment approaches in adolescent chemical dependency. *Pediatric Clinics of North America*, 34:437–447, 1987.
17. Tomb, D.A. *Psychiatry for the House Officer.* Williams and Wilkins, 1984, pp. 108–109, 156.

CHAPTER 21

The Elderly

Older individuals represent an increasing proportion of the U.S. population. In 1900, 4 percent of Americans were 65 or older; in 1977, 11 percent were in this age group; and it is projected that at least 20 percent of our population will be over 65 by the year 2050. It is significant to realize that only about 5 percent of the elderly are living in institutions; this means that 95 percent are living with the rest of society.[1-2]

Of men and women over 65, 86 percent have at least one or more chronic ailment. Thus, elderly people are more likely to take several prescription and over-the-counter medications, as well as to self-medicate with alcohol. Many drugs have the potential for addiction as well as synergistic action among themselves and with alcohol.[1-2]

Pathophysiology of Aging

As a person grows older, physiological changes tend to extend the life of drugs in the body and enable them to have more powerful effects. Pharmacokinetic changes affect drug absorption, distribution, metabolism, and excretion (Table 21.1). Disease, too, often affects these factors.[3-4]

Absorption

Physiological changes that occur within the gastrointestinal tract as the result of aging include increased gastric pH, delayed gastric emptying, reduced small bowel mucosal surface area, and reduced intestinal blood flow. While all of these changes would theoretically influence absorption of oral medications, few significant differences in absorption are seen between younger and older adults. Probably of greater importance is the decline in first-pass elimination of drugs by the liver. Because significant portions of many drugs are metabolized in the liver

Some of the material in this chapter was originally written by H. Thomas Milhorn, Jr., M.D., and published in the July 1990 issue of *Senior Patient* and is issued by permission of McGraw-Hill, Inc.

292 21. The Elderly

TABLE 21.1. Physiological changes in the elderly.

Physiological change	Pharmacokinetic alteration
increased gastric pH	decreased absorption of drugs that are normally nonionized at low pH
increased body fat	decreased fat-soluble drug concentration in the blood
decreased body water	increased water-soluble drug concentration in the blood
decreased serum albumin	increased unbound drug, leading to increased drug activity
decreased cardiac output	decreased metabolism of drugs
decreased renal blood flow	decreased excretion of drugs
decreased splanchnic blood flow	decreased absorption of drugs taken orally, decreased metabolism
decreased liver mass and hepatic blood flow	decreased metabolism of drugs
receptor site change	increased or decreased drug activity

From M. Shlafer and E.N. Marieb, Age and other patient-related factors that alter drug response, in *The Nurse, Pharmacology, and Drug Therapy,* Addison-Wesley, Redwood City, California, 1989, pp. 90–108.

before they enter the systemic circulation, as first-pass elimination rates decline due to aging, a greater quantity of a drug enters the systemic circulation.[3]

Distribution

The lean body mass of an older adult decreases and body fat increases in proportion to total body weight. This change in fat-to-muscle ratio creates a physiological environment in which plasma concentrations of water-soluble drugs are increased, because the drugs are distributed in a smaller relative volume of water. On the other hand, plasma concentrations of lipid-soluble drugs are decreased because of their distribution into a relatively greater fraction of fat. In addition, serum albumin usually decreases about 12 percent in later years. Because many drugs tend to bind to albumin, the decreased number of binding sites leads to a proportionately higher number of unbound drug molecules in the plasma. The unbound portion of a drug is responsible for its pharmacological action.[3]

Metabolism

With increasing age, the body's ability to metabolize drugs declines. The liver, the predominant organ of drug metabolism, loses some of its effectiveness because of a reduction in the effectiveness of its microenzyme system. In addition, liver blood flow is reduced in the elderly, resulting in a decrease in rate of delivery of drugs to the liver.[3]

Excretion

A generalized reduction of renal function occurs with aging. Glomerular filtration rate declines approximately 0.5 percent a year after age 20. As a result, all drugs eliminated by the kidneys have a decreased rate of excretion.[3]

Disease

In addition to physiological alterations, concurrent disease may also alter drugs' effects. A number of abnormalities are common among the elderly, including congestive heart failure, renal disease, dehydration, hypotension, hypertension, diabetes, malnutrition, and cirrhosis. Such disorders can further reduce the functions of vital organs and thereby alter drug absorption, distribution, metabolism, and excretion.[3] In addition, the central nervous system's sensitivity to alcohol and other drugs increases with age.[5]

As a result of physiological and pathological changes, an extreme variability occurs in older adults' responses to drugs. As a general principle, a physician should expect an increased and prolonged drug effect in the elderly.[3]

The Elderly Addict

Few older Americans use street drugs. However, they do have problems with prescription medications and alcohol. Most elderly patients admitted for treatment of chemical dependence are dependent on alcohol alone (86 percent); the remainder are dependent on prescription drugs alone or in combination with alcohol (14 percent).[6]

Alcohol

Prevalence

Alcohol is the number one drug of abuse of older Americans. However, people over age 65 have the lowest rate of alcoholism of any age group. The reasons for the lower prevalence in the elderly are not clear. It may be due to the reduced tolerance to alcohol that is associated with aging, the physiological effects of aging and medical problems that may interfere with the pleasurable effects of drinking, and the increased interactions of alcohol with prescription drugs.[7] In addition, older people today may use alcohol at a lower rate because they lived through Prohibition and the Depression of the 1930s and never became heavy drinkers. Finally, heavier drinkers may die at younger ages, leaving behind those with more moderate drinking habits.[8]

Of the estimated 10 million alcoholics in the United States, probably 3 million of them are over age 60. The male-to-female ratio among elderly alcoholics is about 5 to 1. Women are more likely than men to start drinking heavily later in life, and single women are more likely than married ones to have a drinking problem.[5]

Groups

Elderly alcoholics can be divided into three major groups: survivors, reactors, and binge drinkers. Survivors, who comprise almost two-thirds of older alcoholics, have an early onset of alcohol abuse. Although most alcoholics die at an earlier age, survivors have beaten the odds. Most of them have numerous medical problems, including cirrhosis, organic brain syndrome, and psychiatric problems.

Reactors start drinking relatively late in life. To them, alcoholism is secondary to the stresses of aging—the death of a spouse or other person close to them, retirement, loneliness, reduced income, poor health, or geographic relocation. Because of the late onset of their drinking, reactors show fewer physical consequences and fewer life-style disruptions than other older alcoholics. With abstinence from alcohol and good nutrition, recovery from the physical effects of alcoholism can be complete. Nearly a third of elderly alcoholics fall into this group.[5,7]

Binge drinkers do not drink regularly but occasionally go on binges, drinking relatively large amounts of alcohol over a few days or weeks. Intermittent stress (depression, loneliness, anxiety) is a common ingredient in initiating these episodes. Binge drinkers represent only a small percentage of elderly alcoholics.[5]

Medical Consequences

One of the most important pathological consequences of alcoholism in the elderly is its effect on the cardiovascular system. Alcohol impairs cardiac function, resulting in decreased cardiac output. It may deaden angina pain, a warning sign, leading to myocardial infarction. Alcohol can also cause worsening of hypertension and adversely affect pulmonary function. Alcohol abuse can cause a decrease in respiratory drive, resulting in mental confusion in elderly people with chronic obstructive pulmonary disease. Alcoholism can also lead to adverse nutritional effects in the elderly, including deficiency of thiamine and other nutrients. Gastrointestinal disorders (gastritis, peptic ulcer disease, diarrhea) are common among elderly alcoholics, as are neurological disorders (myopathy, neuropathy, decreased coordination, decreased seizure threshold).[5]

Elderly individuals are more apt to develop cognitive impairment from the use of alcohol than younger ones. They tend to become forgetful and to have more difficulty with reasoning. They may become stubborn because of a lack of understanding or angry and agitated as they become confused. Senile dementia due to alcoholism is of two types—Wernike-Korsakoff syndrome and alcoholic dementia.[1]

Wernike's encephalopathy is an acute stage of brain dysfunction characterized by general cloudiness of the mind and gross confusion. Some ataxia and nystagmus may occur. When treated with thiamine, many of the acute symptoms clear. What is left after about three days is called Korsakoff's psychosis. It is characterized by an inability to learn, a loss of immediate memory, and confabulation. With proper nutrition, absence of alcohol, and time, the condition usually clears or improves. Most improvement is seen in the first three months but may continue up to five years.[1]

Alcoholic dementia is characterized by a gradual intellectual decline due to long-term alcohol abuse and is irreversible. Progression ceases with abstinence from alcohol.[1]

The combined effects of alcoholism and aging are additive, placing older alcoholics at increased risk of premature dementia and decreasing their potential for recovering.[4]

Other Drugs

Older people consume drugs from 400 million prescriptions each year. Although they comprise only 12 percent of the population, they consume about 25 percent of all prescription drugs dispensed. The consequences of drug misuse by the elderly are dramatic. People over 60 account for 40 percent of all drug reactions; one-sixth of hospital admissions for patients over 70 result from adverse drug reactions, and nearly one-fourth of hospital admissions for the elderly are due to their taking prescriptions incorrectly. Factors that contribute to prescription drug misuse among older Americans include poor communication between older patients and physicians, pharmacists, and nurses; complex regimens that require them to take a number of drugs at the same time; treatment by several different physicians, all of whom may be prescribing medicine; a lack of awareness that a drug's effects can be magnified or reduced in aging bodies; an inability to take medicines as prescribed because of vision, hearing, and memory loss or other changes associated with aging; and poor compliance — not taking a prescribed drug at all, discontinuing the drug prematurely, or purposefully altering consumption of it.[9]

Among the elderly, a significant prescription drug abuse problem exists, one that is often referred to as American's hidden problem. The drugs elderly people abuse are almost invariably ones that depress the central nervous system, as these people withdraw from frustrating existences and evade stress rather than seek out new experiences. There is a great variability in the response among older people to mood-altering substances; they may be hypersensitive to even average amounts of chemical substances and suffer mental confusion or fluctuating delirium as a common result.[6,10]

Aging drug addicts can be divided into two groups: surviving street addicts and prescription addicts.[10]

Street Drugs

There are few street addicts over the age of 60. Most have either died from the consequences of injecting unsterile material for years, accidental overdoses, suicide, or trauma. Some opioid addicts over 60 can be found in methadone maintenance clinics.[10]

Prescription Drugs

The prescription drugs the elderly most commonly abuse are opioids, benzodiazepines, and barbiturates. Medical opioid addicts, usually iatrogenic, become addicted from being treated for some painful illness.[10] Those who become addicted during the treatment of an acute self-limiting illness just simply continue to use the pain medication, refilled periodically by their physicians. Those with chronic pain continue to use the medication in belief that if they do not take it they will suffer intense, intolerable pain. The same is true of those who take medication for intermittent pains, such as headaches. In my experience, many of these addicts treat the fear of pain, which is considerably worse than the actual pain, rather than pain itself. Most, when detoxified, find that their pain, if it still exists, can be treated by nonaddicting approaches.

As a result of their complaints about insomnia and anxiety, sleeping pills and minor tranquilizers are the most common of all drugs prescribed for the elderly. These drugs can lead to mental confusion and physical clumsiness. Older patients with marginal mental comprehension are easily pushed into delirium. Sudden withdrawal of the medication can cause them anxiety, vivid nightmares, insomnia, panic attacks, delirium, and seizures. The majority of complaints of insomnia occur because older people are often ignorant about how much sleep they need. Those over 65 may require as little as five hours of sleep a night. Other complaints of insomnia result from nocturnal pain, itching, muscle cramps, depression, or the need to void three to four times a night. Treating the cause of the sleep disturbance or teaching patients nonmedicinal approaches to insomnia in most instances is more appropriate than prescribing sleeping medication.

Signs of prescription drug abuse include requests for drug refills that indicate use out of proportion to objective signs and symptoms or more rapid use than directed; requests for refills of controlled substances prescribed by another physician; requests for refills before the original prescriptions are finished; requests for specific, usually very potent drugs, when other less potent drugs in the same class are said to be ineffective or cause adverse reactions; and undue familiarity with many potent psychoactive drugs, their appearances, side effects and formulations.[11]

Diagnosis

Diagnosing chemical dependence in the elderly can be difficult. Physicians use many rationalizations for not confronting elderly addicts. Family members and physicians may accept an ongoing alcohol or other drug problem as a justifiable response to the stress of aging. Another obstacle to recognizing addiction in the elderly is the stereotype of the skid-row bum. Because elderly patients do not fit this picture, addiction to alcohol or other drugs may not be suspected. In addition, the elderly may not come to the attention of those who might suspect they have a problem.

When behavioral problems develop in the elderly, causes other than drug use are often considered first. The effects of alcohol and other CNS depressants may produce a syndrome indistinguishable from senile dementia (Alzheimer's, multiple infarct dementia).[5]

Drug-related health problems in the elderly may be more difficult to separate from chronic illness and the effects of medication than in younger populations.[12] When elderly patients have problems with controlling gout, diabetes mellitus, hypertension, angina, or incontinence, alcohol abuse should be considered.[9] Temperature regulation may be impaired, increasing the age-related risk of hypothermia. The diuretic effect of alcohol may be significant in the frail elderly. Arrhythmias and decreased left ventricular function are potential cardiac side effects.[8]

Clues in the history and physical examination that may indicate chemical dependence in the elderly include insomnia or changes in sleep patterns, abrupt confusion, inability to function, gastrointestinal problems, palpitations, gait abnormalities and frequent falls, bruises, fractures, burns, or sprains. Self-neglect, poor grooming, or malnutrition may also indicate a problem with alcohol or other drugs. Noticeable behavioral changes, such as social isolation, depression, paranoid behavior, increased family quarrels, or estrangement from family or friends should be investigated.[5-6]

Alcohol withdrawal is commonly overlooked during elderly patients' hospitalizations because transient confusion is so common in this population.[8]

A problem with allowing the elderly to report their own level of drinking is setting a cutoff level for heavy drinking. A few drinks a day may be relatively benign for a healthy young person, but the same intake could be disastrous for any elderly person who is in poor health, has decreased tolerance, and is taking several prescription drugs.

Most measures of substance abuse were standardized on nonelderly men. Such measures include problems with family or friends, employment or legal problems, drinking and driving problems, financial problems, and neglecting responsibilities. Physical aggression, breaking the law, driving a car, and being employed tend to characterize men more than women but characterize the elderly least of all. Some evidence, however, does indicate that the MAST may be an effective screening tool for the elderly.[13]

Indicators of drug use more appropriate for the elderly might include housing problems, falls or accidents, poor nutrition, inadequate personal care or care of clothing or living quarters, lack of physical activity, and social isolation.[12]

Clinical presentations of the chemically dependent elderly are given in Table 21.2.

Being suspicious of and questioning the elderly about chemical dependence can make their care more appropriate and effective.[8]

Treatment

Unfortunately, only a fraction of chemically dependent elderly people ever receive treatment for their disease. Inpatient treatment is often needed to address such issues as detoxification, depression, poor nutrition, weight loss, treatment of acute and chronic medical problems, and polypharmacy. Individual counseling and support are crucial in alleviating patients' guilt, frustration, and depression.

Evaluation

Patients' ability to function and to solve problems must be evaluated early in treatment. If problems are detected in these areas, evaluations should be repeated periodically to look for improvement. Senility may have developed to so great a point in some elderly patients that they simply cannot benefit from treatment—other than by learning to abstain from drugs and to develop better nutrition, and

TABLE 21.2. Clinical presentations of the chemically dependent elderly.

angina	hypothermia
anxiety	incontinence
arrhythmias	injuries
bruises	insomnia
burns	malnutrition
confusion	mood swings
congestive heart failure	myopathy
dementia	noncompliance with medication
depression	palpitations
diabetes mellitus	paranoid behavior
diarrhea	poor grooming
falls	self-neglect
forgetfulness	seizures
fractures	sleep disturbances
gait abnormalities	social isolation
gastrointestinal problems	sprains
	tremor

From H.T. Milhorn, Jr., and L.C. Gardner, The elderly alcoholic: Diagnosis and treatment, *The Senior Patient*, in press. Reprinted with permission of McGraw-Hill.

are better suited for nursing home care. Some may need legal or financial guardians, and their families must make such decisions in these situations. Those with mild or moderate memory impairment should be taught to keep notes and a daily schedule.[1]

Detoxification

Detoxification generally takes longer in the elderly. Benzodiazepines with a short half-life, such as oxazepam (Serax) or lorazepam (Ativan), are preferable to the longer-acting ones such as diazepam (Valium) or chlordiazepoxide (Librium). The dosages should be one-half to two-thirds those used in younger adults.[14]

Thiamine and screening for dietary deficiencies (folate, vitamin B_{12}, magnesium) are advised. Signs and symptoms of concomitant barbiturate, benzodiazepine, or opioid abuse may complicate the picture. Benzodiazepine addiction in particular may prolong the detoxification period.[8]

Rehabilitation

Elderly people, in general, tend to hold very definite ideas. They feel that things should look good on the surface and therefore tend not to make waves but instead comply. They tend to be offended by coarse language, sloppy clothes, and long hair, which are attitudes physicians and counselors should deal with openly and with respect. To them, family secrets should not be aired in public, but what they consider to be personal secrets may not be the same things people of different generations consider to be secret. They may, for example, sometimes consider divorce a secret. The elderly feel that authority should be respected and usually have rigid ideas on male and female roles. Elderly women tend to be dependent and look for people to defend them; elderly men have been taught to be protectors. This rigidity should be recognized. The immorality view of chemical dependence has been deeply engraved in older people. They have been raised to view alcoholism as sinful and the alcoholic as weak, and it is very difficult for them to accept the disease concept of addiction. Finally, many elderly were brought up with deep religious beliefs but have strayed from church over the years. Sometimes their return to church may help their spiritual progress.[1]

The elderly deny abuse much more so than other age groups do. Many of today's elderly grew up at a time when drinking was frowned on, and they may be reluctant to admit even limited consumption.[12]

Frequently, elderly addicts need to deal with deaths, divorces, or other significant losses that happened years ago and that they have not dealt with because of their substance abuse. This is especially true of the late-onset alcoholic, whose heavy drinking may have been initiated by such a loss.[1]

Vocational rehabilitation is generally inappropriate for the elderly. However, social services are especially relevant for older recovering addicts because they often live alone and have few social resources.[14]

Unlike younger people, the elderly are not likely to return to work or to child-rearing. They should be helped to look at the need to improve their physical health and to make sure that their living conditions meet their needs. Reestablishing broken ties with lost family members, and thus improving social support systems, should be pursued.[1]

Counselors should address such relevant issues as retirement, free time, volunteer work, and interactions with grown children. Often, the elderly are concerned about the costs of retirement. They should be told that treatment for chemical dependence is reimbursable under Medicaid and Medicare.[5]

Physical activity is a great healer of depression. Regular walking stimulates people physically, emotionally, and psychologically and should be recommended. Relaxation therapy is well received in this age group and helps to improve their general sense of well-being.[1]

The best approach to treating the elderly is that of gentle support and loving encouragement. Heavy confrontation has no place in this age group. They do not need judgment or punishment, which they tend to provide themselves. They need kind acceptance, gentle support, encouragement that things can change for the better, and reassurance of their importance as people. Treatment programs designed specifically for the elderly are desirable.[1,15]

Treatment issues often encountered in the elderly are summarized in Table 21.3.

TABLE 21.3. Treatment issues in the elderly.

broken family ties	living conditions
death of loved one	medical problems
denial	memory problems
depression	physical condition
detoxification	polypharmacy
embarrassment	poor nutrition
fixed ideas	relaxation
free time	retirement
frustration	shame
guilt	social support system
insomnia	treatment costs
	volunteer work

From H.T. Milhorn, Jr. and L.C. Gardner, The elderly alcoholic: Diagnosis and treatment, *The Senior Patient*, in press. Reprinted with permission of McGraw-Hill.

Aftercare

The goal of planning aftercare is to have elderly patients living at their highest level of functioning and lowest level of care. This may involve living independently at home, living at home with local social support systems, living in halfway houses, or institutionalized care.[1]

In the elderly, long-term addiction often results in feelings of loneliness and isolation that are deeper and stronger than those felt by younger people. The elderly may feel extremely unworthy, needing to have people around them. They need to find creative use of their leisure time and need to revive old interests. Volunteer work serves a need in this age group.[1]

AA and aftercare meetings are very helpful. Daytime meetings are important because many elderly do not like to be out after dark, and night driving is more difficult for many of them. Transportation may be a problem for some; if so, arrangements should be made prior to discharge from treatment.[1,16]

The elderly are more faithful than younger people in attending support group meetings, but they prefer and receive greater benefit from smaller groups. Older patients complain about the noise, rough language, and cigarette smoke that are often associated with larger meetings.[5]

Role of the Physician

Physicians should recognize that pharmacological factors in the elderly tend to prolong and increase the magnitude of effects of drugs. Doses, therefore, need to be reduced. They should be aware that some of their elderly patients have problems with alcohol or prescription medications and should be able to recognize signs and symptoms that may indicate chemical dependence in this age group. Physicians can be instrumental in getting patients into treatment. They should have a basic understanding of treatment issues in the elderly and should play a major role in the long-term recovery of patients. They should realize that the use of mood-altering drugs in recovering elderly patients is, for the most part, not recommended. Occasional questioning about aftercare and/or AA meetings and supporting elderly people's attendance is appropriate.[16]

References

1. Walker B., and P. Kelly. *The Elderly: A Guide for Counselors*. Hazelden, Center City, Minnesota, 1981.
2. Schuckit, M.A. Alcohol, drugs, and the elderly. *Drug Abuse and Alcoholism Newsletter*, vol. 18, no. 3.
3. Shlafer, M., and E.N. Marieb. Age and other patient-related factors that alter drug response. In *The Nurse, Pharmacology, and Drug Therapy*. Addison-Wesley, Redwood City, California, 1989, pp. 90–108.
4. Stirling, J.S., J.W. Largen, and T. Shaw. Interactions of normal aging, senile dementia, multi-infarct dementia, and alcoholism in the elderly. In *Alcoholism in the Elderly: Social and Biomedical Issues*. Ed. by J.T. Hartford and T. Samorajaski. Raven Press, New York, 1984, pp. 227–251.
5. Olsen-Noll, C.G., and M.F. Bosworth. Alcohol abuse in the elderly. *American Family Physician*, 39:173–179, 1989.
6. Abrams, R.C., and G.S. Alexopoulos. Substance abuse in the elderly: Alcohol and prescription drugs. *Hospital and Community Psychiatry*, 38:1285–1287, 1987.
7. Epidemiology. In *Alcohol and Health*. Department of Health and Human Services, Rockville, Maryland, 1987, pp. 14–27.
8. Hesse, K., and J. Savitsky. The elderly. In *Alcoholism: A Guide for the Primary Care Physician*. Ed. by H.N. Barnes, M.D. Aronson, and T.L. Delbanco. Springer-Verlag, New York, 1987, pp. 167–175.
9. The other drug problem. Editorial, *American Family Physician*, 38:90, 1988.
10. Cohen, S. Special groups and situations. In *The Substance Abuse Problems: Volume One*, 1981, pp. 313–363.
11. Cusack, B.J., and R.E. Vestal. Clinical pharmacology: Special considerations in the elderly. In *The Practice of Geriatrics*. Ed. by I.C. Evan, P.J. Davis and A.B. Ford. W.B. Saunders, Philadelphia, 1986, pp. 115–131.
12. Graham, K. Identifying and measuring alcohol abuse among the elderly: Serious problems with existing instrumentation. *Journal of Studies on Alcohol*, 47:322–326, 1986.
13. Whitcup, S.M., and F. Miller. Unrecognized drug dependence in psychiatrically hospitalized elderly patients. *Journal of the Geriatric Association*, 35:297–301, 1987.
14. Bienenfeld, D. Alcoholism in the elderly. *American Family Physician*, 36:163–169, 1987.
15. Kofoed, L.L., R.L. Tolson, R.M. Atkinson, R.L. Toth, and J.A. Turner. Treatment compliance of older alcoholics: An elder-specific approach is superior to mainstreaming. *Journal of Studies on Alcohol*, 48:47–51, 1987.
16. Milhorn, H.T., Jr., and L.C. Gardner. The elderly alcoholic: Diagnosis and treatment. *Senior Patient*, in press.

CHAPTER 22

Ethnic Minority Groups

Definitions

The term ethnic describes a group of people sharing a common background, language, and identity. Members may have similar physical characteristics, but more important, they share beliefs and behaviors that differ from other ethnic groups. When an ethnic group is not allowed full participation in society and reacts to this discrimination, it is classified as a minority group. Population size is not a part of this definition. Women are viewed as a minority group even though they constitute more than 50 percent of the U.S. population.[1]

Ethnic Groups

Blacks, Hispanics, Asian Americans, American Indians, and other ethnic minority groups constitute 40.8 percent of total admissions to treatment programs, even though they represent only 20 percent of the population.[2] Despite this, our knowledge of the use of alcohol and other drugs among America's ethnic minority populations is incomplete, and most of what we know is limited to information about minority youth. Little information exists about ethnic adults, the elderly, and families. Any attempt to deal with chemical dependence in people of a particular culture must show sensitivity to the language, the customs, and the thinking of that culture.[3]

American Indians

In the United States today there are about 1.5 million people of American Indian descent; they comprise less than 1 percent of the total population. They belong to hundreds of tribes representing many distinct cultural traditions. Roughly half of today's Indians remain on reservations; the other half live primarily in cities. Alcohol and drug abuse is believed to be a significant problem among American Indians. Most research on Indian substance abuse has been conducted on reservations—virtually none has been done on urban Indians. We know that Indians began to drink centuries ago after they came into contact with European traders. Alcohol continues to be their drug of choice.[3]

By their ninth birthday, 12 percent of Indian children regularly drink beer, wine, or liquor; 97 percent of them use alcohol by the eleventh grade. Heavy drinking is the main reason why one in two Indian students never finishes high school.[4-5] In some tribes rates of male alcoholism may be as high as 80 to 85 percent and of female alcoholism 35 to 55 percent. Alcohol is a factor in 75 percent of Indian deaths, in 80 percent of suicides, and in contributing to a homicide rate three times the national average. Indians have high rates of cirrhosis and other alcohol-related illnesses.[3] American Indian women appear to be susceptible to alcohol-related problems. Although they drink less than men, they account for nearly half of American Indian cirrhosis deaths and seem to be at particular risk for fetal alcohol syndrome. Although many explanations have been given to explain the high alcoholism rate among Indians, there can be little doubt that for many of their problems alcohol is the cause rather than the effect.[3]

The use of drugs (marijuana, inhalants, heroin, cocaine, minor tranquilizers, sleeping pills) among Indian youth is higher than among non-Indian youth and appears to be increasing.[4]

American Indian values stress the family unit, cooperation, humility, and avoidance of individual recognition. Indians are less likely to talk about their feelings and may be uncomfortable in group therapy. They may view confrontational techniques as hostile acts. They tend to be stoic and, as a result, may underestimate the severity of their problems.[1]

Asian Americans

Asian Americans, who make up less than 2 percent of the population of the United States, have low levels of alcohol and drug use in general.[6] However, Asian American youth appear to use drugs at a rate equal to, if not higher than, the national average.[4] It is often assumed that Asian Americans have similar drinking and drug-using patterns regardless of their national origin. However, Asian Americans have a great diversity of backgrounds, with origins in China, Japan, the Philippines, Korea, India, Vietnam, Cambodia, and other Asian countries. There appear to be significant differences in psychoactive substance use among Asian Americans of different origins.[7]

The diversity of subgroups within this ethnic group adds complexity to the drug abuse effort. Furthermore, findings from a sample of Japanese-Americans who have lived in the United States for several generations are very different from those obtained from a group of recent Korean immigrants. Similarly, findings obtained from a group of Asian-American students in a large university are very different from those obtained from a group of young men of similar age who have recently arrived in the United States as refugees from Southeast Asia.[4] The language problems are formidable.[3]

In general, Asians value academic and occupational accomplishments that bring honor to the family. Failure brings them shame. Asian patients may be uncomfortable expressing emotions openly. They don't like to talk directly about personal problems and may describe these as educational or physical issues.

Gender and age roles tend to be more traditional, and it may take some time for them to become comfortable in family sessions.[1]

The more recent immigrants from Southeast Asia (from Vietnam, Laos, Cambodia) very likely have experienced violence and may have lost family members. They may suffer emotional problems such as posttraumatic shock syndrome. Male Asians who are recent immigrants lose status if they have to assume jobs of lower rank than they had in their original communities; their feeling of shame over this may disrupt their families. Many Asians, therefore, respond well to counseling that has a vocational or educational theme.[1]

Black Americans

The largest ethnic group in the United States, blacks make up about 12 percent of the total population and 92 percent of the nonwhite population.[7] Abuse of alcohol and other drugs is most common among urban black males. Blacks tend to drink heavily or not at all.[3] Among drinkers, black men are less likely to be heavy drinkers than white men; the reverse is true of female drinkers—black women are more likely to be heavy drinkers than white women. However, both black men and women have higher rates of abstention.[7] Black women over 60 use few psychoactive substances of any kind. Black substance abusers often feel uncomfortable at Alcoholics Anonymous meetings dominated by whites, and the AA program is most successful for them when developed within black communities.[2-3]

Twice as many black senior high school students abstain from drugs as white students. Furthermore, black students who do drink consume less alcohol and drink less frequently than white students. However, many more of the black abstainers do report using marijuana than the white abstainers.[7]

Blacks, especially black males, are at high risk for certain alcohol-related illnesses, particularly cirrhosis of the liver, fatty liver, and hepatitis. They have an extremely high incidence of cancer of the esophagus, with incidence rates several times those of whites. Alcohol is considered to be a major causal factor in this type of cancer.[7]

Hispanic Americans

Hispanics comprise more than 6 percent of the population of the United States, and Hispanic youth are the fastest growing ethnic minority age group in America. Hispanic Americans are a heterogeneous group with diverse cultural, national, and racial backgrounds. They come from Colombian, Cuban, Dominican, Puerto Rican, and Mexican backgrounds. Hispanic youth often drop out of school because of substance abuse. Hispanic men have relatively high rates of alcoholism, while Hispanic women have high rates of abstention. Psychoactive drug use among Hispanic women increases with age; those over 60 tend to use minor tranquilizers more than other women and to use them with greater frequency. Mexican American men have both the highest rate of abstention and the highest level of heavy drinking when compared with Hispanics of Cuban, Puerto Rican, or other Latin

American origin. Mexican American women also drink more heavily than women in other groups but also have a high rate of abstention.[7-9]

Diagnosis

Diagnosis of chemical dependence in ethnic minority groups obeys the principles outlined in Chapter 2. It may be somewhat complicated by language barriers and by cultural influences among the various ethnic groups and subgroups. Remember that many of the assessment instruments and psychological tests in use today were developed on white, middle-class adult norms and may not be reliable when used with other populations.[1]

Treatment

Treatment of individuals belonging to ethnic minority groups obeys the principles outlined in Chapter 3. Treatment, like diagnosis, may be somewhat complicated by language barriers and by cultural factors. The use of written assignments may be a problem if a patient's English is poor. The typical family session and group process must be adapted when necessary to cultures in which the young do not speak out in front of elders or in which women and men do not easily discuss their problems together. Many minority members feel strongly about discrimination and prejudice, and their attitudes may influence their interactions with members of the treatment team. Keep in mind that each patient who is a member of an ethnic minority group is an individual. That individual's ethnic beliefs should be assessed and not merely assumed.[1]

Role of the Physician

Physicians should realize that substance abuse is a significant problem in all cultures, be willing to work with patients and their families to get patients into treatment despite the barrier that language difficulty and cultural differences may pose, and be a part of patients' long-term recovery.

References

1. Spicer, J. Counseling ethnic minorities. Hazelden, Center City, Minnesota, 1989.
2. Hanson, B. Drug treatment effectiveness: The case of racial and ethnic minorities in America: Some research questions and proposals. *International Journal of the Addictions*, 20:99–137, 1985.
3. Royce, J.E. Special groups. In *Alcohol Problems and Alcoholism: A Comprehensive Survey*. Free Press, New York, 1981, pp. 103–118.
4. Trimble, J.E., A.M. Padilla, and C.S. Bell. (Eds.). Drug abuse among ethnic minorities. U.S. Department of Health and Human Services, Rockville, Maryland, 1983.

5. Beauvais, F., and S. LeBoueff. Drug and alcohol abuse intervention in American Indian communities. *International Journal of the Addictions*, 20:139–171, 1985.

6. Primm, B.J. Drug use: Special implications for black America. In *The State of Black America 1987*, National Urban League, New York, N.Y., 1987, pp. 145–158.

7. Epidemiology. In *Alcohol and Health*. U.S. Department of Health and Human Services, Rockville, Maryland, 1987, pp. 145–158.

8. Schinke, S.P., M.S. Moncher, J. Pelleja, L.H. Zayas, and R.F. Schilling. Hispanic youth, substance abuse and stress: Implications for prevention research. *International Journal of the Addictions*, 20:809–826, 1988.

9. Matteo, S. The risk of multiple addictions: Guidelines for assessing a woman's alcohol and drug use. *The Western Journal of Medicine*, 149:741–745, 1988.

CHAPTER 23

The Dual-Diagnosis Patient

Dual diagnosis refers to patients who have both a chemical dependence problem and a psychiatric disorder that is independent of the chemical dependence. Patients with chemical dependence and a psychiatric disorder resulting from it are not considered to have a dual diagnosis.

Primary Versus Secondary Psychiatric Disorders

All substances of abuse affect the brain and change patients' level of functioning. Therefore, it is not surprising that such drugs can produce alterations in mood, ability to reason, and content of thinking. Patients abusing alcohol or other drugs are likely to be depressed, anxious, confused, or psychotic. The problem is to decide if these disorders occur secondarily to the substance abuse or if they occur independently of it. Psychiatric disorders occurring independently of substance abuse are said to be *primary* disorders. The distinction between primary and secondary psychiatric disorders is made by history of the time course of the disorders. The one that appeared first is called primary, and the one that appeared second is called secondary. When the first disorder is substance abuse, it is highly likely that psychiatric symptoms will improve rapidly within a few days to weeks after patients stop using drugs.[1-3]

Primary Psychiatric Disorders

Common primary psychiatric disorders that often coexist with chemical dependence include psychotic disorders, mood disorders, organic brain disorders, anxiety disorders, and personality disorders.

Psychotic Disorders

Psychosis describes a degree of severity, not a specific disorder. Psychotic patients have a grossly impaired sense of reality, often coupled with emotional and cognitive disabilities. They are apt to talk and act bizarrely, have hallucinations or have delusional thinking. They may be confused and disoriented. Schizophrenia is the prototype psychotic disorder.[4-5]

Schizophrenia

The typical acute psychosis of schizophrenia displays a variable mixture of disturbances in thought form, thought content, perception, emotion, and behavior.[4-5]

Disturbances of thought form consist of thinking that is frequently incomprehensible to others and appears illogical. Characteristics include loose association, neologisms (made-up words), blocking (sudden ceasing of flow of thought), clanging (senseless rhyming), ecolalia (repeating words or phrases said by others), concreteness, and poverty of speech content.
Disturbances of thought content may include bizarre and confused delusions, persecutory delusions, delusions of grandeur, delusions of influence, and delusions of reference.
Disturbances of perception most commonly take the form of hallucinations, usually auditory but sometimes visual, olfactory, or tactile. These patients may have depersonalization (feeling unreal or detached) and a sense of body change.
Disturbances of emotions include virtually any emotion, and patients may switch from one to another in a short time. Two common affects are blunted (or flat) affect and inappropriate affect. Patients with blunted affect express very little emotion, even when it is appropriate to do so. Patients with inappropriate affect may be intense but are inconsistent in their thoughts or speech.
Disturbances of behavior consists of many bizarre and inappropriate behaviors, including grimacing and posturing, ritual behavior, excessive silliness, aggressiveness, and some sexual inappropriateness.[4-5]

Types of Schizophrenia

Schizophrenia is subdivided into disorganized, catatonic, paranoid, undifferentiated, and residual types.[4-5]

Disorganized type. Patients with disorganized type of schizophrenia have blunted, silly, or inappropriate affects and are frequently incoherent but have no systematized delusions. Grimacing and bizarre mannerisms are common.
Catatonic type. Patients with catatonic type schizophrenia may have any one or a combination of several forms of catatonia. These include catatonic stupor or mutism (no appreciable response to the environment or the people in it), catatonic negativism (resistance to all directions or physical attempt to move them), catatonic posturing (bizarre or unusual postures), catatonic rigidity (physical rigidity), and catatonic excitement (wildly active and excited).
Paranoid type. Patients with paranoid type schizophrenia display consistent, often paranoid delusions that may or may not be acted on. These patients are often uncooperative and difficult to deal with. They may be aggressive, angry, or fearful but rarely display disorganized, incoherent behavior.

Undifferentiated type. Patients with undifferentiated type schizophrenia have prominent hallucinations, delusions, confusion, and incoherence but without the more specific features of disorganized, catatonic, or paranoid type schizophrenia.

Residual type. Patients with residual type schizophrenia are in remission from active psychosis but withdraw socially and have flat or inappropriate affect, eccentric behavior, loose associations, and illogical thinking.[4-5]

Diagnosis of Schizophrenia

To be considered schizophrenic, a patient must have had at least six months of sufficiently deteriorated occupational, interpersonal, and self-supportive functioning and must have been actively psychotic in a characteristic fashion during at least part of that period. Also, physicians cannot account for the patient's symptoms by finding a major affective disorder, autism, or organic mental disorder.[4-5]

Mood Disorders

Mood disorders are common. Two basic abnormalities of mood are recognized—depression and mania. Symptoms in some patients reach psychotic proportions. More severe symptoms are associated with discrete syndromes known as affective disorders, which may be bipolar (manic depression) or unipolar (major depression).[4]

Bipolar Disorder

Mania, at some time severe enough to compromise functioning, is necessary for this diagnosis. Between 80 and 90 percent of bipolar patients also have periods of depression, usually profound. Over 20 percent of manic patients have hallucinations and/or delusions. Severe mania may be indistinguishable from organic delirium.

Unipolar Disorder

These patients have many signs and symptoms of depression, but those symptoms can vary markedly from profound retardation and withdrawal to irritability and agitation. Unipolar patients do not have episodes of mania. Although around 50 percent of chemically dependent individuals are clinically depressed, less than 10 to 15 percent of them have primary depression.[4-5]

Organic Brain Syndromes

Organic brain syndromes are mental disorders of various types caused by a wide range of organic pathology. The most common types are delirium and dementia. These syndromes are common, particularly among the elderly, 10 to 15 percent of whom as inpatients develop a degree of delirium. Delirium is usually brief and reversible; dementia is longer-acting and more apt to be irreversible.[4-5]

Delirium

This is a common condition, particularly among people who are physically ill. These patients may be confused, act bizarre, or even become wild and thus may be mistakenly thought to be suffering from another psychotic illness. They may appear to be normal or somnolent during the day but decompensate dramatically at night. Delirium is a rapidly developing disorder of disturbed attention, which fluctuates with time. Patients may have cloudy consciousness and appear bewildered and confused. They may be very distractible and unable to focus their attention to follow a train of thought or understand what is occurring in their environment. Perceptual disturbances are common and include misinterpretations (they may interpret blowing curtains as someone climbing in a window) and hallucinations (usually visual). Insomnia is almost always present, and symptoms are usually worse at night. Marked drowsiness may occur. Most frequently, disorientation to time occurs, but also to place, to situation, and lastly to person. Patients typically have recent memory impairment and usually deny it. Speech may be confused and unintelligible, and verbal perserveration (persistent repetition of an idea) may occur. Most delirious patients are restless and agitated. Some may be excessively somnolent, and some may fluctuate between somnolence and agitation, usually sleepy during the day and restless at night. Most of these characteristics tend to vary over hours to days.[4-5]

Delirium tends to develop over a period of days and usually lasts less than a week. Change of setting (moving out of familiar surroundings), overstimulation, and understimulation (darkness, sensory deprivation) can all worsen the symptoms, as can stress of any kind.[4-5]

Dementia

Dementia results from a broad loss of intellectual functions due to diffuse organic disease of the cerebral cortex. It has many causes and usually develops slowly. Early on, patients suffer subtle changes in personality, impairment of social skills, a decrease in range of interests and enthusiasms, emotional lability and shallowness of affect, agitation, somatic complaints, vague psychiatric symptoms, and gradual loss of intellectual skills. Later on the full picture emerges: patients lose memory, undergo changes in mood and personality, lose their orientation, and suffer intellectual impairment, compromised judgment, psychotic symptoms, and language impairment.[4-5]

The major treatable forms of dementia are (1) multi-infarct dementia (controlling hypertension may help); (2) normal pressure hydrocephalus (shunt may help); (3) brain tumors; (4) brain trauma resulting in subdural hematoma; (5) infection (pneumonia, urinary tract infection, brain abscess, CNS syphilis, meningitis); (5) metabolic disturbances (hypothyroidism, hyperthyroidism, hyponatremia, hypernatremia, liver disease, Cushing's syndrome, hypoglycemia, hypoparathyroidism, hyperparathyroidism); (6) disorders of the heart, lung or kidneys (congestive heart failure, arrhythmias, subacute bacterial endocarditis, chronic hypoxia and hypercapnia from emphysema, uremia); (7) malnutrition (vitamin B_{12} and folate deficiencies); and (8) ingestion of toxins (lead, mercury, organophosphates).[4-5]

The major untreatable forms of dementia are Alzheimer's disease, Huntington's chorea, and Parkinson's disease. Alzheimer's is a diagnosis by exclusion. It usually begins in the 50s, 60s, and 70s and progresses to death in six to ten years. Ceaseless pacing and a shuffling gait are common. The dementia of Huntington's chorea may precede the chorea and is of an autosomal dominant inheritance. Parkinson's is associated with depression and dementia in some patients.[4-5]

Anxiety Disorders

Anxiety occurs commonly; anxiety disorders do not. Anxiety is an unpleasant sense of apprehension, often accompanied by physiological symptoms (tachycardia, sweaty palms). Anxiety disorder connotes significant distress and dysfunction due to anxiety. An anxiety disorder may be characterized only by anxiety or may involve other symptoms such as phobia or obsession.[4-5]

Adjustment Disorder With Anxious Mood

In this condition, short-lived mild anxiety, apprehension, and mild distractibility occur. It is often related to environmental disorders and usually resolves with the disappearance of the stress. Unfortunately, many patients with this condition are treated chronically with benzodiazepines and develop dependence on them.

Generalized Anxiety Disorder

Generalized anxiety disorder consists of more severe and chronic symptoms (that last longer than six months), including autonomic responses (palpitations, diarrhea, cold clammy extremities, sweating, urinary frequency), insomnia, fatigue, sighing, trembling, hypervigilance, and marked apprehension. Secondary depression is common.

Panic Disorder

Panic attacks have dramatic symptoms lasting minutes to hours. They are self-limited and occur in patients with and without chronic anxiety. Symptoms are characteristic of strong autonomic discharge (heart pounding, chest pains, trembling, choking, abdominal pain, sweating, dizziness, disorganization, confusion, sense of impending doom or terror). Attacks may come out of the blue or be initiated by crowds or stressful situations. They may occur several times daily, weekly, or monthly.

Phobic Disorders

Phobias are fears that are persistent and intense, are out of proportion to their stimuli, make little sense even to sufferers, and lead to avoidance of the feared objects or situations. When sufficiently distressful or disabling, the condition is termed a phobic disorder. Anxiety with ruminations may dominate the day-to-day picture, or anxiety may occur only when patients encounter phobic objects directly. Relief occurs with escape, thus reinforcing avoidance. Three subtypes of phobic disorder have been identified:[4-5]

1. *Agoraphobia* is fear of open or closed spaces, crowded places, unfamiliar places, or being alone. Patients may have other fears and hypochondriacal concerns and may faint, have obsessional thoughts, and suffer depersonalization and derealization (feeling that surroundings are unreal). Most patients with agoraphobia also have panic attacks. Typically, they develop agoraphobia as an extension of panic disorder; that is, unpredictable panic attacks cause them to avoid public places for fear of having attacks.
2. *Social phobia* is fear of public speaking, using public lavatories, blushing, or eating in public. Avoidance of these places and situations can be socially crippling.
3. *Simple phobias* are abnormal fears of things such as animals, thunderstorms, cats, dogs, snakes, insects, and mice. Other simple phobias are fear of closed spaces (claustrophobia) and fear of heights (acrophobia). Fear of air travel is a common simple phobia.[1,4-5]

Obsessive-Compulsive Disorder

Obsessions are repetitive thoughts that patients feel powerless to stop. The thoughts are usually unpleasant, always unwanted, and may be frightening or violent, such as the impulse to leap in front of a car. Patients may develop rituals or compulsions, such as counting or touching, to ward off unwanted happenings or to satisfy an obsession. For example, a patient may develop an obsession with dirt leading to compulsive handwashing rituals. The performance of such behavior temporarily relieves the anxiety of the obsession. A patient's thinking is often magical, such as stamping the foot a given number of times to ward off a dreaded event.

Posttraumatic Stress Disorder

The essential feature of this disorder is the development of characteristic symptoms following a psychologically distressing event that is outside the range of usual human experience, such as a threat to life, to the life of a spouse or child, sudden destruction of one's home, seeing another person killed, or combat or concentration camp experience.

Patients reexperience traumatic events in a variety of ways. They may have disturbing thoughts or nightmares about the traumatic event. Intense psychological stress often occurs when the person is exposed to situations that resemble some aspect of the event or on anniversaries of the event. In addition to reexperiencing the trauma of the event, patients avoid situations apt to precipitate symptoms.

Psychic numbing usually begins soon after the traumatic event. The person feels detached from others, unable to enjoy previously pleasurable activities and unable to feel emotions of any type, especially those associated with intimacy, tenderness, and sexuality. The person may have trouble falling asleep or staying asleep and have an increased startle response, difficulty concentrating, and irritability or frank aggression.[1,4-5]

Personality Disorders

The term personality disorder refers to personality characteristics of a form or magnitude that are maladaptive and cause poor life functioning. Most personality disorders develop in childhood. Patients often resist treatment and change slowly.[4-6]

Antisocial Personality Disorder

Antisocial personality disorder begins in childhood or early adolescence and consists of aggressiveness, fighting, hyperactivity, poor peer relationships, irresponsibility, lying, stealing, truancy, poor school performance, runaway behavior, inappropriate sexual activity, and drug abuse. In adulthood, criminality, assaultiveness, self-defeating impulsivity, promiscuity, unreliability, and crippling drug abuse occur. Such patients fail at work, change jobs frequently, receive dishonorable discharges from the service, become abusing parents and neglectful mates, cannot maintain intimate relationships, and spend time in jails and prisons. They are frequently anxious and depressed and tend to make suicide gestures and have conversion symptoms. This is the most common personality disorder seen in chemical dependence treatment centers.

Histrionic Personality Disorder

Histrionic patients initially seem charming, likable, lively, and seductive but later seem emotionally unstable, egocentric, immature, dependent, manipulative, and shallow. They demand attention, are exhibitionistic, and have a limited ability to maintain stable, intimate, interpersonal relationships with either sex. This disorder occurs predominantly in women. Depression, substance abuse, conversion, somatization, and suicide gestures and attempts are common.

Borderline Personality Disorder

These patients have complex symptoms, including combinations of anger, anxiety, intense and labile affect, chronic loneliness, boredom, a chronic sense of emptiness, volatile interpersonal relationships, identity confusion, and impulsive behavior. Stress can precipitate a transient psychosis.

Narcissistic Personality Disorder

Although often symptom-free, these patients are chronically dissatisfied because of constant needs for admiration and unrealistic self-expectations. They are impulsive and anxious, have ideas of omnipotence, become quickly dissatisfied with others, and maintain superficial, exploitative interpersonal relationships. When their needs are not met they may become depressed, develop somatic complaints, have brief psychotic episodes, or display extreme rage.

Passive-Aggressive Personality Disorder

These patients are irritating and even infuriating. They are oppositional, resentful, and controlling. Thus, they have few friends and have significantly impaired social and occupational functioning. Their hostility is expressed passively by intentional inefficiency, negativism, stubbornness, procrastination, forgetfulness, withdrawal, and somatic complaints. They are overdependent on other people and suffer anxiety, depression, and an inability to cope.

Paranoid Personality Disorder

These aloof, emotionally cold people are typically unjustifiably suspicious, hypersensitive to slights, jealous, and fear intimacy. They tend to be grandiose, rigid, contentious, and litigious and are thus isolated and disliked. They accept criticism poorly, blaming others instead. Psychotic decompensation sometimes occurs.

Schizoid Personality Disorder

These are seclusive people who have little wish or capacity to form interpersonal relationships and derive little pleasure from social contacts. They can perform well in isolated jobs and have a limited emotional range, daydream excessively, and are humorless and aloof.

Schizotypal Personality Disorder

In addition to having features of schizoid personality, these people appear peculiar. They relate strange intrapsychic experiences, reason in odd ways, and are difficult to get to know, yet none of these features reach psychotic proportions.

Obsessive-Compulsive Personality Disorder

These patients, frequently successful men, are inhibited, stubborn, perfectionistic, judgmental, overconscientious, rigid, and chronically anxious individuals who avoid intimacy and experience little pleasure from life. They are indecisive and demanding and are often perceived as cold and reserved. They are at risk for developing obsessive-compulsive disorder and depression.

Avoidant Personality Disorder

These patients are shy, lonely, and hypersensitive. They have low self-esteem. They would rather avoid personal contact than face any potential social disapproval, even though desperate for interpersonal involvement. They suffer from anxiety and depression.

Dependent Personality Disorder

These are excessively passive, unsure, isolated people who become abnormally dependent on others. Their behavior can become very controlling, they may appear hostile and be passive-aggressive. The disorder is more common in women and is likely to lead to anxiety and depression, particularly if dependent relationships are threatened.[4-8]

Secondary Psychiatric Disorders

Psychiatric disorders due to substance abuse occur frequently. In fact, in treatment programs psychopathology is much more often the result of addiction than the cause. Secondary psychiatric disorders due to intoxication, overdose, or withdrawal may mimic primary psychosis, mood disorders, organic brain syndrome, anxiety disorders, and personality disorders.

Psychosis

Hallucinations can occur with intoxication or overdose from CNS stimulants or hallucinogens and with intoxication from phencyclidines. They can also occur as part of the CNS depressant abstinence syndrome, most often during alcohol withdrawal but sometimes during withdrawal from other CNS depressants, such as barbiturates and benzodiazepines. Those that occur during alcohol withdrawal may be of two types. The first occurs as a part of delirium tremens and is always associated with delirium and tremulousness. The second is called hallucinosis; in this type, patients have relatively clear sensoriums and may be aware that their hallucinations are not real.[9]

Cocaine (and amphetamine) psychosis consists of tactile hallucinations—feeling something crawling under the skin (formication) or bugs on the skin (coke bugs). Visual and auditory hallucinations may also occur, as well as a paranoid thought disorder. Stereotyped behavior, such as compulsive behavior or skin picking, may occur. The sensorium is usually clear except in overdose or toxic psychosis. This syndrome is indistinguishable from chronic paranoid schizophrenia.[7]

Phencyclidine psychosis is also indistinguishable from schizophrenia. Agitation, bizarre behavior, persecutory, grandiose, or somatic delusions, and depersonalization may occur. The comatoselike state produced by phencyclidine overdose, with eyes open and muscles rigid, can be confused with catatonia.

Patients with primary schizophrenia are exquisitely sensitive to phencyclidine. Even in small doses it may activate their psychosis.[7]

Psychosis can also occur with high-potency marijuana intoxication and overdose, with CNS depressant intoxication, and with chronic nitrous oxide abuse.[7]

Mood Disorders

Depression can be produced by the chronic use of CNS depressants, CNS stimulants, and phencyclidine. It may also be a prominent part of alcohol, CNS stimulant, and phencyclidine withdrawal.

A maniclike state can be caused by CNS stimulant and phencyclidine intoxication or CNS stimulant overdose.[9]

Organic Brain Syndrome

Delirium can occur with CNS stimulant, phencyclidine, and inhalant intoxication, with overdose of virtually any drug except phencyclidine, which causes coma, and with withdrawal from CNS depressant drugs and opioids.

Dementia most commonly occurs as the result of chronic alcohol abuse but can occur from chronic inhalant abuse. It may be partly or totally reversible with abstinence and good nutrition, but it may be permanent.[9]

Anxiety Disorders

Anxiety occurs with chronic alcohol abuse. It also occurs acutely with CNS stimulant, cannabinoid, and hallucinogen intoxication and with CNS stimulant, cannabinoid, and hallucinogen intoxication and overdose. It is a prominent feature of CNS depressant and opioid withdrawal.[9]

Panic attacks occur with chronic alcohol use and occur acutely with CNS stimulant intoxication and cannabinoid and hallucinogen intoxication and overdose. They are common in CNS depressant withdrawal.[9]

The obsessive-compulsive behavior that sometimes accompanies CNS stimulant intoxication can be confused with obsessive-compulsive disorder.

Some feel that posttraumatic stress disorder may develop from the abuse of alcohol and other drugs.[7]

Personality Disorders

Derangement of personality occurs with chronic use of all drugs. Addictive behaviors (lying, cheating, failure to consider others) that develop as the result of drug abuse can be confused with sociopathic personality disorder. Suspiciousness or paranoia that develops as the result of alcohol, CNS stimulant, cannabinoid, hallucinogen, and phencyclidine use, as well as CNS stimulant and hallucinogen overdose, can be confused with paranoid personality disorder.

Psychiatric disorders resulting from substance abuse are summarized in Table 23.1.

TABLE 23.1. Psychiatric syndromes resulting from substance abuse.

Syndromes	Intoxication							Overdose							Withdrawal						
	CNS depressants	Opioids	CNS stimulants	Cannabinoids	Hallucinogens	Phencyclidines	Inhalants	CNS depressants	Opioids	CNS stimulants	Cannabinoids	Hallucinogens	Phencyclidines	Inhalants	CNS depressants	Opioids	CNS stimulants	Cannabinoids	Hallucinogens	Phencyclidines	Inhalants
Psychosis	X		X	X	X	X	X			X	X	X			X						
Mood disorders																					
depression	X		X							X					X		X			X	
mania			X			X															
Organic brain syndrome																					
delirium			X			X	X	X	X	X	X	X		X	X	X					
dementia	X						X														
Anxiety disorders																					
anxiety			X	X	X					X	X	X			X	X					
panic attacks	X		X	X	X					X	X	X			X						
Personality disorders	X		X	X	X	X				X		X									

Diagnosis

Physicians need to differentiate between primary and secondary disorders because the overall course of the illness is best predicted by its primary diagnosis. Primary alcoholism, for instance, has a better prognosis than primary antisocial personality disorder. In most cases, it is crucial to wait for the secondary disorder to clear before making the definitive diagnosis and initiating treatment. This may take from one week to three months or more. Sleep disturbances and anxiety occurring as part of the benzodiazepine abstinence syndrome, for example, may take up to six months to abate.[7]

Schuckit recommends the following steps when confronted with a patient who fulfills criteria for a psychiatric disorder and who, at the same time, meets the criteria for chemical dependence.[10]

1. Gather the best information possible from the patient and from resource people.
2. Try to establish whether the psychiatric disorder occurred before the onset of the substance abuse or was present during a period of extended abstinence.
3. If the psychiatric disorder is seen only in the context of substance abuse, the chances are 10 to 1 that with abstinence the syndrome will markedly improve within a matter of days to weeks.
4. When the psychiatric disorder does not disappear with time or when there is evidence that it is independent of substance abuse, treatment of the psychiatric syndrome must be considered.
5. Patients with primary psychiatric disorders, such as manic-depressive illness or schizophrenia, will require psychiatric medication for an extended period of time.[10]

Treatment

After making a definitive diagnosis of a primary psychiatric disorder, treatment should be initiated with antidepressants, lithium, or other appropriate drugs. When their psychiatric symptoms are under control, patients can participate in treatment for chemical dependence as outlined in Chapter 3.[9-11]

DSM-III-R Classification System

The DSM-III-R classification system consists of five axes (Table 23.2). Axis I consists of clinical syndromes and V codes. Clinical syndromes are major psychiatric illnesses such as manic-depressive illness, schizophrenia, and chemical dependence. V codes are for conditions not attributable to a mental disorder that are a focus of attention or treatment. These include academic problems, malingering, marital problems, parent-child problems, and uncomplicated bereavement.[1]

TABLE 23.2. DSM-III-R multiaxial classification system.

Axis I	Clinical syndromes, V Codes
Axis II	Developmental disorders
	Personality disorders
Axis III	Physical disorders and conditions
Axis IV	Severity of psychosocial stressors
Axis V	Global assessment of functioning

From *Diagnostic and Statistical Manual of Mental Disorders, Third Edition Revised*, American Psychiatric Association, Washington, D.C., 1987, p. 18.

Axis II consists of developmental disorders and personality disorders. Developmental disorders include mental retardation, autism, and academic skills disorders (learning disabilities in arithmetic, writing, or reading; articulation disorders; expressive or receptive language disorder; and motor skills disorders). Personality disorders include paranoid, schizoid, schizotypal, antisocial, borderline, histrionic, narcissistic, avoidant, dependent, obsessive-compulsive, and passive-aggressive personality.[1]

Axis III consists of physical disorders or conditions, such as alcoholic hepatitis, diabetes, or pancreatitis.[1]

Axis IV indicates the severity of psychosocial stressor, rated on a scale of 1 (none) to 6 (catastrophic). Stressors may be acute events or enduring circumstances. Examples of acute events for adults are breaking up with a boyfriend (2), marital separation (3), divorce (4), rape (5), and death of a child (6). Examples of enduring circumstances are job dissatisfaction (2), serious financial problems (3), unemployment (4), serious chronic illness (5), and concentration camp experience (6). Similar acute events and enduring circumstances are described in DSM-III-R for children and adolescents.[1]

Axis V indicates global assessment of functioning (GAF), rated on a scale of 90 (absent or minimal symptoms) to 1 (persistent danger of hurting oneself or another). GAF is assessed for current situations and overall functioning for the past year.[1]

Axis I and II conditions are assigned coding numbers ranging from 290.00 to 799.90 (Table 23.3); V Codes range from V 15.81 to V 71.09.[1]

As an example of a DSM-III-R classification applied to a dual-diagnosis patient, consider a patient with alcoholism and a primary antisocial personality disorder who has alcoholic hepatitis, has just lost his or her job, and is having some suicide ideations (Table 23.4).

Role of the Physician

Physicians should recognize the existence of primary and secondary psychiatric disorders and should realize that when a psychiatric disorder coexists with chemical dependence, the primary disorder in most cases is the substance abuse. The

TABLE 23.3. Some selected DSM-III-R codes.

295.12	Schizophrenia, disorganized type, chronic
295.22	Schizophrenia, catatonic type, chronic
295.32	Schizophrenia, paranoid type, chronic
295.62	Schizophrenia, residual types, chronic
295.92	Schizophrenia, undifferentiated, chronic
296.24	Major depression, single episode, with psychotic features
296.43	Bipolar disorder, manic, with psychotic features
296.54	Bipolar disorder, depressed, with psychotic features
300.01	Panic disorder, without agoraphobia
300.02	Generalized anxiety disorder
300.29	Simple phobia
300.30	Obsessive-compulsive disorder
301.00	Paranoid personality disorder
301.20	Schizoid personality disorder
301.22	Schizotypal personality disorder
301.50	Histrionic personality disorder
301.60	Dependent personality disorder
301.70	Antisocial personality disorder
301.81	Narcissistic personality disorder
301.82	Avoidant personality disorder
301.83	Borderline personality disorder
301.84	Passive aggressive personality disorder
303.90	Alcohol dependence
304.00	Opioid dependence
304.10	Sedative, hypnotic, or anxiolytic dependence
304.20	Cocaine dependence
304.30	Cannabis dependence
304.40	Amphetamine dependence
304.50	Hallucinogen dependence
304.50	Phencyclidine dependence
304.60	Inhalant dependence
304.90	Polysubstance dependence
305.10	Nicotine dependence
309.24	Adjustment disorder with anxious mood
309.89	Posttraumatic stress disorder

From *Diagnostic and Statistical Manual, Third Edition Revised*, American Psychiatric Association, Washington, D.C., 1987, pp. 509–515.

TABLE 23.4. Example of DSM-III-R classification.

Axis I:	303.90	Alcohol dependence
Axis II:	301.70	Antisocial personality
Axis III:		Alcoholic hepatitis
Axis IV:		Psychosocial stressors – loss of job, severity 3 (moderate, acute event)
Axis V:		Current GAF – suicide ideations (50)
		Highest GAF past year – some difficulty with social functioning (65)

next step is to help get patients into treatment programs for chemical dependence. The definitive diagnosis of the primary disorder can be made only after the effects of the substance abuse have cleared, although a time course of the occurrences of the two conditions can be extremely helpful. Once patients have been treated for chemical dependence and/or primary psychiatric disorders, physicians will play critical roles in the long-term care of patients in the community. Of extreme importance in this role is physicians' judicious use of mood-altering medications.

References

1. *Diagnostic and Statistical Manual of Mental Disorders (Third edition revised)*. American Psychiatric Association, Washington, D.C., 1987, pp. 3–24, 509–515.
2. Merricucii, L.D., L. Wermuth, and J. Sorensen. Treatment providers' assessment of dual-prognosis patients: Diagnosis, treatment, referral, and family involvement. *International Journal of the Addictions*, 23:617–622, 1988.
3. Schuckit, M.A. Dual diagnoses: Psychiatric pictures among substance abusers. *Drug Abuse and Alcoholism Newsletter*, Vista Hill Foundation, March, 1988.
4. Tomb, D. *Psychiatry for the House Officer*. Williams and Wilkins, Baltimore, 1988, pp. 17–64, 73–81, 152–157.
5. Kolb, L.C., and H.K.H. Brodie. *Modern Clinical Psychiatry*. W.B. Saunders, Philadelphia, 1982, pp. 232–519, 593–615.
6. Schuckit, M.A. How relevant are personality disorders? *Drug Abuse and Alcoholism Newsletter*, Vista Hill Foundation, August, 1989.
7. Wilford, B. (Ed.). Psychiatric disorders. In *Review Course Syllabus*. American Medical Society on Alcoholism and Other Drug Dependencies, New York, 1987, pp. 263–272.
8. Rozeneky, R.H., B. Neirick, G.M. Slotnick, and D. Morse. Discriminating between substance abusers with single and dual diagnoses using MMPI Profiles and the MacAndrews Alcoholism Scale: Axis I and Axis II Subtypes. *Psychological Reports*, 63:985–986, 1988.
9. Gallant, D.S. Alcohol and Drug Abuse *Curriculum Guide for Psychiatry Faculty*. U.S. Department of Health and Human Services, Rockville, Maryland, 1982, pp. 59–70.
10. Schuckit, M.A. Evaluating the dual-diagnosis patient. *Drug Abuse and Alcoholism Newsletter*, Vista Hill Foundation, December, 1989.
11. Daley, D.C., H. Moss, and F. Campbell. Dual disorders: Counseling clients with chemical dependence and mental illness. Hazelden, Center City, Minnesota, 1987.

CHAPTER 24

The HIV-Positive Patient

History

In the summer of 1981, a group of physicians in Los Angeles reported 15 cases of *Pneumocystis carinii* pneumonia in young homosexual men. About the same time, physicians in New York, San Francisco, and Los Angeles reported 26 cases of Kaposi's sarcoma, again in young homosexual men. Both of these illnesses were highly unusual in healthy individuals and up to that time had been associated only with patients who had severely compromised immune systems. In 1982 the Centers for Disease Control (CDC) in Atlanta recognized a complex disease in which a defect in cell-mediated immunity occurred. For this reason, it was given the name acquired immune deficiency syndrome (AIDS). The etiological agent, human immunodeficiency virus (HIV), was identified in 1983, and serological tests were subsequently developed. Of the first cases reported in 1981, 90 percent have died.[1-3]

Epidemiology

AIDS has now been reported in all 50 states and in at least 100 countries worldwide.[5] New York, California, Florida, and New Jersey account for 80 percent of the cases in the United States. Within these states, six cities have had the majority of cases: New York (45 percent), Los Angeles (8.2 percent), San Francisco (7.8 percent), Houston (4 percent), Miami (4 percent), and Newark (3.5 percent).[1] By February 1988, 52,256 cases of AIDS had been reported to the CDC.[3] The number had risen to over 102,000 by July 1989 and is expected to reach 270,000 by 1991, resulting in 179,000 deaths. By 1991 an estimated 80 percent of new cases are expected to be distributed in areas outside those that now have the highest incidence.[4] Treatment costs are expected to be between $8 and $16 billion a year.[2] In addition to diagnosed AIDS cases, approximately 1 to 2 million people in the United States have been infected with HIV, and most of them do not know it.[1,4]

The distribution of the syndrome between men and women differs considerably. In the United States, 93 percent of the cases are in men and 7 percent are in women, a ratio of 13 to 1. This distribution is not as dramatic in other countries. In Haiti, for example, the ratio of cases among men and women is 2 to 1. In the United States, whites are affected most often (58 percent), followed by blacks (26 percent) and Hispanics (14 percent).[2]

Of reported cases, 71.9 percent have occurred among homosexual and bisexual men. Intravenous drug users have had the second highest incidence (17.4 percent) and Haitians, the third (4.1 percent). Hemophiliacs account for 2 percent and heterosexuals for 1 percent of cases (Table 24.1).[1] Because about 8 percent of AIDS cases are in homosexual and bisexual men who also have a history of intravenous drug use, one of four AIDS cases (25 percent) involves intravenous drug use.[2]

Why Treatment Centers Should Be Involved

As AIDS infection through the blood supply is eliminated and the rampant spread among homosexuals continues to slow, intravenous drug use will become an even more significant mode of HIV infection. In fact, infected drug users are thought to be the greatest single threat for widespread HIV infection in the general population. This link occurs through heterosexual partners, offspring, and prostitutes. Because there is no cure or vaccine for control of the disease now or in the immediate future, the best hope for control of the spread of the disease is education of high-risk groups, as well as other prevention measures. Unfortunately, drug abusers are much more of a challenge to reach with information than other groups and even more difficult to convince that they need to make behavioral changes. Intravenous drug abusers tend not to understand the threat of AIDS, and those who understand how the virus is transmitted tend to discount the danger. However, evidence suggests that many will change their behavior to reduce their chances of developing AIDS. It is becoming clear that drug treatment programs

TABLE 24.1. Prevalence of acquired immune deficiency syndrome.

Homosexual and bisexual men	71.9%
Intravenous drug users	17.4
Haitians	4.1
Persons who have received blood transfusions (hemophiliacs, etc.)	2.0
Infants born to high-risk mothers	1.4
Heterosexual partners of patients with AIDS	1.0
Others	2.2

From N.M. Amin, Acquired immunodeficiency syndrome, Part 1: Epidemiology, history, and etiology, *Family Practice Recertification*, 9:36–58, 1987.

can play an important role in reaching these individuals. However, for them to be successful, program staff members must overcome their fears of AIDS through education about the disease and all its aspects, sharing feelings with colleagues, learning from other programs, finding and using all available resources, and remembering that fear is usually of the unknown. Practical experience with the feared agent generally reduces the fear or eliminates it.[5]

Official ASAM Policy

The official policy of the American Society of Addiction Medicine (ASAM) on the treatment of patients with alcoholism or other drug dependencies and who have or are at risk for development of AIDS is as follows:

1. ASAM strongly recommends that physicians, other health professionals, and programs for the treatment of alcoholism and other drug dependencies treat these patients.
2. Case-by-case assessment of the medical status of each patient should be made to determine his or her physical capacity to undergo treatment for alcoholism and other drug dependencies. Continuing medical follow-up by a physician familiar with AIDS is recommended.
3. Currently staff and other patients feel anxious about associating with AIDS patients. All personnel, including clinical, dietary, maintenance, and house-keeping personnel, should be educated with the latest medical data.
4. Patients with AIDS do not require isolation any different from that accorded patients with active hepatitis B. Guidelines for protecting staff and other patients from hepatitis B should be followed. Caps, masks, gloves and other kinds of protective wear are not necessary in routine contact, such as for blood pressure checks and group therapy.
5. Continued medical monitoring after the detoxification period is recommended for these patients.
6. Confidentiality, critical to all aspects of alcoholism and other drug dependencies treatment, is particularly important with these patients.[6]

HIV Infection

Individuals infected with HIV may have full-blown AIDS, have an intermediate syndrome known as AIDS-related complex (ARC), or be asymptomatic carriers of the virus.

Human Immunodeficiency Virus

HIV is a retrovirus that initially seems to have been transported from Haiti to the United States in the late 1970s by homosexuals (mostly from New York and San Francisco), for whom the island had become a popular, inexpensive vacation site.[1] The virus has a long latency period, with the incubation period generally varying from 4 to 57 months, although it may be as long as seven to ten years in some. It typically takes from six to eight weeks after HIV enters the body before antibodies to the virus can be detected in the blood. However, this time period is highly variable; it may take as long as eight months for detectable antibodies to develop. The virus is capable of causing severe immunosuppression, leading to widespread opportunistic infection and an increased tendency to develop uncommon malignancies.[1-2]

Human immunodeficiency viruses attack T4 lymphocytes (T helper cells), the master controlling cells of the immune system. These T4 cells normally activate B lymphocytes to produce antibodies against foreign antigens. They also activate or augment the function of T8 cells (T suppressor cells), which stop, suppress, or modulate antibody production by B cells and directly kill virally infected cells, including tumor cells. To function efficiently, T8 cells need the cooperation of intact T4 cells.[1]

Once HIV has gained access to the bloodstream, the first stage of infection occurs when it seeks out and binds to receptors on the surface of T4 lymphocytes. The virus then enters T4 lymphocytes, in the process shedding its coat and exposing its core, which contains RNA. An enzyme, reverse transcriptase, then converts the RNA to a DNA template that the cell inserts into its own chromosomes in the nucleus. The DNA then directs the T4 cells to make copies of the virus. The infected T4 cells eventually die, and the newly formed viral particles attack other T4 lymphocytes, repeating the process. Zidovudine (Retrovir, formerly sold as AZT and still popularly known by that name) works by disrupting the reverse transcriptase enzyme.[1-2]

Healthy individuals have 600 to 1500 T4 cells for every 50 to 700 T8 cells per milliliter of blood. Thus, the ratio of T4 cells to T8 cells is normally 1.0 to 2.0. With severe infection, the ratio tends to fall below 1.0. The absolute number of T4 cells may decline to fewer than 400 per milliliter of blood.[7]

The role of cofactors in progression of the disease is poorly understood. Apparently, conditions that stress the immune system (certain infections, alcohol and other drugs, live vaccines, trauma, poor nutrition, emotional stress) may potentially cause more rapid progression.[8-9]

HIV can be isolated in high concentrations from the blood and semen of infected people and to a lesser extent from breast milk, urine, and cervical and vaginal excretions. The virus can also be detected in saliva and tears, but in fairly low concentrations. In addition, it can be found in the nervous system, particularly in the brains of infected individuals.[1]

HIV is readily destroyed by drying, heat, ultraviolet light, and common detergents and cleansers such as hand soap, household bleach, glutaraldehyde, formaldehyde, ether, ethanol, and isopropyl alcohol. Chlorinated water in swimming pools quickly destroys it. Because it is so easily killed, it is not casually transmitted by nonsexual or non-blood-borne routes, such as shaking hands, touching, talking, kissing, or sitting on a toilet seat previously used by someone with the infection.[1]

TABLE 24.2. Indicator diseases.

Candidiasis of the esophagus, trachea, bronchi, or lungs
Cryptococcus, extrapulmonary
Cryptosporidiosis with diarrhea persisting > 1 month
Cytomegalovirus disease of an organ other than liver, spleen or lymph nodes in a patient > 1 month of age
Cytomegalovirus retinitis with loss of vision
Herpes simplex virus infection causing a mucocutaneous ulcer that persists longer than 1 month; or bronchitis, pneumonitis, or esophagitis for any duration affecting a patient > 1 month of age
Kaposi's sarcoma at any age
Lymphoma of the brain (primary) at any age
Lymphoid interstitial pneumonia and/or pulmonary lymphoid hyperplasia affecting a child < 13 years of age
Mycobacterial disease caused by mycobacteria other than *M. tuberculosis*, disseminated (at a site other than or in addition to lungs, skin, or cervical or hilar lymph nodes)
Mycobacterial disease caused by *M. tuberculosis*, extrapulmonary involving at least one site outside the lungs, regardless of concurrent pulmonary involvement
Pneumocystis carinii pneumonia
Progressive multifocal leukoencephalopathy
Toxoplasmosis of the brain affecting a patient over 1 month of age
HIV encephalopathy
Histoplasmosis, disseminated (at a site other than or in addition to cervical or hilar lymph nodes)
Salmonella (nontyphoid) septicemia, recurrent

HIV wasting syndrome (emaciation, slim disease)

Bacterial infections, multiple or recurrent (any combination of at least two within a 2-year period) of the following types affecting a child < 13 years of age—septicemia, pneumonia, meningitis, bone or joint infection, or abscess of an internal organ or body cavity (excluding otitis media or superficial skin or mucosal abscesses) caused by Haemophilus, Streptococcus (including pneumococcus), or other pyogenic bacteria
Coccidioidmycosis, disseminated (at a site other than or in addition to lungs or cervical or hilar lymph nodes)
Isosporiasis with diarrhea persisting > 1 month
Non-Hodgkin's lymphoma of B-cell or unknown immunological phenotype and the following histological types:
(a) small noncleaved lymphoma (Burkitt's or non-Burkitt's), (b) immunoblastic sarcoma (equivalent to any of the following, although not necessarily all in combination: immunoblastic lymphoma, large-cell lymphoma, diffuse histiocytic lymphoma, diffuse undifferentiated lymphoma, or high-grade lymphoma)

From Revision of the CDC surveillance case definition for acquired immunodeficiency syndrome, *MMWR*, 36:3S–11S, 1987.

Most cases of HIV infection have occurred through one of four routes. The most common mode of transmission is sexual contact, which is responsible for 75 percent of AIDS cases. Transmission by intravenous drug use occurs through contaminated needles or paraphernalia. Blood and blood products can also transmit the infection, as can infected mothers to newborns.[1]

TABLE 24.3. Diagnosing ARC.

Clinical manifestations	Laboratory abnormalities
lymphadenopathy in any two noninguinal sites longer than 3 months	helper T cells $<400/mm^3$
fever $>100°$ for 3 months	T4 helper/T8 suppressor ratio < 1.0
weight loss > 10 percent	leukopenia
persistent diarrhea	thrombocytopenia
fatigue	anemia
night sweats	elevated serum globulins
	anergy to skin tests
	reduced blastogenesis
	positive HIV antibody test

ARC = any two clinical manifestations + any two laboratory abnormalities

From Revision of the CDC surveillance case definition for acquired immunodeficiency syndrome, *MMWR*, 36:3S–11S, 1987.

Diagnosis of AIDS

In the presence of laboratory evidence of HIV infection, any disease in Table 24.2 diagnosed definitively indicates a diagnosis of AIDS. The CDC has also published criteria for the diagnosis of AIDS without evidence of HIV infection, based on presumptive diagnosis of indicator diseases, and with laboratory evidence against HIV infection.[10] A discussion of these criteria is beyond the scope of this chapter.

Diagnosis of ARC

The CDC has also published criteria for diagnosing ARC. The diagnosis is based on the presence of any two clinical manifestations plus any two laboratory abnormalities given in Table 24.3.[10]

HIV Carrier State

The carrier state consists of individuals infected with HIV who do not meet the criteria for AIDS or ARC. They are usually asymptomatic.

HIV Antibody Testing

The body's immune system produces antibodies to fight HIV. The usual tests available commercially detect these antibodies—not the virus itself. Only an antigen test (not yet widely available) or a viral culture, which is complex and expensive, can determine the actual presence of HIV. [2]

The ELISA Test

The most frequently used test currently available for HIV antibodies is the enzyme-linked immunosorbent assay (ELISA). It is manufactured and distributed in slightly different versions by several companies. It works by combining serum drawn from the person being tested with the virus in a test kit to see if binding occurs between the virus and antibodies in the serum. If HIV antibody is present, a chemical reaction occurs that changes the color of the solution. If no HIV antibody is present, the solution remains clear.[2]

False negative results do sometimes occur. Virus characteristics that make false negative results a possibility include the lag time between infection with HIV and production of antibodies (a few weeks to six months), rare individuals never develop HIV antibodies, and in the last stages of AIDS, when the virus almost depletes the immune system, patients may be weakly reactive to the ELISA test or not react to it at all. The best way to make certain that the ELISA test results are not falsely negative is for a patient to avoid all possible exposure to HIV for four to six months and then repeat the test.[2]

False-positive ELISA test results can occur when other antibodies are mistaken for HIV antibodies. Because of this false-positive problem, the results of a single ELISA test should never be considered adequate for determining antibody status. A positive test should be repeated on the same serum sample. If the second test is equivocal or negative, blood should be redrawn and tested anew. However, verification through double testing does not correct all false positive problems. Testing by another method needs to be performed before results can be considered reliable enough to be disclosed.[2]

The Western Blot Test

The most popular test currently used for confirming ELISA results is called the Western Blot Test. Although less sensitive than the ELISA test, it is more specific. It can differentiate between HIV antibodies and antibodies that cross-react with the ELISA antigen and cause most false-positive results. In addition to having a longer turnaround time than the ELISA test, the Western Blot test is considerably more expensive. Future developments will undoubtedly result in improvement of current tests and also yield tests based on new technology. A test for HIV itself appears promising.[2]

Issues in Testing

HIV antibody testing has generated enormous controversy over protecting individual rights and protecting communities against an infectious disease. The American Society of Addiction Medicine (ASAM) has compiled a list of advantages and disadvantages of testing chemically dependent individuals (Table 24.4).[6] These should be helpful in making decisions.

There is currently no medical reason for routine mandatory HIV antibody testing of patients in chemical dependence treatment facilities. The decision to

TABLE 24.4. Advantages and disadvantages of HIV antibody testing.

	Advantages	Disadvantages
Psychological	An HIV negative result may relieve anxiety; an HIV positive result may encourage changes to make remaining life meaningful	Potential for depression, stress, anxiety and suicide exists; in absence of pre- and posttest counseling, reactions to results may be erratic, even dangerous
Economic	Knowledge of status may encourage organizing personal affairs, wills, finances	Potential for job loss and disqualification for health and life insurance is highly possible
Public health	Knowledge of status may increase measures to protect oneself or others	A negative test may discourage modification of risk behavior; a positive test may encourage vindictive or retaliatory behavior leading to further infection
Chemical dependence		Knowledge of positive test may induce relapse or termination of treatment
Social		Ostracism from family and friends is possible; HIV-positive persons lack support of others when they most need it; lack of confidentiality and antidiscrimination policies intensify that risk
Medical	a. Diagnosis Symptomatic patients are at high risk for accompanying disease. Certain AIDS-equivalent syndromes, presumptive diagnoses of opportunistic infections, and other infections now require positive HIV antibody tests to qualify as AIDS level diagnoses. b. Treatment Common infectious diseases may be approached differently in HIV-positive patients. TB, syphilis, hepatitis B, delta infection, bacterial endocarditis, pneumonia, and other infections may require close observation and aggressive treatment in them. c. Intervention Treatments may become available to prevent or delay seropositive individuals from developing AIDS or ARC. Immunosuppressive therapy for another disease may not be indicated for an HIV-positive patient. d. Prevention An HIV-positive woman may consider abortion early in pregnancy or may defer pregnancy.	

From Guidelines for facilities treating chemically dependent patients at risk for AIDS or infected by HIV virus, American Medical Society on Alcoholism and Other Drug Dependencies, New York, 1988.

recommend testing must be individualized, based on a patient's risk factors, desire to be tested, and the potential psychological and social results of a positive test. When testing is deemed appropriate, pretesting counseling should be done, and proper written consent should be obtained. The process should outline what positive and negative tests do and do not mean. The treatment program staff must be trained to deal with the psychosocial effects of such information on patients, on the staff itself, on patients' families, and on other patients should results become known to them.[6]

Treating HIV-Positive and At-Risk Patients

The chemically dependent, HIV-positive patient must deal with two potentially fatal diseases. One cannot be adequately treated without dealing with the other. Standard treatment techniques should be used for chemical dependence. Treatment for HIV infection and those at high risk for acquiring it should include education about AIDS-related conditions, techniques for reducing the risks for those who have not yet acquired the virus, and counseling for the psychosocial impact of HIV infection on patients who test positive.

Education

An extremely important aspect of treating chemically dependent patients who are HIV positive or who are at high risk, education includes a brief history of AIDS, how transmission occurs, how the virus works, the difference between the carrier state, ARC, and AIDS, the progression of the disease, testing information (ELISA and Western Blot), and how to prevent HIV infection.

Risk Reduction

Precautions can be recommended to patients to reduce the risk of their contracting HIV through drug use, sex, and general health practices. Drug-using patients should be encouraged to stay in treatment and lead lives of recovery. If they should relapse, they should avoid intravenous drugs. If they use IV drugs, they should not share needles, syringes, or paraphernalia. If they share needles, they should sterilize them before each use with alcohol or diluted household bleach and rinse them with clean water. They should avoid shooting galleries.[1,4]

Patients should avoid sex with promiscuous individuals, should use condoms for intercourse, should avoid anal sex, and should limit the number of their sex partners.

General health practices include being cautious about exposure to HIV, improving nutrition, getting proper exercise and rest, and reducing stress. Women at high risk for HIV infection, including sexual partners of risk-group men, should avoid pregnancy unless they seek HIV testing and medical advice first.[2]

Counseling

Counseling HIV-positive patients involves assessment, developing treatment goals, treating the psychosocial aspects of the condition, and planning for referral to community resources.

Assessment

Patients who have AIDS-related conditions, or in whom the diagnosis is made after they are admitted to treatment programs should be assessed for their understanding of what their particular condition does and does not mean, their awareness of safe and unsafe interactions with others, and their knowledge of healthy living strategies.[2]

Developing Treatment Goals

Treatment goals for HIV-positive individuals include clarifying their particular AIDS-related condition, impelling change to reduce the risk of their transmitting the virus to others and to reduce the progression of their disease, and instilling in them a hope for lives with some quality.[2]

Psychosocial Treatment

Upon learning of seropositive test results or of confirmed ARC or AIDS, patients tend to progress through three adjustment stages: the initial crisis, a transitional stage, and acceptance.[2]

The *crisis stage* occurs when patients first learn that they are seropositive. This is essentially a state of shock, and denial (an unconscious and normal defense against overwhelming anxiety) is its hallmark. Another characteristic of this stage is the disruptive impact it has on patients' supportive relationships. The diagnosis of HIV infection may force people to disclose previously undisclosed drug abuse, as well as subject patients to the stigma associated with AIDS. For most patients in drug treatment programs, family relationships are already strained, if not severed.[2]

Patients in crisis suffer from disorientation. They tend to have difficulty hearing and retaining information and may distort what they hear about their condition. For this reason, they should be assessed later for how much knowledge about HIV infection they have retained, and the information should be repeated if they have forgotten or confused some of it. The primary treatment goal of the crisis state is to guide patients through denial, allowing it to run its course. The main treatment strategies are empathy, education, and reassurance. For preventive reasons, health care workers address the question of who should be informed about patients' HIV infection; usually this involves patients' sex partners, physicians, and dentists.[2]

The *transitional stage* begins when alternating waves of anger, guilt, self-pity, and anxiety supersede denial. Treatment during this stage focuses on helping patients deal with these reactions. The strategy used is to allow patients to freely ventilate their distress and confusion and be guided through these feelings. Empathy and reassurance continue to be appropriate.[2]

The *acceptance stage* occurs when patients come to accept the limitations that their particular AIDS-related condition impose on them and realize that they can still manage their lives by reacting more with reason than emotion. They accept their condition and begin to integrate it into their lives.[2]

Community Resources

Once patients are in treatment for chemical dependence, begin to plan to get them to needed resources in the community. Consult physicians who specialize in infectious diseases, arrange mental healthcare for patients suffering severe depression or suicidal tendencies, and help AIDS patients arrange for financial assistance through Supplemental Security Income (SSI) (patients with ARC are not currently eligible for SSI). In addition, many patients upon discharge will need help with housing, and some will need legal counsel. For example, anxious divorced or separated partners may deny patients child visitation rights or ignorant employers may dismiss them on learning of test results even if patients can perform their jobs and have acceptable work histories. Finally, patients should be put in touch with various community support groups for AIDS-related conditions.[2]

Involving the Family

Family includes not only conventional members by virtue of blood or legal connection but also such others as ongoing sexual and/or drug-using partners, living mates, and friends with whom patients have established meaningful bonds. These individuals will be affected by a patient's condition. Issues will center around patient needs for family support and family needs resulting from a patient's condition.[2]

Patient Needs

Critical to patients' progress is their significant others' knowledge about AIDS-related conditions, the course of the disease, how the virus is transmitted, and practices to ensure safe contact. Family members may need to make behavior changes to support patient treatment goals for a patient's continued health. They should be assessed for their potential for understanding a patient's condition, making needed behavioral changes, coping with the array of adjustment reactions, capabilities of supporting the treatment plan outlined for the patient, and assisting with medical and other community resources. A primary strategy is to involve a key support person at the earliest possible opportunity.[2]

Family Needs

Needle-sharing associates and sex partners of HIV-infected patients should be assessed for likely risk of past exposure and HIV antibody testing. If their test results are positive, they should become involved in local community support groups and may need treatment for chemical dependence as well.[2]

All people close to HIV-infected patients, including estranged family members, when they learn of patients' condition, are likely to experience considerable distress. Young drug-abusing significant others will be as ill-prepared as patients to deal with this reaction. Older and more conventional family members, such as parents, typically react with shame and guilt and may reject patients. Treatment goals for the family include promoting behavioral change toward healthy, nonrisk practices and developing the ability to cope psychosocially with a patient's condition and their response to it.[2]

Precautions in Treatment Programs

People caring for HIV-infected patients should protect themselves against getting blood or fluids of others into their own bodies through cuts, abrasions, or other openings. Washing their hands before caring for patients helps protect patients who are susceptible to infection; washing their hands after caring for patients helps protect themselves. To protect their patients, healthcare workers should be free of disease, fever, abscesses, diarrhea, and yeast infections.[6] Universal blood and body fluid precautions, based on the principle that all individuals are potentially infectious to others in healthcare settings, are highly recommended and should be used.[11] Specific recommendations for treatment program personnel are given in Table 24.5.[6]

Role of the Physician

Treatment program physicians and referring physicians have important roles to play in treating patients with AIDS-related conditions and chemical dependence.

Treatment Program Physicians

The responsibilities of treatment program physicians include educating staff members, educating patients about AIDS-related conditions, and caring for HIV-positive patients medically. Physicians are likely initially to be the only staff members with adequate knowledge of AIDS and related conditions. Educating treatment program staff can involve lectures and small groups to discuss fears and anxieties about treating patients. Educating patients can involve lectures to all patients as a group and counseling individual patients. Patient care involves detoxification, treating usual medical problems, and working with physicians specializing in infectious diseases for the complication of HIV infection.

Referring Physicians

The roles of referring physicians, other than helping to get patients into treatment, are to monitor patients' progress in treatment and provide follow-up care

TABLE 24.5. Precautions in treatment programs.

1. Wash your hands. If there is likely to be contact with body fluids or if your hands have scrapes or scratches, wear gloves.
2. Gloves are not required for handling patient clothing and other unsoiled articles; they are not required for touching a patient's intact skin or giving backrubs.
3. Wear disposable gloves when handling any body fluids, especially blood. Avoid touching blood with your bare hands.
4. Keep your hands away from your mouth and face while working and wash your hands before eating.
5. It is safe to use the same bathroom as someone with AIDS, but, as you would in any living situation, follow good sanitary practices. Do not spill excrement on toilet seats, clean the bathroom regularly, wash your hands after using the facilities, and clean surfaces visibly soiled with blood, fecal material or other body secretions. A good bathroom and kitchen disinfectant for soiled surfaces is household bleach (5.25%) mixed with one part to ten parts of water. Bleach is also useful on the shower floor to control the fungus that causes athlete's foot.
6. Dishes used by people with AIDS may safely be used by others after they have been washed in hot soapy water. Allow to drain dry.
7. Wear a water-resistant gown, lab coat, or smock when your clothing is likely to come in contact with secretions, excretions, or blood.
8. Use plastic bags to dispose of soiled tissues, dressings, Band-Aids, and soiled gloves. Close and secure bags tightly when discarding.
9. Wash soiled linens and towels in a washing machine using hot water and detergent. Dry on high heat.
10. Bedpans and urinals should be handled in a sanitary manner. Excrement need not be treated before being flushed down the toilet.
11. Use gloves to clean up patients' diarrhea or vomit. Clean up patient and their linens immediately, rinse soiled surfaces with soapy water, and put soiled linens into plastic bags until ready to launder.
12. After completing care, WASH YOUR HANDS and use lotions on clean hands. Lotion replaces the natural oil removed by handwashing and helps prevent the dry chapped condition that may allow disease-causing organisms to get through the skin. Such areas may also develop mild infections that could be transmitted to patients.
13. Hepatitis B vaccination is recommended for all hepatitis B antibody negative people who come in contact with blood or body fluids from patients with potential HIV disease. This is to protect against both hepatitis B and hepatitis delta infections.
14. Yearly PPD skin testing (with appropriate medical prophylaxis if a new conversion should occur) is recommended for people caring for patients with HIV spectrum disease.

From Guidelines for facilities treating chemically dependent patients at risk for AIDS or infected by HIV virus, American Medical Society on Alcoholism and Other Drug Dependencies, New York, 1988.

for both AIDS-related conditions and chemical dependence once patients return to the community.

References

1. Amin, N.M. Acquired immunodeficiency syndrome, Part 1: Edpidemiology, history, and etiology. *Family Practice Recertification*, 9:36–58, 1987.
2. Sulima, J.P. *What Every Drug Abuse Counselor Should Know About AIDS*. Manisses Communications Group, Washington, D.C., 1987.

3. Battjes, R.J., C.G. Leukefeld, R.W. Pickens, and H.W. Haverkos. The acquired immunodeficiency syndrome and intravenous drug abuse. *Bulletin on Narcotics*, 40:21–34, 1988.

4. Jewell, M.E., and G.S. Jewell. How to assess the risk of HIV exposure. *American Family Physician*, 40:153–161, 1989.

5. DesJarlais, D.C., and S.R. Friedman. AIDS 2 (Supplement):65–69, 1988.

6. Guidelines for facilities treating chemically dependent patients at risk for AIDS or infected by HIV virus. American Medical Society on Alcoholism and Other Drug Dependencies, New York, 1988.

7. Kaplin, M.H. The AIDS epidemic and the drug substance abuse patient. *Journal of Substance Abuse Treatment*, 4:127–136, 1987.

8. Kaslow, R.A., W.C. Blackwelder, D.G. Ostrow, D. Yerg, J. Palenicek, A.H. Coulson, and R.O. Valdiserri. No evidence for a role of alcohol or other psychoactive drugs in accelerating immunodeficiency in HIV-1-positive individuals. *Journal of the American Medical Association*, 261:3424–3429, 1989.

9. MacGregor, R.R. Alcohol and drugs as co-factors for AIDS. *Advances in Alcohol and Substance Abuse*, 7(2):47–71, 1987.

10. Revision of the CDC surveillance case definition for acquired immunodeficiency syndrome. *Morbidity Mortality Weekly Report*, 36:3S–11S, 1987.

11. Recommendations for prevention of HIV transmission in health-care settings. U.S. Department of Health and Human Services, Rockville, Maryland, 36 (Supplement):3–14, 1987.

CHAPTER 25

The Impaired Physician

The Impaired Physician

Prevalence

Chemical dependence is a leading occupational hazard for physicians. Precise information on its prevalence is not available; however, it is believed to be no greater than that of the general public.[1-2]

Characteristics of the Impaired Physician

Identifying impaired physicians is difficult, primarily because of two factors: the conspiracy of silence among professionals and other people in physicians' lives, and self-deception in impaired physicians. Talbott and Benson presented six areas in impaired physicians' lives where clues to their chemical dependence can be found: community involvement, family life, employment patterns, physical status, office conduct, and hospital duties (Table 25.1). The areas become involved sequentially, although two or three may seem to be involved simultaneously. The last area affected is the medical setting—hospitals, staff rounds, emergency rooms, and medical society meetings.[3]

Community Involvement

Isolation and withdrawal from the community and its activities often signal the onset of chemical dependence in physicians. Talbott and Benson describe the "target syndrome," in which successive rings of involvement (community activities, leisure activities, church, friends, peers, distant family, nuclear family) are peeled away until only the center of the target, the physician, remains. The community and friends gradually lose respect for the physician and lose confidence in his or her emotional stability.

Family Life

As part of the target syndrome, impaired physicians withdraw from family activities, relationships, and communication. Family fights erupt, and child abuse

336

TABLE 25.1. Clues to chemical dependence in six areas of the impaired physician's life.

Community Isolation and withdrawal from community activities, leisure activities and hobbies, church, friends, peers Embarrassing behavior at club or parties Arrests for driving while intoxicated, legal problems Unreliability and unpredictability in community and social activities Unpredictable behavior; i.e., inappropriate spending, excessive involvement in political activities **Family** Withdrawal from family activities, unexplained absences from home Fights, child abuse Development in spouse of disease of "spousaholism" Abnormal, antisocial, illegal behavior by children Sexual problems—impotence, extramarital affairs, contracultural sexual behavior Assumption of surrogate role by spouse and children Institution of geographic separation or divorce proceedings by spouse **Employment** Numerous job changes in past five years Frequent geographic relocations for unexplained reasons Frequent hospitalizations Complicated and elaborate medical history Unexplained intervals between jobs Indefinite or inappropriate references Working in job inappropriate for qualifications Reluctance of job applicant to let spouse and children be interviewed Reluctance to undergo immediate preemployment physical examination	**Physical status** Deterioration in personal hygiene Deterioration in clothing and dressing habits Multiple physical signs and complaints Numerous prescriptions and drugs Frequent hospitalizations Frequent visits to physicians and dentists Accidents Emotional crises **Office** Disruption of appointment schedule Hostile, withdrawn, unreasonable behavior to staff and patients "Locked-door syndrome" Excessive ordering of supplies of drugs from local druggists or by mail Complaints by patients to staff about doctor's behavior Absence from office—unexplained or due to frequent illness **Hospital** Making rounds late, or inappropriate, abnormal behavior during rounds Decreasing quality of performance; i.e., in staff presentations, writing in chart Inappropriate orders of medications Reports of behavioral changes from hospital personnel ("hospital gossip") Involvement in malpractice suits and legal sanctions against hospital Reports from emergency department staff of unavailability or inappropriate responses to telephone calls

From G.D. Talbott and E.B. Benson, Impaired physicians: The dilemma of identification, *Postgraduate Medicine,* 68:58–64, 1980.

(physical or emotional) may occur. The best way to identify impaired physicians is not to ask who drinks alcohol or uses other drugs addictively but instead to look at those physicians who are separated from their families or whose children have serious emotional, legal, or scholastic problems.

Employment Patterns

As the disease evolves, impaired physicians typically seek employment in a new location. Numerous job changes and frequent relocations (the geographic cure) are indicative of chemical dependence. Unexplained intervals between jobs can also be a significant clue. Inappropriate jobs for a person's level of training may be another clue.

Physical Status

Next, physical signs and symptoms of the disease become evident. Poor personal hygiene and unkempt appearance in a previously well-dressed physician are strong clues. Numerous and constant physical complaints, frequent visits to fellow physicians, multiple medications (often self-prescribed), and frequent hospitalizations may provide additional clues. Repeated automobile accidents or accidents while on vacation or involved in hobbies or leisure activities may also provide evidence of chemical dependence, as may wide mood swings and emotional crises.

Office Conduct

Impaired physicians may arrive late or have unexplained and lengthy absences from their offices. They may become angry, hostile, and inconsistent, prompting complaints from patients and, later, office staff. Physicians may give inappropriate orders and frequently lock themselves in their offices or bathrooms to use drugs. Talbott and Benson call this the "locked-door" syndrome.

Hospital Duties

The last place impaired physicians' problems become apparent is in the hospital. Making rounds at midnight, writing inappropriate orders, going into the wrong rooms, reading the wrong charts, writing more illegibly than usual can all be signs of chemical dependence. Physicians' behavior frequently changes, and they may be slow in responding to emergency room calls or not answer them at all. Hospital staff may notice slow, slurred speech, and may report smelling alcohol on physicians' breath. Impaired physicians may become involved in malpractice suits and legal sanctions against hospitals.[3]

The Impaired Woman Physician

Several studies have examined chemically dependent women in medicine. Bissell and Skorina examined the patterns of diagnosis, referral, and help-seeking behaviors of 95 alcoholic women in AA who had at least a year of sobriety. Addiction to drugs other than alcohol were common: Only 40 percent reported addiction to alcohol alone. Nearly 77 percent reported serious suicide ideation prior to sobriety, 27.4 percent reported it after stopping drinking, and 40 percent had actually made suicide attempts—15.8 percent more than once. Treatment experiences ranged from AA only (21 percent) to long-term residence treatment of 15 weeks or more (23 percent). Most had reached treatment by means other than referral by therapists or by impaired-physician committees.[4]

Martin and Talbott studied 37 female physicians who had been in treatment in the Georgia Impaired Physicians Program. This represented only 4.6 percent of all physicians in the program, despite the fact that nationally women make up 13.4 percent of all physicians. The physicians tended to be high academic achievers, and many had mates who expected them to fit into traditional social and family roles. Many identified with self-effacing and nonassertive roles rather than with more powerful postures male physicians often identify with.[5-6] Many of the issues of female physicians in treatment are the same as those of nonphysician women discussed in Chapter 19.

State Medical Society Programs

Early Efforts

The American Medical Association provided early leadership in the area of physician impairment. In 1972 the AMA house of delegates adopted a policy statement declaring that any physician who became aware of an apparent problem in a colleague had an ethical responsibility to take affirmative action—that is, to seek treatment or rehabilitation for that physician. The AMA defined impairment as "the inability to practice medicine with reasonable skill and safety to patients by reason of physical or mental illness, including alcohol or drug dependence."[7]

In 1974 the AMA drafted model legislation that state legislatures could use in modifying individual medical practice acts to provide for the treatment and rehabilitation of impaired physicians. The response of state medical societies to these initiatives was dramatic. Today, every state has established impaired physician programs.[8-9]

The Programs

State medical society programs typically offer impaired physicians confidential and nonpunitive assistance. If they refuse to cooperate in their own rehabilitation, some state medical associations report them to the state board of medical examiners.[8]

Medical societies usually have mechanisms for confidential reporting of impairment, such as a 1-800 telephone number. Reports may come from colleagues, hospital administrators, nurses, patients, or physicians' families. Once the information is verified, it is given to a committee member or members who are responsible for confronting physicians with evidence of their impairment and persuading them to enter treatment.[8,10]

Medical Society of Georgia Study

In 1987, Talbott et al. reviewed the first 1,000 physicians treated in Georgia's impaired physician program. Because this is the largest group reported in the literature, we will briefly review the findings. The mean age of physicians in this study was 45.3 years. Most were married (65.2 percent), some were separated (14.2 percent), and 9.9 percent had never been married. Marital discord was reported in 80.2 percent of those who were or who had been married. Only 5.9 percent had a primary psychiatric disorder. In the study population, 74.4 percent were in practice, 15.1 percent were unemployed or retired, and 9.5 percent were residents.[11]

Of the physicians studied, 63 percent had intact medical licenses, while 32.9 percent had problems with theirs. A small fraction (0.9 percent) had never had a license (interns), and the status of 3.2 percent was unknown. In the same group, 74 percent had intact DEA licenses, while 20.8 percent had problems with theirs. Again, a small percentage had never had a DEA license (1.7 percent) or their status was unknown (3.5 percent).[11]

Of the study group, 28.4 percent had legal problems, 68.1 did not, and 3.5 percent were unknown. Most of the physicians who were unemployed had many of the license and legal problems. Only 49.9 percent of the group had neither a legal nor a license problem.[11]

Two specialties—anesthesia and family practice—were overrepresented in the study group, suggesting that physicians in these two specialties are at higher risk for developing chemical dependence than those in other specialties. Anesthesiologists were more likely than other specialty groups to abuse narcotics and to use more than one drug. They were also more apt to use drugs intravenously. Family practitioners were more likely than physicians in other specialties to be in solo practice and to be from rural areas. They were also found to be preponderantly alcohol-dependent as compared to physicians in other specialties. As a result, they were more likely to have more severe physical sequelae than physicians in any other specialty.[11]

Physicians in the study had used a variety of drugs. Alcohol was the drug most commonly abused, followed by meperidine and diazepam. Using more than one drug was frequent, particularly among younger physicians; only 28.0 percent of the physicians in the study reported the use of just one drug. Cocaine abuse was not reported prior to 1980, but afterwards it was given as the drug of choice by 28.6 percent of the physicians. Parenteral drugs were abused by 38.8 percent of the physicians.[11]

The authors concluded that several factors play a role in the development of chemical dependence in physicians: genetic disposition and environmental exposure; stress and poor coping skills; lack of education about the various kinds of impairment that affect a physician's ability to practice medicine with reasonable skill and safety to patients; the absence of effective prevention and control strategies; drug availability in a permissive professional and social environment; and denial of chemical dependence.[11]

TABLE 25.2. Most frequently abused drugs by impaired physicians.

All physicians[a]		Anesthesiologists[b]	
Drug	Percent	Drug	Percent
alcohol	70.18	alcohol	52.74
meperidine	25.72	fentanyl	45.21
diazepam	16.54	meperidine	34.93
amphetamines	10.24	diazepam	19.86
cocaine	10.24	cocaine	15.75
marijuana	9.79	morphine	14.38
oxycodone	9.10	marijuana	9.59
codeine	7.21	oxycodone	9.59
fentanyl	6.53	amphetamines	4.11
pentazocine	6.53	codeine	4.11
propoxyphene	4.55	pentazocine	4.11
morphine	4.10		

[a] Based on K.V. Gallegos, F.W. Veit, P.O. Wilson, T. Porter, and G.D. Talbott, Substance abuse among health professionals, *Maryland Medical Journal,* 37:191–197, 1988.
[b] Based on K.V. Gallegos, C.H. Browne, F.W. Veit, and G.D. Talbott, Addiction in anesthesiologists: Drug access and patterns of substance abuse, *Quarterly Review of Biology,* April, 1988, pp. 116–122.

In two follow-up studies from the same program, Gallegos et al. identified the most commonly abused drugs among impaired physicians as a whole and among anesthesiologists (Table 25.2). Alcohol was the drug of choice of both groups, although a smaller percentage of anesthesiologists reported alcohol abuse. The most striking difference between these two groups is the fact that fentanyl was reported as an abused drug by 45.21 percent of anesthesiologists but only by 6.53 percent of the physicians as a whole. This was undoubtedly due to anesthesiologists' easy access to fentanyl.[1,12]

Intervention

Defined

A process that culminates in confrontation, intervention is often necessary because impaired physicians have difficulty reaching out for help. It involves convincing them of the seriousness of their drug problem and helping them enter treatment, while protecting their dignity, preserving their anonymity, and sparing them embarrassment. It is not an easy or pleasant task, but it is a necessary one.[8,13] The two main types of intervention are professional and nonprofessional. Nonprofessional intervention is done most often by family members and/or close friends and was discussed in Chapter 5. Professional intervention is discussed below.

The Intervention Team

The intervention team should consist of at least two persons. The team concept allows the confronters to give each other emotional support. At least one member of the team should be someone in the same specialty, of the same sex, and, if possible, recovering from chemical dependence. Members of the team should have nonjudgmental and supportive attitudes and should have experience or training in intervention strategies.[8]

Members of the intervention team must have no professional or social associations with the impaired physician. Because of the impaired physician's denial, he or she would use such a relationship to destroy the effectiveness of the intervention.[13]

Preparing for the Confrontation

Training of the intervention team begins by examining their attitudes and instilling desirable ones in them. These attitudes include:

1. Understanding, appreciating, and accepting that chemical dependence is a biopsychosocial disease, not a bad habit, moral or ethical fault, or psychological disorder.
2. The impaired physician program is an advocacy program; it is not a program for punishment.
3. It is a program of the state medical association, not a private or local effort.
4. Chemical dependence is a disease involving the family, which needs to be included and helped.
5. Response to the intervention team may be anger, threats, hostility, or massive denial; the team must be prepared for this.[9]

The intervention team should have clearly defined goals and objectives for the confrontation. Regardless of its outcome, the team should have a plan of action when they leave the confrontation. Members should anticipate and be prepared to deal with denial, hostility, and other defenses. They should have documentation on paper of the impaired physician's destructive behavior and actions resulting from chemical dependence, and they should mobilize support systems, including the spouse and older children and the physician's partners, peers, nurses, or hospital administrator. The team may have to meet two or three times before actually confronting the impaired physician.[13]

The Confrontation

When the team feels it is adequately prepared, they contact the impaired physician by telephone, telling him or her that the caller represents the state medical society and that they need to see him or her immediately on professional business, which is too personal to discuss on the phone. The physician is given a choice of meeting with the team in his or her office, home, or in the state medical society office. A date, time, and place for the meeting are then arranged.[13]

At the time of the confrontation, the following procedure is followed:

1. The leader of the intervention team introduces himself or herself and the other members of the team and explains that they represent the state medical society.
2. The leader explains the medical society's program for impaired physicians and its advocacy role. The physician is told that the team is there to help, not hurt.
3. The team member who is also a recovering physician discusses his or her disease and recovery, pointing out that chemical dependence is a treatable disease and that the behavior, actions, emotions, and consequences are secondary to the illness. Members emphasize that the impaired physician is suffering from a disease and is not bad, evil, weak or crazy.
4. Members present the specifics of the physician's drug-abusing behavior in a factual, nonjudgmental manner.
5. Members anticipate the physician's responses, such as denial, anger, or rationalization. They should never argue with the physician, get angry or defensive, even in the face of personal or professional attack.
6. The team should not let the physician sidetrack the discussion.
7. The intervention team shares its assessment of the seriousness of the physician's problem.
8. Members explain what will happen if the physician does not enter treatment.
9. The impaired physician is given specific treatment plans and programs, both local and out of state, but is not allowed to arrange for a friend to treat him or her. Members advise him or her that the treatment plans and programs presented are the only ones acceptable to the state medical society.[13-14]
10. Once a mutually acceptable treatment source is agreed upon, arrangements are made for the physician to enter treatment. He or she is presented a contract that states that he or she will not practice again until cleared according to the advocacy position of the state medical society as it relates to licensure, medical staff positions, and medical standing in the community.[13]

If the team is unsuccessful, it returns again in a day or two. If it is still unsuccessful, a second team makes a visit, repeating the visit in a day or two if it too is unsuccessful. Each team reports to the intervention committee, which, in turn, reports to the impaired physician's committee, which is responsible to the state medical society.[13]

If the intervention fails and members believe that the impaired physician is a danger to patients, he or she is told that the intervention committee will abandon its advocacy role and make a report to the impaired physician committee, which in turn may file a report with the state medical association, which can then notify the state examining and licensure board of the physician's state.[13]

Treatment of the Impaired Physician

Chemically dependent physicians are often seriously ill by the time they enter treatment. Typically, they are more dysfunctional (physiologically, psychologically, socially, spiritually) than nonphysicians. They often have been so absorbed in their practices that they have become isolated from other people. Because elaborate denial and defense mechanisms are part of the disease of chemical dependence, they go to great lengths to deny that they have a problem and to prove that their lives are under complete control. Another problem with treating physicians is that they adamantly reject the role of patient.[8]

Although there is a relatively low incidence of primary psychiatric disorders among chemically dependent physicians, secondary depression is common. This usually clears in a few days to weeks. Physicians tend to minimize their drug use. Whereas street addicts tend to congregate in a drug culture, physicians tend to use drugs privately for fear that their drug abuse will be discovered.[8]

Because of most physicians' high level of denial, inpatient treatment is almost always indicated. Treatment programs vary considerably throughout the country. The format for the Medical Association of Georgia's Impaired Physician Program has become a model for many. Treatment is divided into three phases. The first phase is inpatient treatment, which lasts about 28 days and obeys the same principles outlined in Chapter 3. In addition, problems specific to physicians, such as practice and licensure issues, are discussed in groups for impaired health professionals.[15]

During the second phase, physicians live in half-way houses with other impaired health professionals. During the day, they attend a partial hospitalization (day program). Several evenings a week they attend AA meetings, and once or twice a week they attend a Caduceus meeting, which is a support group for health professionals. This phase is about a month long.

In phase three physicians participate in a process called mirror imaging. As part of treatment they may work in treatment centers as associate counselors, but not as physicians. Mirror imaging is a method of allowing patients to see other patients whose disease is more advanced than theirs and to realize that "there, but for the grace of God, go I." They continue to live in half-way houses, to attend evening AA meetings, and to attend some evening group sessions. This phase may last one to two months or more.

Aftercare

At the time of discharge from treatment, physicians sign aftercare contracts that may require them to attend three to four AA meetings a week, as well as weekly meetings of local Caduceus clubs. Random drug screens are an integral part of aftercare, which usually lasts two years. During this period, and afterwards, Caduceus clubs serve as physician advocates in issues such as licensure and DEA registration.[15-16]

Recovery

Recovery for physicians progresses through the same stages as for nonphysicians — pretreatment, stabilization, early recovery, middle recovery, and late recovery. Recovering physicians may also be caught up in partial recovery, and factors contributing to their relapse are also the same as for other addicts. Many physicians face a temptation nonphysicians do not have to deal with—such as returning to a profession in which mood-altering and addicting drugs are abundant. The anesthesiologist whose drug of choice was fentanyl, for example, must return to the operating room after treatment and actually administer the drug to patients. When relapse does occur, physicians should follow the procedures outlined in Chapter 4.

The recovery rate for physicians is high. In one study, at two years and four years, it was 93 percent and 86 percent, respectively.[3] For married physicians, spouses usually play major roles in detection, intervention, treatment, and recovery. Families can be physicians' most important resources in recovery. Al-Anon and Alateen can be exceptional sources of information and support for spouses and other family members.[17-19]

References

1. Gallegos, K.V., F.W. Veit, P.O. Wilson, T. Porter, and D. Talbott. Substance abuse among health professionals. *Maryland Medical Journal*, 37:191–197, 1988.
2. Southgate, M.T. Prevalence of alcohol and other drug problems among physicians. *Journal of the American Medical Association*, 255:1913–1920, 1986.
3. Talbott, G.D., and E.B. Benson. Impaired physicians: The dilemma of identification. *Postgraduate Medicine*, 68:56–64, 1980.
4. Bissell, L., and J.K. Skorina. One hundred alcoholic women in medicine. *Journal of the American Medical Association*, 257:2939–2944, 1987.
5. Martin, C.A., and G.D. Talbott. Women physicians in the Georgia impaired physicians program. *Journal of American Medical Women's Association*, 42:115–121, 1987.
6. Martin, C.A., and G.D. Talbott. Special issues for female impaired physicians. *Journal of the Medical Association of Georgia*, August, 1986, pp. 483–488.
7. American Medical Association Council on Mental Health: The sick physician: Impairment by psychiatric disorders, including alcoholism and drug dependence. *Journal of the American Medical Association*, 233:684–687, 1973.
8. Wilford, B.B. (Ed.). The drug-abusing physician. In *Drug Abuse: A Guide for the Primary Care Physician*. American Medical Society, Chicago, 1981, pp. 285–298.
9. Conner, S.L. Comparison of impaired physician programs nationwide. *Maryland Medical Journal*, 37:213–215, 1988.
10. Spickard, W.A. The impaired physician. In *Alcoholism: A Guide for the Primary Care Physician*. Ed. by H.N. Barnes, M.D. Aronson, and T.L. Delbanco. Springer-Verlag, New York, 1987, pp. 188–193.
11. Talbott, G.D., K.V. Gallegos, P.W. Wilson, and T. Porter. The Medical Association of Georgia's impaired physicians program: Review of the first 1,000 physicians: Analysis of specialty. *Journal of the American Medical Association*, 257:2927–2930, 1987.

12. Gallegos, K.V., C.H. Browne, F.W. Veit, and G.D. Talbott. Addiction in anesthesiologists: Drug access and patterns of substance abuse. *QRB*, April, 1988, pp. 116–122.
13. Talbott, G.D. The impaired physician and intervention: A key to recovery. *Journal of the Florida Medical Association*, 69:793–797, 1982.
14. Robertson, J.J. (Ed.). Confrontation techniques. In *The Impaired Physician Proceedings of the Third AMA Conference*. American Medical Association, Chicago, 1979.
15. Arnold, W.P., M.A. Smith, R.F. Bedford, and L. Garner. Drug-impaired physicians: Identification, intervention, treatment. *Virginia Medical*, 114:467–472, 1987.
16. Haynes, T.L. The physician and chemical dependence. *Michigan Medicine*, 87:326–328, 1988.
17. Talbott, G.D. The impaired physician: The role of the spouse in recovery. *Journal of the Medical Association of Georgia*, March, 1987, pp. 190–192.
18. Samkoff, J.S., and J.R. Krebs. Families and physician impairment. *Pennsylvania Medicine*, 92:38–39, 1989.
19. Samkoff, J.S., and J.R. Krebs. Treating the chemically impaired medical family. *Pennsylvania Medicine*, 92:33–34, 1989.

Terminology

Abstinence. Living without the use of psychoactive substances.

Abstinence syndrome. The unpleasant signs and symptoms following discontinuation of a drug upon which a user has become dependent.

Acetaldehyde. Substance produced in the liver by oxidation of alcohol.

Acid head. A habitual heavy user of LSD.

ACOA (Adult Children of Alcoholics). A support program aiding adults with problems resulting from having had alcoholic parents.

Acquired immune deficiency syndrome (AIDS). A disorder of the immune system resulting from infection with human immunodeficiency virus (HIV); specific criteria must be met to make the diagnosis.

Active smoking. Smoking a cigarette.

Addict. A person who is presently, or has been in the past, dependent on one or more drugs, including alcohol.

Addiction. *See* chemical dependence.

Affinity. Tendency of a drug to bind to specific receptor sites.

Aftercare. A structured recovery program after treatment; it may be a few months to two years in length.

Agonist. A drug that binds to receptor sites and produces a response.

Agonist-antagonist. A drug such as pentazocine (Talwin) that possesses both agonist and antagonist properties.

AIDS-related complex (ARC). A lesser disorder of the immune system than AIDS; caused by HIV infection.

Alcohol dehydrogenase pathway. Pathway in which alcohol is oxidized to acetaldehyde; the reaction is catalyzed by alcohol dehydrogenase.

Alcoholic. An addict whose dependence is on alcohol.

Antagonist. A drug that binds to receptor sites and does not produce a response; it may block the effect of another drug.

Al-Anon. A self-help organization for family and close friends of alcoholics.

Alateen. A self-help group for teenage children of alcoholics.

Alcoholic. A person with the disease of alcoholism.

Alcoholics Anonymous (AA). The prototype, and largest, of the support groups.

Alcoholism. A chronic, progressive disease characterized by significant impairment that is directly associated with persistent and excessive consumption of alcohol. Impairment may involve physiological, psychological, or social dysfunction.

Amotivational syndrome. A state of passive withdrawal from usual work, school, and recreational activities, usually accompanied by failure in school, at work, and at home, due to chronic, heavy marijuana use.

Bad trip. A frightening reaction after the use of a hallucinogenic drug.

Bag. A measurement of heroin (usually containing about five grains of diluted heroin, 1–5 percent pure) or marijuana (usually containing 1/7–1/5 oz.).

Bagging. Breathing fumes from a paper bag in which a solvent soaked piece of cotton or rag has been placed.

Balloons. Drugs (heroin or cocaine) are sometimes packaged for sale in balloons.

Bang. The act of injecting a narcotic.

Basing. Using freebase cocaine.

Bender. Being on a drug spree.

Bible. The *Physician's Desk Reference* (PDR). Also called the "book."

Big Bags. Bags of heroin that cost $5 or $10.

Big book. Book written by active members of Alcoholics Anonymous describing the behavior and characteristics of alcoholics.

Big man. The person who supplies a pusher with drugs.

Blackout. A temporary loss of memory caused by alcohol or other drug intoxication.

Blood alcohol level (BAL) or concentration (BAC). Concentration of alcohol in the blood. It is expressed in various units of measurement (0.10 gm/100 ml = 100 mg/100 ml = 100 mg%].

Bomb. A large-size marijuana cigarette; also, high-quality heroin that has been diluted very little.

Bombed out. Feeling the effects of a drug.

Bong. A water pipe used to smoke marijuana; the smoke bubbles through the water and eliminates some of the harshness.

The Book. The *Physicians' Desk Reference*; also called "the Bible."

Boost. To shoplift. A common way for an addict to obtain money to support an addiction.

Booting. Attempting to prolong the initial effects of a heroin injection by injecting a small amount, then withdrawing blood back into the syringe and repeating the process.

Bottoming-out. When a person has reached a level of emotional, spiritual, and physical harm, due to drug abuse, that he or she can no longer tolerate.

Brick. A pressed block of marijuana, opium, or morphine; in the case of marijuana, it weighs one pound.

Bummer. A frightening reaction after taking a drug.

Burn. Cheating or being cheated in drug deals.

Burned out. Refers to a chronic drug user who is too weary of the hassle of obtaining drugs or to heavy marijuana smokers, particularly young people, who become dull and apathetic and withdraw from their usual activities.

Buzz. Feeling the effects of a drug, usually alcohol or marijuana.

Buzz bomb. Pipe for smoking nitrous oxide.

Candy. Drugs.

Candy man. A person who sells drugs.

Carrier state. State in which an individual is infected with HIV but asymptomatic; he or she can pass the etiological agent on to others.

Cent. In drug language a cent refers to a dollar, a nickel is $5, a dime is $10.

Chemical dependence. A chronic, progressive disease characterized by significant impairment that is directly associated with persistent and excessive use of a psychoactive substance. Impairment may involve physiological, psychological, or social dysfunction.

Chief enabler. The primary person in the addict's life who makes it easier for him or her to continue drinking or using.

Chipping. Using drugs irregularly and infrequently.

Clean. Not using or possessing drugs.

Coast. To experience the drowsy, somnolent effects of heroin.

Cocaine anonymous (CA). Support group similar to AA but for cocaine addicts.

Codependent. One who lets another person's behavior affect him or her and who is obsessed with controlling that person's behavior.

Coke head. A heavy user of cocaine.

Coke whore. A person who sells sex to get cocaine.

Cold turkey. Quitting using a drug without the benefit of medication.

Come down. Returning to a normal state after drug effects have worn off. For heroin addicts this state signals the beginning of withdrawal symptoms.

Competitive inhibition. One drug competes with another at receptor sites.

Confirmatory test. A second line test for verifying a positive screening test.

Confronting. A technique of challenging another person's behavior and perception of reality.

Conning. To lie, persuade, or cajole for the purpose of manipulation or deception.

Conversion. The expression of emotional conflict through physical symptoms.

Cook. Heating heroin powder with water until it dissolves and is ready for injection.

Cop. The act of purchasing a drug.

Crack. Freebased form of cocaine HCl; so named because of the crackling sound it makes when it is smoked.

Crack house. A house whose main purpose is the smoking of crack cocaine.

Crash. Suddenly falling asleep after the heavy use of stimulants or to rapidly return to a normal state when the drug effects have worn off.

Cross-addiction. An addict dependent on one drug in a class is considered to be addicted to all drugs in the class; alcohol and diazepam (Valium) are considered cross-addictive.

Cross-reactivity. Drugs in the same class giving a false positive screening test result; for example, phenylpropanolamine read as amphetamine.

Cross-tolerance. The development of tolerance to drugs in the same class as the abused drug.

Crossing the wall. Passing from the abuse stage into the dependence stage; thought to involve central nervous system neurotransmitter derangement.

Deal. To sell illicit drugs.

Dealer. A person who sells drugs, particularly narcotics.

Delirium tremens. Severe form of alcohol withdrawal; occurs in Stage 4 of the alcohol abstinence syndrome.

Delusion. A false, irrational, and persistent belief.

Denial. Symptom of chemical dependence characterized by the subconscious lack of recognition of a problem even in the face of significant adverse consequences, and despite the fact that the problem is evident to others.

Dependence. *See* chemical dependence.

Designer drug. Substance resulting from minor changes in the molecular structure of a parent drug to avoid prosecution for the manufacture of a scheduled drug. The psychoactive properties are retained.

Detoxification. The process by which a drug-addicted person returns to normal physical and mental functioning; this may be accomplished by the abrupt end of drug use (cold turkey), or by gradual discontinuation of the drug under medical supervision.

Dime. In drug language a dime refers to $10.

Dirty. Having drugs in one's possession (opposite of clean).

Dispositional tolerance. Tolerance due to an increased rate of metabolism.

Distillation. Process by which beverages with an alcohol content greater than 14 percent are produced; the fermentation product is heated to boil off the alcohol, which is condensed and collected.

Disulfiram (Antabuse). Medication to help support recovery from alcoholism.

Dollar. In drug language a dollar refers to $100.

Dope. Narcotic drugs.

Down regulation. Development of decreased numbers of postsynaptic receptors in response to prolonged receptor stimulation.

Drug. A substance that exerts a mood-altering effect on the central nervous system and that has the potential to produce dependence; includes alcohol.

Drug addict. A person with the disease of chemical dependence resulting from drug use other than alcohol.

Dried out. Detoxified from a drug.

Drug addiction. *See* chemical dependence.

Druggies. People who frequently experiment with a wide variety of drugs; also, high school or college youth who use drugs regularly.

Dry drunk. Attitudes and behaviors of the abstinent alcoholic or drug addict that seem identical to attitudes and behaviors seen during periods of active drinking or drug use.

Dual-diagnosis. Patient with both a chemical dependence and a primary psychiatric disorder.

Efficacy. Ability of a drug to produce a response.

Eight ball. Approximately 3 grams of cocaine.

ELISA Test. Screening test for antibodies to HIV.

Enabler. An individual who provides the means, or opportunity, for the alcoholic or drug addict to continue psychoactive drug use.

Factory. A secret place where drugs are diluted, packaged, or prepared for sale.

Fermentation. The process by which ethanol is produced by action of yeasts on natural vegetable sugars.

Fetal alcohol effect (FAE). Lesser degree of adverse fetal effects from alcohol than FAS.

Fetal alcohol syndrome (FAS). Severe birth defects resulting from alcohol use during pregnancy.

First-order kinetics. The metabolism of a drug occurs at a rate proportional to its concentration.

First-pass effect. The initial metabolism of a drug administered orally as it passes from the intestine through the liver to the blood.

Fix. The injecting of heroin or the heroin itself (also applies to using any drug intravenously).

Flashback. The recurrence of a previous drug-induced experience that occurs despite the absence of that drug.

Flashing. A term applied to sniffing glue.

Floating. Being under the effects of a drug.

Freak out. A bad, panicky reaction to a drug; or simply to take a drug.

Freebase. Smokable form of cocaine.

Front. To sell drugs to another person on credit.

Fruit salad. A game, usually played by teenagers, in which one pill is swallowed from each bottle in a medicine cabinet.

Garbage head. A person who will use any drug available to get high.

Get off. To experience the effects of a drug; also, to take a heroin injection.

Geographic cure. Moving to another location (city, state) in an attempt to "cure" one's addiction by the move alone.

Getting on. To feel the effects of marijuana.

Glow. To feel the euphoric effects of a drug.

Grower. A person who grows marijuana.

Half-life. Time required for the serum concentration of a drug to fall to 50 percent of its previous level.

Half-way house. A structured transitional living situation between inpatient treatment and returning home.

Hallucination. A visual, auditory, olfactory, or tactile perception that does not exist outside of one's mind..

Hallucinosis. Visual hallucinations occurring with a relatively clear sensorium.

Head. A person who favors a particular drug, as in pot head.

Head shop. Shops that sell drug paraphernalia.

Hero. The child, usually the oldest, in the family who assumes many of the responsibilities given up by the addict; works hard for positive recognition.

Higher power. The "God as we understood him" of Alcoholics Anonymous.

Hit. To take a drug, particularly heroin or marijuana.

Holiday syndrome. Tendency to relapse on special occasions, such as Thanksgiving, Christmas, birthdays, or anniversaries.

Hooked. Addicted to a drug.

Huffing. The act of inhaling the fumes of solvents or aerosols.

Human immunodeficiency virus (HIV). Virus that suppresses the immune system, usually leading to ARC or AIDS.

Hypnotic. A drug that induces sleep.

Intervention. A process designed to speed up the occurrence of a crisis situation to get the addict into treatment earlier than normally would occur.

Isolation. The deliberate avoiding of relationships and communication with others that might threaten the ability to use drugs.

Junk. Drugs, particularly heroin.

Junkie. A heroin addict.

Kick. To break a drug addiction, as in "kicking the habit."

Kindling. Phenomenon of developing a symptom only after regular use of a drug over a period of time.

Knockout drops (Mickey Finn). A mixture of alcohol and chloral hydrate.

Lid. A measurement of weight used for marijuana; ranging from 3/4 to 1 ounce, it is enough for approximately 40 marijuana cigarettes.

Light up. To smoke marijuana.

Loaded. To be heavily intoxicated, whether from alcohol or another drug.

Loss of control. Inability of addicts to stop alcohol or drug use once it is initiated; for example, ending up drunk when the intent was only to have a few drinks.

Lost child. The child in the chemically dependent family who withdraws from the family in a quiet way.

Mainstream smoke. Smoke that is inhaled directly from the cigarette by the smoker.

Mascot. The child in the chemically dependent family who assumes the role of joker or clown.

Microsomal enzyme oxidation system (MEOS). Pathway for oxidizing ethanol to acetaldehyde; it is catalyzed by microsomal enzymes.

Minimizing. Reducing drug use to the smallest possible significance, extent, or degree. A defense mechanism.

Minor tranquilizers. Benzodiazepines used for sedation.

Monkey on my back. A person's drug dependence.

Mood altering drug (MAD). A drug that makes a person feel different. Psychoactive substance.

Naltrexone (Trexan). Medication to help support recovery from opioid addiction.

Narc. A narcotics police officer.

Narcotic. Term used to designate drugs with morphine-like actions. Comes from the word narcosis.

Narcotics Anonymous (NA). Similar to AA, but designed for narcotic addicts.

Needle habit. Some addicts, often referred to as needle freaks, are not particular about what drug they inject but get their thrills simply from the act of injecting.

Neurotransmitter. Chemical substance in the brain whose purpose is interneuron transmission of nerve signals.

Nickel. In drug language a nickel refers to $5.

Nickel bag. A package, usually of marijuana or heroin, that is worth $5.

Nod. To feel the effects of a heroin injection (pleasurable drowsiness and peacefulness), probably so called because the head nods forward.

Noncompetitive inhibition. A drug that binds in a distorted manner to receptors, preventing normal interaction between another drug and its receptors.

O.D.. Overdose.

Opiate. A term used to designate drugs derived from opium, as well as their semisynthetic cogeners.

Opioid. A term used to designate all drugs (natural, semisynthetic, synthetic, agonist-antagonist) with morphine-like actions.

Paraphernalia. The equipment needed to inject heroin, smoke pot, or freebase cocaine.

Partial recovery. Low-quality sobriety resulting from failing to progress in recovery.

Partition coefficient. Measure of the relative solubility of a drug.

Passive smoking. Passively inhaling smoke in the local atmosphere from another's smoking.

Pharmacodynamic tolerance. Tolerance that takes place at the cellular level in the brain.

Pharmacodynamics. Study of how drugs exert their effects.

Pharmacokinetics. Branch of pharmacology that is concerned with drug absorption, distribution, metabolism, and excretion.

Physical dependence. Dependence on a drug that is characterized by an abstinence (withdrawal) syndrome.

Pill head. A person who frequently uses amphetamines and barbiturates or is addicted to prescription drugs.

Potency. The dose of a drug needed to produce a given response when compared to the dose of another drug required to produce the same response.

Popping. To take a pill; also, the subcutaneous injection of heroin.

Postacute withdrawal syndrome. Characterized by continued lesser withdrawal symptoms for months to years past acute withdrawal.

Pot head. A heavy user of marijuana.

Primary psychiatric disorder. A psychiatric disorder not resulting from drug use.

Projection. Blaming others for one's own failings and inadequacies.

Psychedelic drugs. Drugs that induce altered states of perception, thoughts, and feelings that are not experienced otherwise except in dreams or at times of religious experience. Hallucinogenic drugs.

Psychological dependence. Dependence on a drug that is characterized by the absence of an abstinence (withdrawal) syndrome.

Pusher. A dealer who sells drugs directly to an addict; a person who is one step below the wholesaler in the drug-distribution system.

Rationalization. Using socially acceptable but untrue explanations for inappropriate behavior.

Receptors. Specific sites, usually on the outer membrane of cells, where drugs interact.

Recovery. Process in which the physiological, psychological, and social damage caused by chemical dependence is healed; a lifelong process.

Relapse. A process leading back to drinking or using; the act itself.

Regression. The reverting to a level of emotional maturity appropriate to an earlier stage in life.

Repression. The unconscious exclusion from one's own conscious mind of unbearable thoughts, experiences, or feelings.

Residential treatment. A form of treatment that is longer and less intense than inpatient treatment; therapeutic communities and half-way houses are forms of residential treatment.

Reverse tolerance. Phenomenon of requiring less and less drug to get high after tolerance has developed. In the case of alcohol, reverse tolerance may be due to progressive liver damage with reduced ability to metabolize alcohol.

Rig. Apparatus for injecting heroin or smoking pot.

Ripped. To be highly intoxicated by a drug.

Roach. A marijuana cigarette when it has burned down too far to be held with the fingers.

Roach clip. An instrument (pin, tweezers) used to hold a roach.

Rock cocaine. Freebase form of cocaine produced by combining cocaine HCl with baking soda and heating; so-named because this form resembles small rocks.

Run. A period of heavy and prolonged use of a particular drug, usually referring to amphetamines or cocaine.

Rush. The initial euphoric effects occurring after a heroin, cocaine, or amphetamine injection.

Scapegoat. The child in the chemically dependent family who uses delinquent and rebellious behavior to gain attention.

Score. To buy a drug.

Screening test. A test for the presence of drugs, usually in the urine, used to screen a population.

Script. A prescription for a drug; an abbreviation of the word prescription.

Script doc. A physician who deliberately over prescribes or misprescribes psychoactive substances for profit, or who is so easily duped that he gains a reputation for gullibility.

Secondary psychiatric disorder. A psychiatric disorder resulting from drug use.

Sedative. A drug that relaxes and calms.

Sedative-hypnotic. A drug that relaxes and calms but also induces sleep, depending on the dose.

Set. The emotional and mental state of a person before he or she uses a drug.

Setting. The conditions and circumstances surrounding a drug user when he or she uses the drug.

Shooting gallery. A location where addicts inject heroin.

Shoot up. To inject a drug, particularly heroin.

Sick. To experience the beginning of withdrawal symptoms.

Sidestream smoke. Smoke that enters the local atmosphere from the lit end of a cigarette.

Slip. A brief, short-lived relapse followed by an immediate return to abstinence.

Snow lights. Flickering bright lights at the periphery of the visual fields that are seen after cocaine use.

Sober. A term reserved for alcoholics who work a program of recovery that includes the twelve steps of AA and emphasizes spiritual values, positive thinking, and a productive life-style.

Speed freak. A heavy user of amphetamines.

Spoon. A measurement of heroin (1/16 of an ounce), or cocaine (1/4 of a teaspoon).

Stash. A cache of hidden drugs.

Stoned. Being high on a drug.

Straight. A person who doesn't use drugs; a square; also a term for a regular cigarette.

Strung out. An addict who has a severe addiction; or an addict's physical appearance because of a severe addiction.

Substance abuse. Persistent and excessive use of a psychoactive substance, not resulting in significant impairment from physiological, psychological, or social dysfunction.

Substance use. Regular or intermittent, but not excessive, use of a psychoactive substance, such as social drinking or recreational drug use.

Support group. A group of people recovering from some form of drug addiction who agree to assist each other in recovery.

Suppression. The conscious pushing away of feelings and events into the background.

Target syndrome. Successive rings of involvement (community activities, leisure activities, church, friends, peers, distant family, nuclear family) are peeled away until only the center of the target, the addict, is left.

Teetotaler. One who totally abstains.

Telescoping. The phenomenon of addiction developing more rapidly in women and adolescents than in men.

Therapeutic community. A form of residential treatment in which a minimum of professional staff is used; treatment may be confrontational.

Tight. A person who is intoxicated by alcohol or other drugs.

Toke. To smoke a marijuana cigarette; the term refers to both smoking the whole cigarette and just taking a puff.

Toke pipes. Pipes used to smoke marijuana.

Toke up. To light a marijuana cigarette.

Tolerance. The necessity to use, over a period of time, larger and larger doses of a drug to get high.

Toot. To snort or sniff cocaine.

Tough love. Allowing an addict to suffer the consequences of his or her own behavior; an ultimate path to help.

Tranquilizer. *See* sedative.

Trip. The act of taking a hallucinogen, particularly LSD; or the effects of its ingestion.

Turn on. To take a drug or encourage another to do so; to feel the effects of a drug.

Upregulation. Development of increased numbers of postsynaptic receptors in response to prolonged receptor blockade.

User. A person who uses drugs.

Volume of distribution. Ratio of the amount of a drug in the body divided by the concentration of the drug in the plasma at time zero.

Wasted. To lose consciousness from drug intoxication.

Wernicke-Korsakoff syndrome. A form of dementia produced in part by thiamine deficiency secondary to alcoholism; neurological signs and psychosis occur.

Western Blot Test. Confirmatory test for antibodies to HIV.

Whippit. Whipped cream dispenser containing nitrous oxide as the propellant.

Wiped out. Acute drug intoxication.

Wired. A person who is feeling the high effects of amphetamines; the term also applies to a heroin addict.

Withdrawal syndrome. *See* Abstinence Syndrome.

Works. The apparatus for injecting narcotics, particularly heroin.

Yen. Restless sleep that occurs during narcotic withdrawal. Also, drug craving.

Zero-order kinetics. The metabolism of a drug occurs at a constant rate.

Zonked. Acutely intoxicated by a drug.

Street/Slang Names for Drugs

A-bomb (marijuana + heroin)
Acapulco gold (marijuana)
Acid (LSD)
Adam (MDMA)
Amies (amyl nitrite)
AMP (marijuana + formaldehyde)
Amys (amyl nitrite)
Angel dust (phencyclidine)
Angel hair (phencyclidine)
Angel mist (phencyclidine)
Animal tranquilizer (phencyclidine)

Bad seed (mescaline/peyote)
Banaple gas (butyl nitrite)
Barbs (barbiturates)
Base (cocaine)
Beans (barbiturates, mescaline/
    peyote)
Bennies (amphetamine sulfate)
Bernice (cocaine)
Bhang (hashish)
Big chief (mescaline/peyote)
Big D (LSD)
Big H (heroin)
Bindweed (morning glory seeds)
Black beauties (Biphetamine)
Black birds (Biphetamine)
Black hash (hashish)
Black mollies (Biphetamine)
Black pills (opium)
Black Russian (hashish)
Black stuff (opium)

Blockbusters (barbiturates)
Blond hash (hashish)
Blotter (LSD)
Blotter acid (LSD)
Blue acid (LSD)
Blue bullets (Amytal)
Blue devils (Amytal)
Blue dolls (Amytal)
Blue heaven (LSD)
Blue heavens (Amytal)
Blue mist (LSD)
Blue star (morning glory seeds)
Blue tips (Amytal)
Blue velvet (paregoric)
Bluebirds (Amytal)
Blues (Amytal)
Booze (alcohol)
Brew (alcohol)
Brown dots (LSD)
Business man's LSD (DMT)
Business man's lunch (DMT)
Buttons (mescaline/peyote)

C (cocaine)
C.J. (phencyclidine)
Cactus (mescaline/peyote)
Cactus buttons (mescaline/peyote)
Cadillac (phencyclidine)
Canned satira (hashish)
CB (Doriden)
Charas (hashish)
Charlie (cocaine)

China white (fentanyl)
Chlorals (chloral hydrate)
Christmas trees (Tuinal)
Cibas (Ritalin)
Coca (cocaine)
Cohoba (mappine)
Coke (cocaine)
Cola (cocaine)
Copilots (dextroamphetamine)
Crack (cocaine)
Crank (methamphetamine)
Crosses (amphetamines)
Crystal (methamphetamine, phency-
    clidine)
Crystal joints (phencyclidine)
Cubes (LSD)
Cyclones (phencyclidine)

D (Dilaudid, LSD)
Deeda (LSD)
Dexies (dextroamphetamine)
Dillies (Dilaudid)
Dollies (methadone)
Dolls (methadone)
Doobie (marijuana)
Dots (LSD)
Double crosses (amphetamines)
Double trouble (Tuinal)
Downers (barbiturates)
Dreamer (morphine)
Dust (phencyclidine)
Duster (tobacco + heroin)

Ecstacy (MDMA)
Elephant tranquilizer (phencyclidine)
Embalming fluid (phencyclidine)
Eve (MDEA)

Flake (cocaine)
Flying saucers (morning glory seeds)
Foolpills (barbiturates)
Footballs (dextroamphetamine,
    Dilaudid)
Fours (Dilaudid, Tylenol + codeine)
Freebase (cocaine)

Ganga (marijuana)
Geronimo (alcohol + barbiturates)
Giggleweed (marijuana)
Girl (cocaine)
Glass (methamphetamine)
Goofballs (barbiturates)
Goofers (barbiturates + ampheta-
    mines)
Goon (phencyclidine)
Gorilla biscuits (phencyclidine)
Grass (marijuana)
Green and whites (Librium)
Green dragons (barbiturates)
Gum (opium)

H (heroin)
Hairy (heroin)
Harry (heroin)
Hash (hashish)
Hay (marijuana)
Haze (LSD)
Hearts (amphetamines)
Heaven (cocaine)
Heaven dust (cocaine)
Heavenly blue (morning glory
    seeds)
Hemp (marijuana)
Hog (phencyclidine)
Hop (opium)
Horse (heroin)
Horse tranquilizer (phencyclidine)

Ice (methamphetamine)
Indian hay (marijuana)

J (marijuana)
Jane (marijuana)
Jelly beans (amphetamines)
Jet fuel (phencyclidine)
Joc aroma (butyl nitrite)
Joint (marijuana cigarette)
Joy powder (heroin)
Joy stick (marijuana cigarette)
Juice (alcohol)
Junk (heroin)

K.J. (phencyclidine)
K.W. (phencyclidine)
Kay jay (phencyclidine)
Kick (butyl nitrite)
Kiff (tobacco + marijuana)
Killer weed (marijuana, phencyclidine)
Knock-out drops (chloral hydrate + alcohol)
Krystal joint (phencyclidine)

L (LSD)
Lady (cocaine)
Laughing gas (nitrous oxide)
Lebanese (hashish)
Line (cocaine)
Locker popper (butyl nitrite)
Locker room (butyl nitrite)
Lords (Dilaudid)
Love drug (Quaaludes, MDA, MDMA)
Lovely (phencyclidine)
Ludes (Quaaludes)
Lysergide (LSD)

M & M (MDMA)
M (morphine)
M.J. (marijuana)
M.S. (morphine)
Magic mushrooms (psilocybin/psilocyn)
Mahjuema (hashish)
Mary (marijuana)
Maryann (marijuana)
Maryjane (marijuana)
Mellow yellows (LSD)
Mesc (mescaline/peyote)
Mescal (mescaline/peyote)
Meth (methamphetamine)
Mexican brown (heroin, marijuana)
Mexican locoweed (marijuana)
Mexican reds (Seconal)
Mickey Finn (chloral hydrate + alcohol)
Microdots (LSD)

Mint weed (phencyclidine)
Miss Emma (morphine)
Mist (phencyclidine)
Monkey dust (phencyclidine)
Moon (mescaline/peyote)
Morph (morphine)
Mud (heroin)
Mujer (cocaine)
Mushrooms (psilocybin/psilocyn)

Nebbies (Nembutal)
Nimbies (Nembutal)
Nose candy (cocaine)
Nose powder (cocaine)

O (opium)
Op (opium)
Orange cubes (LSD)
Oranges (dextroamphetamine)

P (mescaline/peyote)
Pajoa roho (barbiturates)
Paper acid (LSD)
Paradise (cocaine)
PCP (phencyclidine)
Peace (phencyclidine)
PeaCe pill (phencyclidine)
Peachies (amphetamine sulfate)
Pearls (amyl nitrite)
Pearly gates (morning glory seeds)
Pellets (LSD)
Pep pills (amphetamines)
Perico (cocaine)
Peruvian flake (cocaine)
Peter (chloral hydrate)
Peyoti (mescaline/peyote)
Pink ladies (barbiturates)
Pinks (barbiturates, Seconal)
Pinks and grays (Darvon)
Polvo blanco (cocaine)
Poppers (amyl nitrite)
Pops (codeine)
Pot (marijuana)
Purple hearts (Luminal)

Quads (Quaaludes)
Quartz (methamphetamine)
Quas (Quaaludes)

R.D. (Seconal)
Ragweed (marijuana)
Rainbows (Tuinal)
Red devils (Seconal)
Redbirds (Seconal)
Reds (Seconal)
Reds and blues (barbiturates)
Reefer (marijuana cigarette)
Roach (butt end of marijuana
    cigarette)
Roaches (Librium)
Rock (cocaine)
Rocket fuel (phencyclidine)
Root (marijuana cigarette)
Rope (marijuana)
Rush (butyl nitrite)

Sacred mushrooms (psilocybin/
    psilocyn)
Satan's scent (butyl nitrite)
Schoolboys (codeine)
Scuffle (phencyclidine)
Seccies (Seconal)
Selma (phencyclidine)
Sherman (phencyclidine)
Shrooms (psilocybin/psilocyn)
Silly putty (psilocybin/psilocyn)
Sleeping pills (barbiturates)
Smack (heroin)
Smash (acetone extract of cannabis)
Snappers (amyl nitrite)
Snorts (phencyclidine)
Snow (cocaine)
Soapers (Quaaludes)
Soles (hashish)
Soma (phencyclidine)
Sopes (Quaaludes)
Speed (methamphetamine)
Speedball (cocaine + heroin)
Spirits (alcohol)
Splash (amphetamine sulfate)

Stick (marijuana cigarette)
STP (DOM)
Stumblers (barbiturates)
Sugar (LSD)
Sugar cubes (LSD)
Supercools (phencyclidine)
Supergrass (PCP + marijuana, high
    potency marijuana)
Superweed (phencyclidine)
Surfer (phencyclidine)

T (phencyclidine)
Tabs (LSD)
TAC (phencyclidine)
Tar (opium)
Tea (marijuana)
Ten-8-20 (methadone)
Texas tea (marijuana)
The champagne of drugs (cocaine)
Thing (heroin)
Thrust (butyl nitrite)
TIC (phencyclidine)
Toilet water (butyl nitrite)
Tooies (Tuinal)
Toot (cocaine)
Topi (mescaline/peyote)
Tranks (phencyclidine)
Trees (Tuinal)
Ts and Blues (Talwin + pyribenza-
    mine)

Uppers (amphetamines)

Wackey weed (phencyclidine)
Wafers (methadone)
Wake-ups (amphetamines)
Water (methamphetamine)
Wedding bells (morning glory
    seeds)
Wedges (LSD)
Weed (marijuana)
White stuff (heroin)
Whites (amphetamine sulfate)
Window panes (LSD)
Woobie weed (phencyclidine)

X (MDMA)
XTC (MDMA)

Yellow bullets (Nembutal)
Yellow dolls (Nembutal)

Yellow jackets (Nembutal)
Yellows (Nembutal)
Yopo (mappine)

Zombie dust (phencyclidine)

Index

363